Feb 1995.

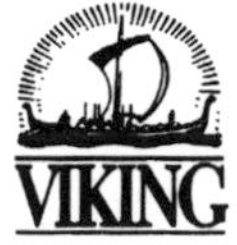
VIKING

The Penguin Book of SYMPTOMS AND EARLY WARNING SIGNS

A Comprehensive New Guide to Self-Diagnosis

Dr Michael Apple and Dr Jason Payne-James
Editor: Dr Roy Macgregor

VIKING

VIKING

Published by the Penguin Group
Penguin Books Ltd, 27 Wrights Lane, London W8 5TZ, England
Penguin Books USA Inc., 375 Hudson Street, New York, New York 10014, USA
Penguin Books Australia Ltd, Ringwood, Victoria, Australia
Penguin Books Canada Ltd, 10 Alcorn Avenue, Toronto, Ontario, Canada M4V 3B2
Penguin Books (NZ) Ltd, 182-190 Wairau Road, Auckland 10, New Zealand

Penguin Books Ltd, Registered Offices: Harmondsworth, Middlesex, England

First published 1993
1 3 5 7 9 10 8 6 4 2
First edition

Typeset by Duncan Petersen Publishing Ltd; film output by Cooling Brown

Printed in England by The Bath Press

A CIP catalogue record for this book is available from the British Library

ISBN 0-670-85314-3

The ideas, procedures and suggestions in this book are not intended to replace the services of doctors; they are intended to enable patients to collaborate more effectively with professionals in combating illness and disease. All matters regarding health require some degree of medical supervision, and any applications of treatments set forth in this book are at the reader's own risk.

The Authors

Dr Roy Macgregor, the editor, is the presenter of ITV's popular medical programme, *The Treatment*. He read medicine at Cambridge and is a family doctor at the model Kentish Town Health Centre in north London, where he has been a partner for ten years. He has presented *Doc Spots* on breakfast television, made successful videos on health and fitness, is the author of *A Handbook for 300 Common Ailments*, and has written numerous health education publications and magazine articles.

Dr Michael Apple read psychology at Liverpool University, graduating with first class honours. He worked in merchant banking before returning to university in 1971 to study medicine, graduating from Birmingham with a distinction in psychiatry. After surgical, medical and paediatric posts, he joined a general practice in Watford, Hertfordshire, in 1980. He is especially interested in children's diseases, general medicine and psychological problems. His articles, often humorous, are published in the *British Medical Journal*, the *Daily Telegraph* and *General Practitioner*.

Dr Jason Payne-James read medicine at London Hospital Medical College and afterwards held various hospital appointments in medicine, surgery, orthopaedics, accident and emergency and gastroenterology. He is now a forensic medical examiner and a researcher, writer and lecturer with a particular interest in clinical nutrition, home care and home therapy. He has been a radio doctor; has produced, written and directed medical videos and published many learned papers in medical journals.

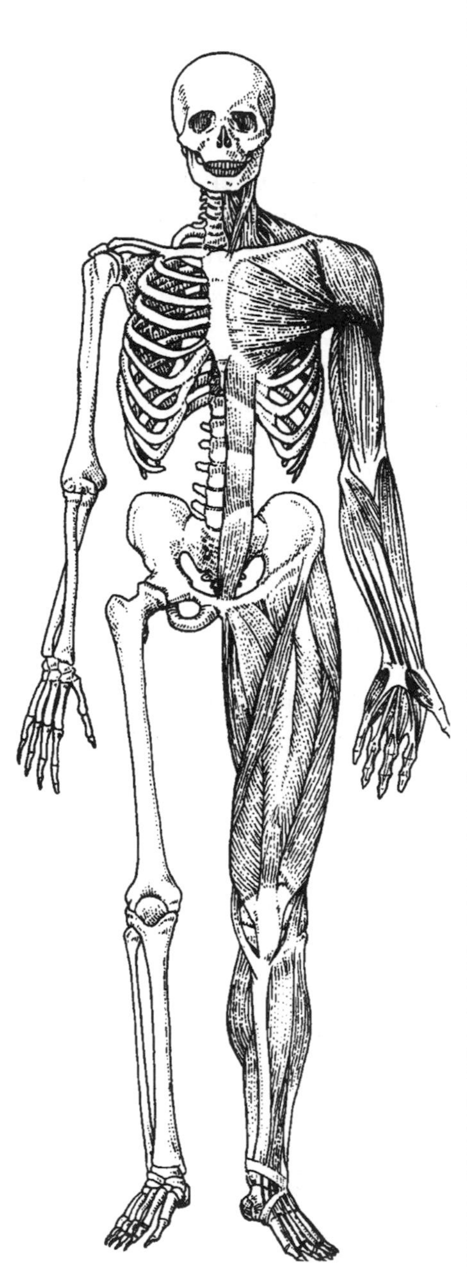

CONTENTS

An explanation of how the contents are ordered is given on page 9. The book's main sections are:

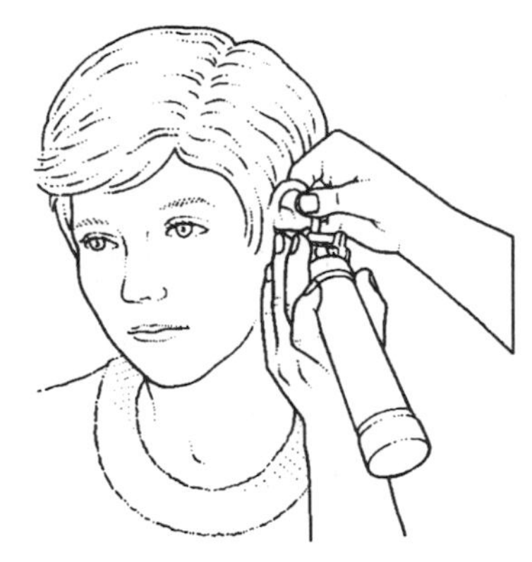

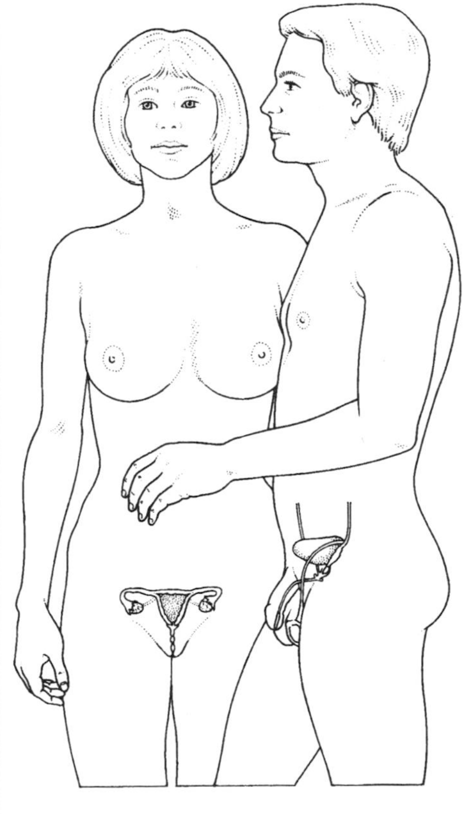

INTRODUCTION

This book sets out to tell you more about symptoms and self-diagnosis than any other guide: an ambitious goal.

It also tries to reveal how a doctor thinks when faced by a patient reporting symptoms. We believe that understanding how a doctor arrives at a diagnosis is fundamentally important to the patient. We have therefore provided a complete and intelligent picture of your symptoms, informing you what *is* likely to be happening to your body as well as what is *not* likely.

Considering diagnoses in order of probability helps you to go through the same process of elimination and decision-making as a doctor.

This is a book which will enable you to question your doctor and to reach a conclusion together with him or her — to participate actively in diagnosis and treatment, rather than to receive passively.

Symptoms and Early Warning Signs is not a book about avoiding doctors altogether. Rather, the aim is to help you approach a visit to the doctor with the knowledge necessary to put your illness in perspective.

We also hope that the book will arm you with the know-how to make important decisions about your health — yourself.

All of us, doctors included, are hypochondriacs at times. We hope that you will find ***Symptoms and Early Warning Signs*** a hypochondriac's dream, not a nightmare.

Dr Roy Macgregor

The approach

For the first time ever in a popular medical guide, all the symptoms you could reasonably expect to encounter are put into perspective. A diagnosis may be possible in the presence of only some of the starred features. It is not necessary to experience all the features in order to confirm a diagnosis.

We divide the diagnoses into:

■ What is **probable**: the common causes of the symptom such as would immediately spring to a doctor's mind. Most of these probable diagnoses occur commonly: doctors see them regularly.

■ What is **possible**, once the probable causes have been excluded. Some of these diagnoses are not uncommon, but they may well require testing to establish them without doubt.

■ **Rare** causes: it would be misleading to define *how* rare. The frequency of these diagnoses is extremely variable. Unless your symptoms happen to match closely the features listed, these diagnoses are unlikely. Extensive testing may be required to establish these diagnoses and in some cases doubt may remain.

Using this book

1 Always start with your symptom or symptoms. (Often you will have a combination of symptoms rather than just one.) If it is easy to put a name to the symptom, such as headache or painful wrist, look for this in the index, which lists all the symptoms, and which will refer you straight to the relevant page number.

2 If your symptom is not quite so obvious, or easily defined, you need to decide if it can be isolated to a single part of the body — such as the knee, or abdomen — or whether it is a 'general', whole-body symptom, such as fever, or weight loss.

In the case of symptoms clearly occurring in one part of the body, or in one system of the body, for example the digestive system, turn straight to the relevant section and look through it. You will find that:

■ Each part of the body has its own section, clearly identified with a heading.

■ The sections are arranged in a logical order, starting at the top of the body (with the eyes) and moving downwards towards the feet. It ends with 'general' symptoms which cannot be easily isolated to any one part of the body or any one of the body's systems.

The abdominal symptoms are an exception to this rule.

Using This Book

■ Within each section, the order generally echoes that of the book as a whole: the specific come first, and the general come last. Also, symptoms which are obvious to others — revealed by clear visual signs such as a rash or a limp — are put first. Inwardly experienced symptoms, or those which only you are likely to know about, such as loss of sense of smell, come last within a section.

The psychological and nervous symptoms in *The Brain and Nervous System* are an exception to this rule, following an alphabetical sequence.

In addition, symptoms are grouped like with like, so that, for instance, a common cold, shivers, chills and sweating all occur within the same few pages.

Simply browse through the relevant section looking for the symptom, or combination of symptoms that fits your condition; and if necessary follow the cross-referencing, which has been introduced to avoid too much unnecessary repetition.

3 If your symptom or symptoms cannot be isolated to a single part of the body, go to the 'general' symptoms section, which comes last in the book. (We use single quotes around the word general because although such symptoms may appear to be general, they may well, on closer inspection, be specifically related to a problem in one part of the body, or one of the body's systems.)

Within this last section of the book, symptoms are again ordered like with like, and as far as possible they proceed to from the obvious and noticeable to the 'internal' and private. But this classification is not so easy to apply to general symptoms and to give additional help with symptom-finding in this section, the black bands up the edges of each page give extra help to what is covered on these pages.

Medical terms

Certain medical or neo-medical terms are used so often in this book that explaining their meaning every time would be too space-consuming. They are:

Acute
Occurring now; a sudden appearance or exacerbation.

Anxiety
'Fear spread thin'; feelings of dread and worry.

Benign tumour
A lump which is not cancerous.

Chronic
A disease or illness either lasting a long time or present for years.

Circulatory disease
Disease of the arteries or veins which carry blood around the body.

Cyanosis
Bluish skin colouration caused by lack of oxygen in the tissues.

Cyst
A sac within the body, usually fluid-filled; may also appear as a swelling in or on the body.

Diagnostic
Unique to; aiding the diagnosis.

Follicle
Glandular structure under skin from which a hair grows.

Immunosuppression
The immune system is the body's defence system against infection and other insults; if it is supressed, by either illness or drugs, its normal function is limited or rendered less effective.

Indigestion, acidity
Both terms are used to describe discomfort after eating.

Lesion
A mark; a cut; a wound.

Malaise
Feeling generally unwell.

Malignant
Cancerous.

Nodule
A lump or swelling generally felt on the body's surface.

'Non-specific'
Usually describes a symptom which does not signify any disease in particular.

Palpable
Can be felt by hand.

Phlegm
Sticky mucous, produced typically in the lungs as a response to infection.

Rigor
A sudden shaking episode, typically accompanied by a fit of shivering.

Sepsis
Infection.

Systemic
Affecting all of the body's systems; widespread rather than local.

Tumour
A growth, often a lump, either benign or malignant.

Accents

Words spelt out in capitals do not carry accents in this book. They include Sjögren's disease; Ménière's disease and Guillain-Barré syndrome.

THE EYES, NOSE AND EARS

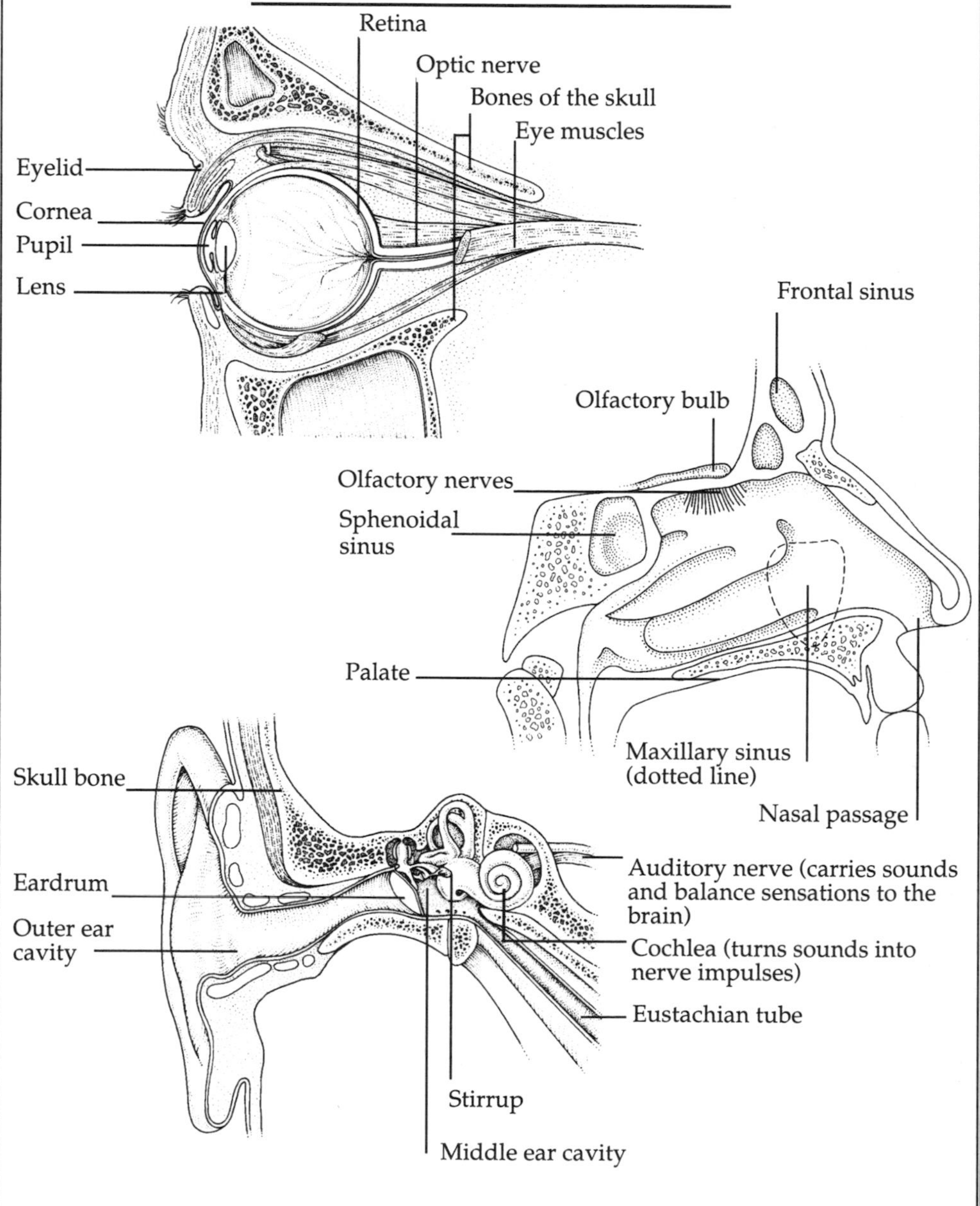

THE EYES INTRODUCTION

The eyes are extraordinary structures: delicately built, yet durable, and highly sensitive. Just as interesting are the mechanisms within the brain that interpret the visual impulses travelling to it from the eyes.

Even now, our understanding of how the eyes work is only sketchy. The study of the eyes is one of the most specialized branches of medicine. There are, however, only a few common symptoms of eye disease — symptoms such as blurred vision or a red eye. Most family doctors have just a working knowledge of eye disease, enough to make a confident diagnosis of everyday problems, but not to assess anything out of the ordinary, which will automatically be referred to an eye specialist. Eye problems are common in modern life. Children are prone to eye infections; adults to eye irritation; and the elderly to deteriorating eyes.

Report all but the most trivial eye problems to your doctor, especially pain or blurred vision. If there is eye disease such as glaucoma in your family, you should have regular eye checks.

SKIN CHANGES AROUND THE EYE

Brief colour changes are probably due to minor infections. Here are other possibilities to explain more long-lasting colour changes.

PROBABLE
INJURY

POSSIBLE
ECZEMA
XANTHELASMA

RARE
RODENT ULCER

PROBABLE

■ INJURY
Any injury causing bruising of the forehead, or above the eye, will result in a blue/black eye, as the blood in the bruise tracks down the face to settle around the eye. In other words, a black eye need not be caused by injury directly to the eye area.
* At first, redness and pain.
* Black eye appears after a few hours.
* Fades over seven to ten days.

THE EYES

POSSIBLE

■ ECZEMA
The skin of the eyelids and below the eyes is sensitive to many agents.
* Red, itchy skin.
* Dry and flaky.

Those suffering from eczema elsewhere on the body are prone to this problem. Sometimes it is caused by an allergy to face make-up, nail varnish or soap. Often, an allergy test is needed to pinpoint the cause.

■ XANTHELASMA
* Yellowish, slightly raised nodules underneath or to the corners of the eyes in adults.
* Painless.
* Grow very slowly.
* Similar nodules may be found on elbows, hands, knees.

If you notice these, have a cholesterol check, since xanthelasma are often a sign of raised blood fats.

RARE

■ RODENT ULCER
A slow-growing skin cancer found on the face, by the bridge of the nose or the outer margin of the eye's orbit. Usually on an elderly person.
* Begins as a slightly raised spot.
* Crusts as it grows.
* May bleed.

Cure can be virtually guaranteed if treated early.

RING AROUND CORNEA

PROBABLE
ARCUS SENILIS

POSSIBLE
IRON RING

RARE
COPPER RING

PROBABLE

■ ARCUS SENILIS
A white circle around part or all of the cornea, common in the over-60s. If seen in a younger person, it may be associated with raised blood cholesterol, which should be checked. Otherwise it is of no significance.

POSSIBLE

■ IRON RING
A brown ring may be left after an iron filing has been removed from the cornea.

RARE

■ COPPER RING
Also called Kayser-Fleischer ring. A brown or green ring associated with the rare condition of Wilson's

Disease, in which copper builds up in the body. A childhood disease.
* Liver disease (swelling, easy bruising, jaundice).
* Tremor of the limbs.
* Dementia.

Early detection and treatment means a good outlook.

RED AND PAINFUL EYE

Never ignore this symptom, which may be a sign of sight-threatening disease. Seek immediate medical attention.

PROBABLE
SEVERE CONJUNCTIVITIS

POSSIBLE
ACUTE IRITIS
ACUTE KERATITIS

RARE
ACUTE GLAUCOMA

PROBABLE

■ SEVERE CONJUNCTIVITIS
Conjunctivitis is inflammation of the white of the eye, giving rise to a mass of red blood vessels running over the eyeball. It is highly contagious, so tends to spread rapidly around a family.
* Initially, itching.
* Both eyes become red.
* The redness is greatest around the outer part of the eyeball.
* Bright light is mildly irritating.
* A yellow discharge.
* Crusted eyelids.

Antibiotic eyedrops are the widely used remedy. Sometimes the symptoms are confined to one eye only; in such cases a doctor will look very carefully to exclude other diseases.

POSSIBLE

■ ACUTE IRITIS
This is inflammation of the coloured part of the eye, the iris, or associated structures. Iritis is not a final diagnosis in itself, since it can be caused by many diseases, in particular arthritic disorders and connective tissue disorders.
* Usually only one eye is affected.
* Moderately painful and red.
* Redness is greatest around the coloured iris.
* The pupil is smaller on the affected side.
* Vision is reduced, blurred.
* The pupil may appear irregular after repeated attacks.

Appropriate eye drops will reduce inflammation and dilate the pupil.

■ ACUTE KERATITIS
Once again, this is not a final diagnosis, but a complication of several diseases affecting the cornea of the eye. The commonest are an ulcer on the cornea, or injury.

THE EYES

* Rapid onset of symptoms.
* One eye affected.
* No change in vision.
* Profuse watering; blinking.
* Light irritates the eye.

There are now highly effective anti-viral drugs to counter the herpes virus which is the usual cause of this problem, and early treatment is needed.

RARE

■ ACUTE GLAUCOMA
The eyeball contains fluid which circulates via tiny channels. In glaucoma, this fluid builds up pressure, causing changes in the field of vision. However, the changes usually happen so gradually that nothing is noticed until a late stage in the disease. For this reason, screening for glaucoma is strongly advisable in anyone with a family history of the problem, and in anyone over the age of 60. Sudden, rapid rise in pressure can, on rare occasions, occur because of blockage in the channels, or perhaps if a drug constricts the pupils. This is acute glaucoma.

The early symptoms of glaucoma are:
* None at all.
* Possibly vague aching in the eyeball.
* Haloes around lights at night.
* Tunnel vision — *see page 43.*

Acute glaucoma is a medical emergency causing:
* Sudden, excruciating pain in the eye.
* Vomiting as a result of the pain.
* Redness around the iris.
* A hazy cornea.
* Vision severely reduced.

Urgent treatment is needed to reduce pressure within the eye and to save sight.

SLIGHTLY REDDENED EYE, OR RED EYE WITHOUT PAIN.

These are unlikely to signify any serious underlying cause, unless there is also blurred vision, or light hurts the eyes.

PROBABLE
CONJUNCTIVITIS
ALLERGY

POSSIBLE
SUBCONJUNCTIVAL HAEMORRHAGE
FEVERISH ILLNESS

RARE
SCLERITIS/EPISCLERITIS
MENINGITIS

PROBABLE

■ CONJUNCTIVITIS
An infection of the conjunctiva, the thin membrane that covers the white of the eye.
* Eyes feel itchy and sore.
* Redness appears rapidly, due to many dilated blood vessels.
* The redness is least next to the

coloured iris, greatest at the sides of the eyeballs.
* Yellow pus in the corners of the eyes.
* Eyelids may be crusted.

Conjunctivitis is usually a straightforward diagnosis, but be cautious if redness affects one eye only, when other possibilities need to be considered. Antibiotic eye-drops are effective.

Contact lenses are frequently a cause of eye problems. Keeping soft lenses in your eyes for prolonged periods means you are 17 times more likely to have an eye infection or conjunctivitis. It is much better to use short-use, hard, gas-permeable lenses.

Another frequent cause of infection is inadequate cleaning of lenses or — equally important — the lens case.

■ ALLERGY

Recurrent, mildly red eyes raise the possibility of allergy. Common causes of allergies (allergens) are pollen, smoky atmospheres and air pollution. Sometimes, contact lenses, or the solutions used to clean them, are to blame.
* Mildly red, itchy eyes.
* May be seasonal, plus sneezing and a runny nose.
* May be related to exposure to allergens as listed above.
* Discharge, if any, tends to be white and not yellow.
* Under-surface of eyelids may appear grainy.

Several effective anti-allergy treatment can help, though for some this becomes a long-term problem.

POSSIBLE

■ SUBCONJUNCTIVAL HAEMORRHAGE

An extremely satisfying condition for a doctor to diagnose, since the patient can usually be totally reassured that no harm will come of it.
* Painless, so the condition is often pointed out by someone else.
* One eye has a bright red patch.
* The patch may cover half or more of the white of the eye.
* Stops short at the iris.
* Fades away towards the sides of the eye.

It may look alarming, but it is simply due to bleeding from a tiny blood vessel and will fade away over a couple of weeks. In the elderly, it may call for a check on blood pressure.

If, however, it occurs after a blow to the head, expert assessment is needed to check whether there is damage to the eye further back in its socket.

■ FEVERISH ILLNESS

Any such illness will give slightly red eyes; measles is notorious for this effect — but now occurs infrequently.

RARE

■ SCLERITIS/EPISCLERITIS

* One part of the white of the eye is red.
* Prominent blood vessels are seen to cause the redness.

* Slight discomfort.
* Recurrent.

This condition is notable since it tends to be associated with other diseases, especially joint problems. It needs further investigation.

■ MENINGITIS
A few red flecks suddenly appearing on the whites of the eyes may be the earliest signs of meningitis in a baby or child. There may also be:
* A high-pitched cry.
* Drowsiness.
* Photophobia.
* A bulging, soft spot (fontanelle) on the baby's scalp.
* A red rash elsewhere on the body.

This is a medical emergency: rush the baby or child to hospital.

ABNORMALLY SMALL PUPILS

The pupils are the apertures through which light enters the eyes. Their size is controlled by nerves which make the pupils open and close. Those nerves are affected by changes within the brain and, surprisingly, within the chest. It is not always obvious whether one pupil is abnormally small or the other pupil is abnormally large.

It is normal for both pupils to become smaller in bright light. The pupils of children and of the elderly tend to be smaller than those of adults. A young person, unconscious, and with pupils like pin points, arouses the immediate suspicion of a narcotic drug overdose.

PROBABLE
LONG-SIGHTEDNESS

POSSIBLE
DRUGS
IRITIS

RARE
HORNER'S SYNDROME

PROBABLE

■ LONG-SIGHTEDNESS
Small pupils are normal in the long-sighted.
* Both pupils are small.
* The pupils react briskly to light and dark.

POSSIBLE

■ DRUGS
Many drugs, and typically pilocarpine and timolol used to treat glaucoma (*page 45*), constrict the pupils by affecting the nerves controlling them. Small pupils may also be a side effect of the powerful narcotic painkillers such as morphine, dihydrocodeine and pethidine or drugs of misuse such as heroin.

■ IRITIS
See page 36. Suggested by finding:
* Small, irregular pupil in one eye only.
* Pain.
* Redness around the iris

RARE

■ HORNER'S SYNDROME
A combination of:
* One abnormally small pupil.
* Drooping eyelid on that side.
* The eye bulging forward slightly.
* Decreased sweating on that side of the face.

The significance of Horner's syndrome is that it reflects irritation of one of the nerves controlling the pupil somewhere along its route from the brain, down into the chest and up again to the eye. The irritation could be caused by a lung tumour; enlarged glands within the chest; multiple sclerosis; or brain disease. So although Horner's syndrome is uncommon, its significance is great and all the more so if there are associated symptoms such as:
* Chest pain.
* Coughing blood.
* Unsteadiness of gait.
* Blurred vision, numb hands.

ENLARGED PUPILS

PROBABLE
EMOTION
DRUGS

POSSIBLE
THIRD NERVE PALSY
INJURY
COMA
ADIE'S PUPIL
BLINDNESS

RARE
IRRITATION OF NERVES TO EYE

PROBABLE

■ EMOTION
Both pupils will dilate in response to emotional triggers such as fear, excitement and anxiety. Accompanying symptoms include:
* Rapid pulse.
* Thumping heart beat.
* Dry mouth.
* 'Stars' in the eyes; but this is controversial.

■ DRUGS
Commonly prescribed eyedrops, such as atropine and homatropine, are used to treat iritis and are intended to dilate the pupil.

POSSIBLE

■ THIRD NERVE PALSY
See page 28. The third nerve is one of several controlling eye movements. If the nerve becomes paralysed:
* The eye turns outwards.
* The eyelid droops.
* The pupil enlarges.

The Eyes

■ INJURY
A blow to the eye severe enough to damage its internal structure will upset movement of the pupil. This is not uncommon in games using a small ball such as squash.
* Probably bruising around the eye.
* Enlarged pupil, unreactive to light.
* Blurred vision is likely.

Clearly, this needs immediate treatment.

■ COMA
A severe head injury or other serious disease affecting the brain, such as a stroke, may cause dilated pupils.
* Deep unconsciousness.
* Breathing irregular and shallow.
* No response to painful stimulus.

At the worst, dilated pupils in both eyes which do not respond at all to light signal brain death.

■ ADIE'S PUPIL
A harmless condition, generally in a young woman with:
* One enlarged pupil, which constricts in reaction to bright light, but more slowly than usual.
* Vision and health otherwise normal.

■ BLINDNESS
The pupil in a blind eye will be larger than its companion because the normal reflex response to bright light is absent.

RARE

■ IRRITATION OF NERVES TO EYE
The same process which produces Horner's Syndrome (*page 19*) can, in its early stages, stimulate the nerve, causing a dilated pupil.

Accompanying symptoms which raise suspicion therefore include:
* Chest pain.
* Coughing blood.
* Unstead gait.
* Blurred vision, numbness of hands.

IRREGULAR PUPILS

Normal pupils are round or slightly oval, but minor irregularities are common. Their significance depends on the individual's overall state of health.

PROBABLE
NORMAL VARIANT

POSSIBLE
IRITIS

RARE
MULTIPLE SCLEROSIS
SYPHILIS
BRAIN TUMOUR

PROBABLE

■ NORMAL VARIANT
Minor degrees of irregularity are almost certainly of no importance and may well be hereditary.
* No pain or visual disturbance.
* No change with passing of time.
* Otherwise sound health.

POSSIBLE

■ IRITIS
See page 36. A small, irregular pupil is a particular feature of this painful condition, especially after repeated attacks.

RARE

■ MULTIPLE SCLEROSIS
A neurological disease usually beginning in early adult life.
* Sudden loss or blurring of vision in one eye.
* Numbness and weakness of different parts of the body.
* Tremor, unsteady gait.

It is rarely posssibe to make a definite diagnosis of multiple sclerosis until several years have passed.

■ SYPHILIS
Not long ago, small, irregular pupils would immediately have brought syphilis to mind. Other features would be:
* Brief, severe limb pains.
* Unsteady gait.
* Loss of pain sensation in joints, leading to gross distortion of knees, ankles.
* Drooping eyelids on both sides.

■ BRAIN TUMOUR
Might be possible if an irregular pupil is found together with:
* Severe and increasing headaches.
* Change of personality.
* Progressive weakness of one side of the body.

ENLARGED EYEBALL

PROBABLE
HYPERTHYROIDISM

RARE
TUMOUR
THROMBOSIS
CONGENITAL GLAUCOMA

PROBABLE

■ HYPERTHYROIDISM
Strictly speaking, this causes not enlargement but protruberance of the eyeballs.
* Both eyeballs affected.
* Sweating, weight loss.
* Fine tremor, hyperactivity.

Though treatment controls the general effects, the eyes often remain a little protuberant.

THE EYES

RARE

■ TUMOUR
* Progressive swelling of one eyeball. (Children or adults.)
* Squint, loss of vision, pain.

Only after expert assessment can treatment be decided.

■ CONGENITAL GLAUCOMA
Raised pressure inside the eye gives rise to a child with
* 'Calf eyes'.
* Cornea appears to bulge.

■ THROMBOSIS
A risk in cases of meningitis and severe dehydration. Blood clots in the structures behind the eyes rapidly causing:
* Painful protruding eyes.
* Restricted eye movements.
* Eyes that look swollen.

COLOURED PATCHES ON EYEBALL

Doctors often check the eyes as a matter of routine because the eye may be an indicator of disease elsewhere in the body, for example jaundice or anaemia.

The POSSIBLE and RARE causes of coloured patches and are really very infrequent.

PROBABLE
PTERYGIUM
PINGUECULA

POSSIBLE
SCLERITIS

RARE
GROWTHS

PROBABLE

■ PTERYGIUM
A sheath of blood vessels and accompanying tissue grows out along the white of the eye towards the cornea. The term derives from the Latin for a wing — to which the 'path' does have a superficial resemblance.
* Commonest in the middle-aged.
* Small, triangular-shaped white tissue, blood vessels within.
* The broad base points away from the cornea.

A pterygium rarely causes anything other than a cosmetic problem, or possibly slight irritation; but can be removed if it threatens to grow over the cornea.

■ PINGUECULA
The name derives from a term meaning 'to do with grease'. These yellowish discolourations are again little more than a cosmetic nuisance. Usually only found in the elderly.
* Yellow, opaque raised lumps in the white of the eye.
* Triangular-shaped, with the broad base closest to the cornea.

POSSIBLE

■ SCLERITIS
In between episodes of inflammation, these groupings of blood vessels simply form a flat, discoloured area to one side of the eyeball. *See page 17.*

RARE

■ GROWTHS
Any of the lumps and bumps — warts, cysts, moles and cancers — that grow on skin anywhere in the body may appear on the white of the eye. Diagnosis is a specialist matter. Report any recently noticed spot to your doctor. Remember, the appearance of any of these on the eye is very rare. Much more common are pterygium and pinguecula, above.

DISCHARGE FROM EYES

Eyes may discharge tears or pus, or often a combination of both.

PROBABLE
CONJUNCTIVITIS
ALLERGY

POSSIBLE
BLOCKED TEAR DUCT
ECTROPION

RARE
GONORRHOEA

PROBABLE

■ CONJUNCTIVITIS
* Red, itchy eyes develop over a day or so.
* Constant discharge of small amounts of yellow pus.
* Eyelids stick together in the mornings.

Minor infections settle by bathing the eyes with tepid water; severe infections, especially in children, need antibiotic drops. *See also page 16.*

■ ALLERGY
Suggested by a combination of:
* Eyes that run depending on the season.
* Itching, depending on the season.

See also page 17.

POSSIBLE

■ BLOCKED TEAR DUCT
In babies, this is a common cause of eyes constantly running with tears and of repeated episodes of conjunctivitis. The tear duct is too narrow for tears to drain normally into the nose.
* Usually only one eye is affected.
* Eye runs tears even when the baby is perfectly well.

Most babies grow out of this by their first birthday. If necessary, it is possible to dilate the tear duct surgically — a minor operation.

■ ECTROPION
A lower eyelid turns outwards so that tears spill over; common in the elderly.

RARE

■ GONORRHOEA
Not long ago, gonorrhoea was common enough to consider it as the reason for a baby to develop a heavy discharge from the eyes. Now it is a rarity in the developed world. It affects new-born babies.
* Profuse yellow pus surrounding the eyes and under the eyelids.
* Swollen eyelids, making it difficult to open the eyes.
Untreated, it causes blindness.

CONSTANT TWITCHING MOVEMENTS OF THE EYES

Technical term: nystagmus. It is not always an abnormality, as some people show a few beats of nystagmus if they look to the extreme of their gaze. This apparently minor symptom has been the subject of extensive research.

PROBABLE
VESTIBULITIS

POSSIBLE
UNCORRECTED POOR VISION
MULTIPLE SCLEROSIS
ALCOHOLISM

RARE
TUMOURS
CONGENITAL BLINDNESS

PROBABLE

■ VESTIBULITIS
A viral illness that upsets the organs of balance within the ear.
* Abrupt giddiness.
* Nausea; vertigo on attempting to move.
* Nystagmus may be noticed by an observer.
Though alarming, it is a harmless condition that gradually fades away. *See also page 391.*

There is also a natural nystagmus which some people are born with. This is not a sign of any illness.

POSSIBLE

■ UNCORRECTED POOR VISION
An eye test is recommended if nystagmus is noticed in an otherwise well child.

■ ALCOHOLISM
Alcoholics with poor diets become deficient in vitamin B1, thiamine.

The result is damage within the brain, causing:
* Nystagmus.
* Poor memory.
* Disorientation.
* Weak, tingling limbs.

■ MULTIPLE SCLEROSIS
Nystagmus is not an early sign of multiple sclerosis, but is found in more advanced cases.
* Muscular weakness.
* Tremors.
* Stiff limbs.
* Blurred vision that comes and goes.

RARE

■ TUMOURS
Nystagmus of recent, otherwise unexplained onset suggests that the individual should be checked for brain tumours, of which other features may be:
* Change of personality.
* Severe headaches.
* Unilateral deafness, tinnitus.
* Unsteady gait.

■ CONGENITAL BLINDNESS
The eyes of those born blind frequently show searching movements, that is, a constant slow shifting of the gaze.

CLOUDY CORNEA OR LENS

Disease in either of these structures gives rise to a clouded, opaque appearance. Without the right equipment it may be difficult to decide whether the opacity is in the normally clear cornea, or whether it is in the deeper lens.

PROBABLE
CATARACT
INJURY

POSSIBLE
CONGENITAL

RARE
TRACHOMA
VITAMIN A DEFICIENCY
INFECTION
ACUTE GLAUCOMA
TUMOUR

PROBABLE

■ CATARACT
The clouded appearance of a cataract causes:
* Circular, grey appearance over–lying the pupil.
* Gradually worsening, indistinct vision.

A disease of later life. Standard treatment is to replace the cataract with an artificial lens.

■ INJURY
Any serious injury to the cornea will leave an opaque patch, which may obscure vision, depending on its position.

THE EYES

POSSIBLE

■ CONGENITAL
Several unusual inherited conditions can cause a cataract or lead to deterioration of the cornea during childhood. Diagnosis only established by a specialist examination.

RARE

■ TRACHOMA
Though rare in developed countries, this infection is one of the commonest worldwide causes of blindness.
* Swollen eyelids.
* Under surface of eyelids is granular.
* Gradual opacity of the cornea.

■ VITAMIN A DEFICIENCY
Or keratomalacia. Worldwide, this is a serious and avoidable cause of blindness, especially in children. Rare in developed countries.
* Hazy cornea with a thickened, coarse appearance.
* Night blindness.
* Coloured whites of the eyes.

■ INFECTION
Yet another hazard to vision now confined mainly to undeveloped countries. Possible sources of infection are parasites, gonorrhea and syphilis, complications of each giving rise to a clouded cornea.

■ ACUTE GLAUCOMA
Gives a clouded cornea, but in a red, excruciatingly painful eye *(see page 45)*.

■ TUMOUR
In children, the earliest sign of a tumour within the eye may be that the lens appears opaque.
* Often both eyes are affected.
* May be hereditary.
* A newly-appeared squint is also cause for suspicion.

CATARACTS

A cataract is an opaque patch within the lens of the eye. It cuts down the amount of light that can enter the eye and whatever light does enter is made hazy and blurred. An early cataract will not cause any symptoms and will only be spotted on examination of the eye; but a mature cataract is visible as a whitish haze on the lens. Between these two stages there will be variable symptoms.

Most cataracts are the result of ageing. Occasionally they occur following injury or disease. On rare occasions, a child is born with a cataract because of disease within the womb.

PROBABLE
AGEING
INJURY

POSSIBLE
DIABETES
STEROID USE

RARE
CONGENITAL RUBELLA
METABOLIC OR CONGENITAL DISEASE

PROBABLE

■ AGEING
Most people over 60 will have some opacity of the lens, but if a cataract forms, it will be relatively obvious.
* No other general disease.
* Vision deteriorates slowly.
* Eyes are pain free.

Cataract surgery is an ever-improving cure for this common problem.

■ INJURY
Any but the most superficial injury to the cornea or lens leaves a permanent scar. This includes burns and infections, of which trachoma is the most common.
* The size of the opacity remains unchanged.
* Disturbance of vision depends on its size.

POSSIBLE

■ DIABETES
Those suffering from this condition have an increased risk of developing cataracts in later life.

■ STEROIDS
Steroids are invaluable drugs, used in the treatment of many diseases including severe asthma, joint diseases and inflammatory eye diseases such as iritis (*see page 36*). However, their long-term use can cause many side-effects, including early formation of cataracts. So don't use steroid eye-drops without specialist advice and monitoring. Otherwise, there is a risk of causing cataracts and of allowing infections to run wild over the cornea.

RARE

■ CONGENITAL RUBELLA
Rubella — German measles — caught during the first four months of pregnancy will cause multiple abnormalities in the developing baby. These include:
* Cataracts.
* Mental retardation.
* Heart disease.
* Deafness.

These tragic consequences are avoided by routine vaccination of girls against the disease.

■ METABOLIC OR CONGENITAL DISEASE
Several unusual conditions may explain cataracts in children, usually in association with:
* Failure to thrive.
* Developmental delay.

TWITCHING EYELID

For some reason this symptom generates much anxiety. It is not clear why this should be so. Although Hollywood uses it as

cinematic shorthand for an impending nervous breakdown, it is harmless.
* Brief, repeated twitching.
* Same lid is affected.
* Worse when tired or stressed.
* Rarely lasts for longer than a few days.

DROOPING EYELIDS

PROBABLE
ECTROPION

POSSIBLE
BELL'S PALSY
CONGENITAL

RARE
THIRD NERVE PALSY
MYASTHENIA GRAVIS
SYPHILIS

PROBABLE

■ ECTROPION
Sagging of the lower eyelids, very common in the elderly.
* The red under-surface of the lid is exposed.
* Tears spill out easily on to the cheek.
* Increased risk of conjunctivitis.

Really bad cases can be tightened up by a simple operation.

POSSIBLE

■ BELL'S PALSY
A paralysis of the facial nerve.
* One lower eyelid droops.
* Sudden onset.
* The eye cannot be completely closed.
* The face sags on that side.

Recovery takes time and is often incomplete. Medical examination is advisable to exclude a stroke, giving a similar picture, but with subtle differences.

■ CONGENITAL
The probable diagnosis in a child with drooping upper eyelids.
* Normal eye movements.
* Normal muscular power.

RARE

■ THIRD NERVE PALSY
Refers to the third cranial nerve which is damaged (for example by pressure).
* Paralysis involves one eye only.
* Drooping upper lid.
* Eye turns outwards.
* Enlarged pupil.

Specialist investigation is needed to determine the underlying cause, which may be a brain tumour, or an enlarged artery in the brain.

■ MYASTHENIA GRAVIS
A treatable condition causing rapid tiring of the muscles. Drooping eyelids are an early feature.
* Both upper eyelids are affected.
* Muscles elsewhere grow fatigued abnormally fast.

■ SYPHILIS
The late stage of syphilis, which may be 20 years after the first infection, causes widespread nerve disorders.
* Tingling feet.
* Brief shooting pains in the limbs.
* Unsteady movements.
* Pain sensation is diminished.
* Drooping eyelids on both sides.

EYELIDS INFLAMED OR ITCHY

Localized inflammation probably due to infection. More generalized itching is usually allergic.

PROBABLE
BLEPHARITIS
ALLERGY

POSSIBLE
INSECT BITES
PUBIC LICE

RARE
TRACHOMA

PROBABLE

■ BLEPHARITIS
An irritating condition in which the margins of the eyelids just by the roots of the hairs become chronically inflammed.
* Constant raw appearance.
* Crusting near the roots of the eyelashes.
* Flaking skin on eyelids.
* Intense irritation.

The problem is often associated with eczema elsewhere on the body. All doctors have their favourite treatments, a sure sign that none works, but antibiotic ointments may help.

This common condition may be thought of as a type of dandruff affecting the eyelids. Some people find it helps to wash their eyelids nightly with a diluted solution of shampoo on a cotton bud.

■ ALLERGY
The upper eyelid is involved, causing a persistent mild irritation and desire to rub.
* Skin is slightly reddened.
* Dry, flaking skin all over upper eyelid.
* Often eczema elsewhere.

This is another minor but annoying condition, presumably due to an allergic reaction. Possible triggers are hair spray, new eye make-up or nail varnish, but the reason often remains obscure even after allergy testing.

POSSIBLE

■ INSECT BITES
A common reason in the summer and autumn.
* Localized, raised red bump.
* Itchy for a few hours.

■ PUBIC LICE
Lice will happily make a home in any hairy area, including the eylids.. A diagnosis to be

delivered with tact.
* Tiny round insects seen adhering to root of eyelashes.
* May also inhabit the eyebrows.
* Will also be present in the pubic area.

Treatment is straightforward.

RARE

■ TRACHOMA
A Third World infection causing
* Swollen eyelids.
* Grainy red under-surfaces of the eyelids.

One of the most common preventable causes of blindness.
See also page 26.

LUMPS ON EYELIDS

PROBABLE
STYE
INFECTED MEIBOMIAN CYST

POSSIBLE
MOLLUSCUM CONTAGIOSUM

RARE
DACROCYSTITIS
RODENT ULCER

PROBABLE

■ STYE
Infection at the root of a single eyelash.
* Often preceded by a day of mild discomfort.
* Swelling appears at root of hair.
* Pus appears.

Antibiotic drops help, as does removing the hair to allow drainage of pus.

■ INFECTED MEIBOMIAN CYST
The meibomian glands are helpful little structures which produce a greasy lubricant for the eyelashes. Infection reaches them via hair roots.

The important difference between this condition and a stye is that the lump is behind the root of the eyelash, on the flat part of the eyelid. It can be felt and seen as a small, pea-like lump below the skin.
* Pain, redness inside an eyelid.
* Small, tender lump appears.

Treatment same as for a stye, although antibiotic pills may be required. Often an unsightly lump remains, which may need to be removed later.

POSSIBLE

■ MOLLUSCUM CONTAGIOSUM
A long name for a benign, wart-like condition, that appears in mini-epidemics among children.
* Small, rounded, slightly raised lumps.
* The centre of the lump dips inwards.
* Other, similar lumps likely elsewhere on body.

Harmless, though cosmetically a nuisance; can be removed.

RARE

■ DACROCYSTITIS
Infection in the tear-producing glands, which are tucked away at the corners of the eyes.
* Pain, swelling near bridge of nose.
* Skin becomes red and tender.
* Pus discharges from eye.

A fairly serious condition that needs early treatment. *See also page 33.*

■ RODENT ULCER
A slow-growing form of skin cancer, commonest in the elderly who have led an outdoor life.
* Begins as a small, pearly lump.
* Grows slowly.
* Centre ulcerates and bleeds.

Considered curable, but needs attention as early as possible. *See also page 14.*

SWOLLEN EYELIDS

The loose skin of the eyelids easily swells to an alarming degree, but rarely for any serious reason.

PROBABLE
ALLERGY
STYE
BLEPHARITIS (CHRONIC)

RARE
ORBITAL CELLULITIS
NEPHROTIC SYNDROME

PROBABLE

■ ALLERGY
An allergic reaction of the skin of the eyelids to soap, hair spray or some other agent, though frequently the cause remains unknown. Usually both eyes are affected.
* Painless.
* Mild itching, flaking skin.
* Looks worse after sleep, because swelling worsens when a person lies flat.

■ STYE
Though a stye is a boil at the root of an eyelash, large ones do cause generalized swelling of the rest of the eyelid. *See also page 30.*
* Only one eye affected.
* Treatment as for a stye.

■ BLEPHARITIS (CHRONIC)
Prolonged inflammation of this kind, described on *page 29*, eventually makes the eyelids permanently swollen and roll-edged.

RARE

■ ORBITAL CELLULITIS
A spreading infection involving the skin of the eyelids and the surrounding parts of the face.
* Confined to one eye.
* May begin in a scratch or a stye.
* So much swelling that the eyelids cannot be opened.
* Red, tender eyelids.
* Malaise, temperatures.

Needs vigorous and immediate treatment with antibiotics to

prevent it spreading into the eye or elsewhere in the face.

■ NEPHROTIC SYNDROME
A kidney disorder due to a variety of causes, as a result of which fluid builds up in several parts of the body. Usually in boys around two to three years.
* Gradual onset.
* Swelling of abdomen, ankles, and face.
* Breathlessness.

PAIN OR ACHING IN EYE AREA (even if slight)

PROBABLE
EYE STRAIN
NASAL CONGESTION
CONJUNCTIVITIS

POSSIBLE
GLAUCOMA
DACROCYSTITIS
FLU-LIKE ILLNESS
SINUSITIS

RARE
TUMOUR

PROBABLE

■ EYE STRAIN
This familiar symptom arises after hours of close work, especially under poor or glaring light.
* Vision is undisturbed.
* Aching in and around eyes.
* Relieved by a few hours' rest.

Recurrent eye strain means that you should have an eye test, or consider adjustment to the lighting where you work.

■ NASAL CONGESTION
Along with a common cold there is often:
* Aching behind and around the eyeball.
* Blocked, runny nose.
* Mild headache.

The symptoms settle after a few days.

■ CONJUNCTIVITIS
Gives a prickling sensation, together with:
* Red eyes, worst around the margins.
* Mildly irritated by light.
* No loss of vision.
* Often a crusty deposit on the eyelashes.

POSSIBLE

■ GLAUCOMA
See page 45. This serious, but treatable condition frequently causes no other symptoms than a vague ache in and around the orbit.

It is easily detected with a simple eye check by an optician.

■ DACROCYSTITIS
An infection in the tear duct at the inner corner of the eye.
* Pain and swelling.
* A red lump appears.
* Eye runs with tears and pus.

Early treatment with antibiotics is advisable.

■ FLU-LIKE ILLNESS
Aching in the eyes is a frequent accompaniment to a feverish illness, including the common cold, or flu.
* Vision unaffected.
* Slight redness of eyes.
* Fever, aching muscles.

Within a few days, the underlying causes shows itself.

■ SINUSITIS
A very common cause of aching in and around the eyes.
* Usually develops after a common cold.
* Pain or pressure felt across the forehead or under the eyes.
* Worse on leaning forward and in the morning.

Sinusitis responds to aromatic inhalations and antibiotics.

RARE

■ TUMOUR
Needs to be considered in cases of persistent pain, especially with:
* Children
* Bulging eye.
* Disturbed vision.
* Newly appeared squint.

DRY EYES

* A constant feeling of irritation in the eyes.
* Frequent, mild conjunctivitis.

PROBABLE
AGEING

POSSIBLE
DRY ATMOSPHERE

RARE
SJOGRENS' SYNDROME

PROBABLE

■ AGEING
It seems that the eye's natural ability to lubricate itself with tears decreases with age. 'Artificial tears' in the form of eye-drops are effective, but have to be used regularly.

Prolonged use of a VDU (visual display unit) can cause uncomfortable or dry eyes. There is static electricity between the eyes and the screen. Dust is attracted to the eyes and can cause irritation. Tip: have your own duster and use it to keep the area around your work-station as free from dust as possible.

THE EYES

POSSIBLE

■ DRY ATMOSPHERE
Many people complain of dry eyes during the winter, when central heating systems are on.

RARE

■ SJOGREN'S SYNDROME
A general term for a group of disorders in which membranes in the eyes and in the salivary glands dry out, leading also to a dry mouth. It may be associated with rheumatic disorders or with auto-immune disorders, giving rise to:
* Joint pains.
* Swollen joints.
* Rashes.

Blood tests can pin down the underlying cause.

FEELING SOMETHING IN THE EYE

Considering how much dust flies around the average street, it is remarkable how rarely anything gets into the eyes.
* A sudden, pricking feeling in one eye.
* Rapid blinking.
* Tears, aversion to light.
* Mild discomfort.
* The feeling that you must get something out of your eye.

PROBABLE
FOREIGN BODY
CONJUNCTIVITIS

POSSIBLE
INGROWING EYELASH
ALLERGY
STYE

RARE
CORNEAL ULCER

PROBABLE

■ FOREIGN BODY
Typically dust. Often a helper can see and remove the foreign body. But beware of a foreign body involving high-speed fragments, for example, while hammering concrete or drilling. Continuing symptoms, or signs of infection, deserve specialized examination in case a foreign body has lodged deeper in the eye.

■ CONJUNCTIVITIS
It is common, during the early stages of conjunctivitis before the redness is noticeable, to feel that something is lodged in the eye. No doubt many cases of conjunctivitis do actually begin with a small foreign body, which then creates infection.

POSSIBLE

■ INGROWING EYELASH
A constant feeling of irritation in one part of the eye suggests that you should scrutinize the eyelids for this frequently overlooked cause.

■ ALLERGY
A recurrent feeling of irritation may be caused by allergy:
* Mild redness.
* Itching, rather than pain.
See also page 17.

■ STYE
An infection at the root of one of the eyelashes.
* Visible as a yellow swelling.
* Thet eye becomes red.
* Swelling of the eyelid is common.

Pulling out the eyelash, if you can face it, allows drainage of the infection, otherwise antibiotic ointment treatment will be necessary.

RARE

■ CORNEAL ULCER
A possibility if only one eye is inflamed. These uncommon infections begin with:
* Itching in one eye.
* Intense photophobia.
* Redness, mainly around the coloured iris.

A doctor will check for an ulcer using a fluorescent stain. The usual cause is the herpes virus. Vigorous treatment with anti-viral eye drops is necessary.

MODERATE TO SEVERE PAIN IN EYE

With the exception of an obvious foreign body, any such degree of eye pain needs expert assessment since neglect may damage sight.

PROBABLE
FOREIGN BODY
ULCER OR ABRASION OF CORNEA

POSSIBLE
IRITIS
EPISCLERITIS
SHINGLES

RARE
ACUTE GLAUCOMA
RETROBULBAR NEURITIS
THROMBOSIS

PROBABLE

■ FOREIGN BODY
Dust, grit or in-growing eyelashes cause irritation out of all proportion to the size of the foreign body.
* One eye affected.
* Sudden onset, feeling something in the eye.
* Intense irritation and watering.
* Light irritates the eye.
* Vision unaffected, though may be blurred by tears.

The eye's own protective mechanisms sweep out the foreign body in most cases.

■ ULCER OR ABRASION OF CORNEA
An ulcer can quite easily occur on the delicate cornea, due to damage from a foreign body or from infection. The symptoms are:
* Intense discomfort in one eye.

The Eyes

* Builds up over a few hours.
* Light causes much discomfort.
* Redness around the iris (the coloured part of the eye).

POSSIBLE

■ IRITIS
An inflammation of the iris; it may be associated with a variety of rheumatic disorders, which need to be considered in recurrent cases.
* One eye affected.
* Redness, greatest around the coloured area.
* Marked aversion to light.
* Blurred vision.
* Small pupil on affected side.
Treatment with eye drops, though quite straightforward, is necessary to prevent permanent damage to the iris.

■ EPISCLERITIS
Irritation in one part of the eye:
* Redness in one obvious area of the white of the eye.
* Prominent blood vessels.
* Pain is moderate.
* Moderate aversion to light.
* Vision is unaffected, apart from blurring due to tears.

■ SHINGLES
Every doctor has a tale to tell of being fooled by the early stages of this condition, which is caused by the chicken pox virus.
* At first, discomfort around one side of the face with no skin changes.
* After five to ten days, a rash appears.
* Crusting sores develop over the eyelids, side of the nose and cheek.
* Accompanied by severe pain.
* If spots appear on the tip of the nose, there is an increased chance of the eye being affected.
The worry about this otherwise harmless condition is ulceration of the cornea. Fortunately, there are now powerful anti-viral drugs which reduce this possibility, but they need to be given early in the illness.

RARE

■ ACUTE GLAUCOMA
See page 45.

■ RETROBULBAR NEURITIS
Inflammation of the optic nerve, especially associated with multiple sclerosis.
* Rapid loss of vision in one eye.
* Moderate pain when the eye is moved.

■ THROMBOSIS
A blood clot in the skull behind the eyes, causing:
* Sudden pain behind both eyes.
* Eyes to protrude.

EYES ABNORMALLY SENSITIVE TO LIGHT

Any existing irritation of the eyes will cause some discomfort in bright light. Persistent or severe sensitivity to light is termed photophobia, and can be a symptom of:

PROBABLE
CONJUNCTIVITIS
ALLERGY

POSSIBLE
IRITIS
CORNEAL DAMAGE
MEASLES

RARE
MENINGITIS
ALBINISM

PROBABLE

■ CONJUNCTIVITIS
Mild redness around the outer parts of the whites of the eyes,plus:
* Sticky discharge.
* A mild, gritty feeling in eyes.
Antibiotic eye treatment is usually advisable. *See page 15.*

■ ALLERGY
Recurrent photophobia suggests an allergy, especially in someone with other signs of an allergic constitution, such as:
* Eczema.
* Runny nose: sneezing on exposure to pollens, animal hair.
* Itching eyes on exposure to dust or in specific environments.
* Vision is not affected, other than by the watering produced by the allergy.

Treatment is typically a combination of anti-histamine tablets and anti-allergic eye-drops.

POSSIBLE

■ IRITIS
See page 36.

■ DAMAGED CORNEA
A picture similar to iritis, but with:
* Less severe pain.
* Redness around the cornea.
* History of abrasion or ulcer in the eye.

Needs appropriate treatment.

■ MEASLES
An increasing rarity in developed countries, where vaccination programmes are leading to its eradication, measles is still found in the Third World, where it can kill up to 20 per cent of children.

Aversion to light is a prominent feature in the days before the rash appears.
* High fever for four days.
* Bloodshot eyes.
* Runny nose, cough.
* Blotchy red rash appears behind the ears and spreads over whole body.
* Temperature remains high for another three to four days.

RARE

■ MENINGITIS
Aversion to light is a significant symptom of meningitis, but there will usually be associated symptoms, including:
* Headache.
* Resistance and pain on attempting to bend the neck.
* Nausea.
* Drowsiness, or confusion.

* In babies, a bulging, soft spot on top of the skull.

If you suspect meningitis, don't delay seeking medical advice.

■ ALBINISM

Due to lack of pigment, albinos have a special sensitivity to bright lights. Nystagmus (abnormal eye movements, *see CONSTANT TWITCHING MOVEMENTS OF THE EYES, page 24)* and squint are also common features.

BLURRED VISION

The everyday experience of the world being somewhat out of focus can nearly always be put down to just that — in other words, you need spectacles.

Temporary blurring will result from any eye irritation causing tears to flow, for instance conjunctivitis. Persistent or recurrent blurring may result from the following:

PROBABLE
UNCORRECTED VISION

POSSIBLE
MACULAR DEGENERATION
CATARACT
EFFECTS OF DRUGS

RARE
DIABETES

PROBABLE

■ UNCORRECTED VISION

With time, the power of the lens of the eye changes, as does that of the muscles that change its shape in order to focus in on objects at different distances from the eye.

* A very gradual change.
* Can be corrected with spectacles.

Adults are aware of the process. This may not be so in children, who may not realize that they have a problem: hence the importance of eye tests in childhood.

POSSIBLE

■ MACULAR DEGENERATION

A process of deterioration of part of the retina in the elderly, causing loss of fine vision to a variable degree, not correctable with glasses. *See page 44.*

■ CATARACT

The interference with light caused by the cataract may be misinterpreted as blurred vision. *See page 25.*

■ EFFECTS OF DRUGS

Many drugs affect the muscles in the eye, causing blurred vision. It is a question of relating the symptom to taking the drug. Common culprits include those drugs given to control bladder function, and anti-depressants.

RARE

■ DIABETES
Swings in the bloodstream's sugar level can cause blurred vision.
* A temporary symptom, fading within minutes.
* Undiagnosed diabetes causes thirst, excess urine production, tiredness.

DISTORTION OF VISION

Objects look too small, or too large, and straight lines appear curved. Not a common symptom and, if persistent, needs expert assessment.

PROBABLE
UNKNOWN CAUSE

POSSIBLE
DETACHED RETINA

RARE
DISTORTION OF THE RETINA

PROBABLE

■ UNKNOWN CAUSE
The sensation of distortion of size or shape sometimes happens for just a brief moment. An object may suddenly seem to be distant.
* Vision otherwise unaffected.
* Recovers within moments.

POSSIBLE

■ DETACHED RETINA
Light falling on the crinkled, detaching retina is seen as distorted.
* Preceded by many floaters — *see page 42*
* The classic symptom is often described as a 'curtain coming down to obscure the sight'.
* Many flashing lights.

Seek medical help immediately, since early intervention can prevent loss of vision. *See page 47 for further details.*

RARE

■ DISTORTION OF THE RETINA
Just as distortion of a screen distorts the film projected on it, so distortion of the retina has the same effect. This may be caused by tumours, bleeding or inflamation. Other symptoms, if any, include:
* Symptoms of retinal detachment, *above.*
* A bulging eye.
* Loss of vision.
* In children, a white appearance to the lens.

DOUBLE VISION

Movements of the eyes are delicately co-ordinated by an automatic process of the brain. The process has to be learned, accounting for the alarming gyrations of the eyes that occur in new-born babies until they have

THE EYES

developed the necessary co-ordination. Once achieved, we experience stereoscopic vision beyond the dreams of Hollywood. When things go wrong, we start seeing two of everything since the brain is no longer able to merge the output from the two eyes into one image. Don't confuse this symptom with blurred vision, which raises quite different possibilities.

PROBABLE
USING EXTREMITIES OF GAZE
PARALYSIS OF EYE MUSCLES

POSSIBLE
MULTIPLE SCLEROSIS

RARE
DISPLACEMENT OF EYE BALL
MYASTHENIA GRAVIS
DISEASE OF ONE LENS

PROBABLE

■ USING EXTREMITIES OF GAZE
It is normal to experience double vision if the eyes are swivelled to the extreme left or right, up or down.

■ PARALYSIS OF EYE MUSCLES
The eye is moved by six muscles, each of which turns the eye in a particular direction. Paralysis of any of those muscles results in double vision because the affected muscle is unable to move the eye as well as the other eye can move. The pattern of weakness gives a clue as to which muscles are affected, being some combination of:
* The affected eye turning inwards or outwards.
* Eyelid may droop.
* Pupil on that side may be wider than on the unaffected side.

Many cases are unexplained. A head injury is a common cause and will be obvious. Other possibilities are meningitis, infections and botulism, but these give rise to further dramatic symptoms which overshadow the double vision, for instance:
* Severe headache.
* Confusion, drowsiness.
* The eye hurt by light.

POSSIBLE

■ MULTIPLE SCLEROSIS
A disease of the nervous system often beginning in early adult life. Double vision results from partial weakness of the eye muscles.
* Vision may also be blurred.
* Slight discomfort in the eye.
* Unsteadiness in walking.
* Tremor or weakness in the arms or legs.
* Numbness of the limbs.

The double vision usually recedes over a few weeks.

RARE

■ DISPLACEMENT OF EYEBALL
Caused by something pushing the eye forwards and interfering with

its movements. Bleeding behind the eye, or thrombosis, would be suggested by:
* Sudden onset.
* Pain in eye(s).
* Eye(s) suddenly protruding.

Graves' disease, associated with an overactive thyroid gland, or a tumour behind the eye, would produce:
* Slower onset of symptoms.
* Gradual protrusion of one or both eyes.
* Sweating, rapid pulse and weight loss.

■ MYASTHENIA GRAVIS
An unusual disease in which muscles anywhere in the body tire rapidly. Eye symptoms are an early feature.
* Eyelids droop.
* Double vision may occur in any direction of gaze.
* Both eyes are affected.

The diagnosis is established by the individual's reaction to certain injected drugs.

■ DISEASE OF ONE LENS
The apparently impossible symptom of double vision affecting one eye may, in fact, though rarely, be due to disease in one lens which splits the image as a prism does.

FLASHING LIGHTS

Caused by individual light receptors firing off in the retina.

PROBABLE
NORMAL

POSSIBLE
MIGRAINE

RARE
DETACHED RETINA

PROBABLE

■ NORMAL
Flashing lights are frequently experienced after a blow to the head or after suddenly getting up from a squatting position, when blood flow is briefly disturbed.
* Both eyes affected.
* You feel light-headed, briefly.
* Return to normal within seconds.

POSSIBLE

■ MIGRAINE
Flashing lights shimmering in one section of the field of vision are a typical warning of the onset of migraine.
* Usually both eyes are affected.
* Nausea.
* Headache.

See also page 112.

THE EYES

RARE

■ DETACHED RETINA
See page 47.
* One eye affected.
* A shower of flashes.
* Numerous floaters.

These symptoms need urgent specialist attention

FLOATERS - FLOATING SPOTS BEFORE THE EYES

The interior of the eye is a liquid, in which it is normal for clumps of cells to float around, hence the term 'floaters'. An alternative medical term is muscae volitantes, meaning 'flying flies'.

PROBABLE
NORMAL

POSSIBLE
SEVERE SHORTSIGHTEDNESS

RARE
DETACHED RETINA
DAMAGE TO RETINA

PROBABLE

■ NORMAL
A floater is probably harmless if:
* There are only one or two.
* Vision is otherwise normal.
* The eye is painless.

POSSIBLE

■ SEVERE SHORT-SIGHTEDNESS
This can cause the release of more than usual numbers of floaters.

RARE

■ DETACHED RETINA
See page 47. Before complete detachment, warning signs include:
* Large numbers of floaters.
* Showers of lights.

If you have these symptoms, you need urgent specialist attention.

■ DAMAGE TO RETINA
Inflammation or bleeding within the eye causes:
* Many floaters in one eye.
* Blurring of vision.
* Pain.
* Redness.

Treatment depends on the cause.

SEEING HALOES AROUND LIGHTS

This happens if the cornea becomes waterlogged, as in glaucoma, or if something within the lens is scattering light.

PROBABLE
GLAUCOMA

POSSIBLE
CATARACT

PROBABLE

■ GLAUCOMA
See page 45.
* Haloes, seen especially at night.
* Tunnel vision.

Untreated, glaucoma progressively destroys sight, producing little by way of symptoms until the disease is well advanced. So it is important to have your eyes checked if a close relative suffers from glaucoma, while those over 60 should be checked anyway from time to time.

POSSIBLE

■ CATARACT
See page 25. The haziness in the lens acts like a prism: it scatters light so that objects appear to be surrounded by haloes and rainbows.

TUNNEL VISION

Loss of the outer field of vision: you seem to look at the world through a tube. The brain is so adaptable that the condition can progress remarkably far before you notice a problem.

PROBABLE
GLAUCOMA

POSSIBLE
RETINITIS PIGMENTOSA
MIGRAINE

RARE
BRAIN TUMOUR
SYPHILIS

PROBABLE

■ GLAUCOMA
Suggested by the combination of:
* Tunnel vision.
* At night, bright lights appear to be surrounded by haloes.
* Sometimes, aching in eyes.
See page 45.

POSSIBLE

■ RETINITIS PIGMENTOSA
See page 46.

■ MIGRAINE
* Symptoms develop over a few minutes.
* Visual field appears to shrink.
* Followed by severe headache, nausea.
* Vision recovers.

THE EYES

RARE

■ BRAIN TUMOUR
Can cause tunnel vision by increasing the pressure inside the brain, or by a direct destruction of the parts of the brain required to interpret vision. There are likely to be other symptoms such as:
* Severe headache, typically on waking at night.
* Persistent nausea.
* Change of personality.
* Altered awareness.

■ SYPHILIS
Years after infection, the widespread damage wrought by this disease also causes a multitude of symptoms including:
* Severe shooting pains in limbs.
* Unsteady gait.
* Drooping eyelids.
* Loss of pain sensation in limbs, leading to grossly deformed joints.
* Some degree of mental disturbance.

BLINDNESS

There can be no glossing over the fact that many causes of blindness remain untreatable. It is, therefore, of little consolation — but nonetheless important — to know which causes of blindness are treatable, or at any rate controlable. People with high blood pressure, diabetes or a family history of glaucoma should take special care of their eyes and heed any warning signs, including flashing lights, pains in the eyes and pain in the temples.

BLINDNESS, GRADUAL

Gradual, permanent loss of vision.

PROBABLE
CATARACT
MACULAR DEGENERATION
DIABETIC EYE DISEASE
GLAUCOMA

POSSIBLE
HIGH BLOOD PRESSURE
CHOROIDITIS
RETINITIS PIGMENTOSA

RARE
TRACHOMA

PROBABLE

■ CATARACT
A white patch seen in the lens of the eye and nearly always due to the ageing process.
* Very gradual loss of clear vision.
* The awareness of light is not lost, only clarity.

Cataract surgery is surely one of modern medicine's unqualified successes. *See page 25.*

■ MACULAR DEGENERATION
The retina of the eye is made up of a sandwich of light-sensitive elements. The macula is a small area of the retina where these elements are most concentrated

and where the sharpest vision is achieved.

'Degeneration' means, literally, decrease in function — part of the natural process of ageing. This is the commonest cause of deterioration of eyesight in the elderly. Disease in the macula has a serious effect on vision, but does not cause total loss of sight. The usual reason for it is deterioration in the blood supply or the nerves to or in that area. Unfortunately, little can be done to halt established degeneration, but sometimes it is possible to seal blood vessels with a laser.

* Gradual, painless loss of vision.
* Central vision deteriorates.
* Vision, especially close vision, is blurred and not improved with spectacles.
* Outer vision is unaffected.
* Objects may look distorted or small.

There is never complete loss of vision, because the outer parts of the retina are spared.

■ <u>DIABETIC EYE DISEASE</u>
One long-term effect of diabetes is degeneration of blood vessels within the retina. This causes loss of vision that can be gradual or sudden, depending on the pattern of degeneration. Diabetics, therefore, need regular checks on their retinas. It is possible to treat blood vessels which appear diseased with a laser beam. There are no symptoms of this condition: it has to be assessed by an expert.

■ <u>GLAUCOMA</u>
Raised pressure inside the eye, a common condition, which should be screened for in the elderly and earlier in those with a family history of glaucoma. The features of blindness caused by this insidious disease are:

* Painless.
* Peripheral vision is lost, giving rise to tunnel vision.
* Occasionally, aching in eyes.
* At night, bright lights appear to be surrounded by a halo.

POSSIBLE

■ <u>HIGH BLOOD PRESSURE</u>
This may increase the likelihood of macular degeneration (*see above*) and should be treated. Mild to moderate high blood pressure has no symptoms. Very high blood pressure over a long period may cause:

* Severe headaches.
* Symptoms due to strain on the heart such as breathlessness, ankle swelling, palpitations or chest pain.

■ <u>CHOROIDITIS</u>
The choroid is one of the layers in the sandwich that makes up the retina. Inflammation in the choroid results in a gradual, but permanent, loss of vision corresponding to the site of damage. The reason for most cases of choroiditis is unknown, although there is a proven association with toxoplasmosis, an infection that causes an illness similar to glandular fever.

Syphilis used to be a more common cause.

* You may recall an episode of disturbed vision in one eye.

THE EYES

* You then become aware of an area of blindness in that eye.
* Only one eye affected.
* The area is fixed, and neither grows nor shrinks.

■ RETINITIS PIGMENTOSA
A degenerative condition affecting the retina and so called because of the dark pigment that is visible over the retina through an opthalmoscope. This tends to be an inherited condition and nothing can be done to stop it.
* Symptoms begin in adolescence.
* Gradual loss of the peripheral field of vision, leading eventually to tunnel vision.
* Night blindness.

RARE

■ TRACHOMA
Worldwide, trachoma is a common cause of blindness, but it is rare in the developed world. The infection causes:
* Extremely sore, puffy eyes.
* Running eyes.
* Scarring of the cornea, resulting in partial or total blindness.

SUDDEN BLINDNESS

Unusual, but when it does occur, this usually has a serious underlying cause.

PROBABLE
BLOCKAGE OF CENTRAL RETINAL ARTERY
BLOCKAGE OF CENTRAL RETINAL VEIN
DETACHED RETINA
AMAUROSIS FUGAX – MINI-STROKE
STROKE

POSSIBLE
TEMPORAL ARTERITIS
MIGRAINE
OPTIC NEURITIS
VITREOUS HAEMORRHAGE
ACUTE GLAUCOMA

RARE
METHYL ALCOHOL POISONING
INJURY
HYSTERIA

POSSIBLE

■ BLOCKAGE OF CENTRAL RETINAL ARTERY
This artery supplies blood to the back of the eye. Blockage may occur because of a tiny blood clot or because the artery constricts to the point where it cuts off blood flow:
* Sudden, total blindness.
* No pain.
* One eye affected.

If the blockage is a result of spasm of the artery, there is a chance of vision returning after an hour or so. Otherwise, there is no treatment. It is important to search for causes that may threaten the sight of the other eye, for example, a source of blood clots in the heart, or temporal arteritis (*see below*).

■ BLOCKAGE OF THE CENTRAL RETINAL VEIN
This vessel carries blood away from the eye. Blockage is usually caused by pressure from a diseased retinal artery, which runs very close to the vein.
* The elderly, and those with diabetes or high blood pressure, are at increased risk.
* Loss of vision is rapid, but not instant, as in arterial blockage.
* Usually, light can still be seen. Sometimes partial vision returns, though this can take a few weeks.

■ DETACHED RETINA
It may come as a surprise to know that the retina is not firmly attached to the back of the eye, but is held in place by the pressure of fluid within the eye. The retina can tear, allowing fluid to leak behind it and to peel it off the back of the eye. A blow to the head may also dislodge the retina, or, rarely, a tumour growing at the back of the eye.
* Most common in the very short-sighted.
* Multiple flashing lights may be a warning of detachment.
* A shadow appears to fall over the field of vision. Sometimes described as a curtain descending over the field of vision.

With early treatment, the retina can often be anchored back into place.

■ AMAUROSIS FUGAX — MINI-STROKE
This is, in fact, a blockage of the central retinal artery; however, the blood clot rapidly dislodges.
* Sudden, painless loss of vision in one eye.
* Vision returns after a few minutes.

Your doctor must search for the site where the blood clots originate. It is usually in the carotid artery, which runs up the neck.

■ STROKE
A stroke is caused by blockage of blood flow within the brain. If the blockage happens to involve the part of the brain that processes the information from the eyes, the result is blindness.
* Sudden, painless onset.
* Vision is usually lost in both eyes at once.
* Sudden paralysis of one side of the body.
* In severe strokes, unconsciousness follows.

The exact nature of the loss of vision can give a clue as to where in the brain damage has occurred.
See also BLIND SPOTS, page 49.

POSSIBLE

■ TEMPORAL ARTERITIS
This cause of blindness should be better known because it is treatable. It is associated with a condition known as polymyalgia rheumatica *(see also page 271)* and occurs in the elderly.
* Gradual appearance of a vague weakness and malaise.
* Muscular tenderness, especially

The Eyes

around shoulders and neck.
* Tenderness over the temples: a very significant symptom.

The condition responds dramatically to steroid drugs, which can save sight if the condition is recognized in time.

■ MIGRAINE
Visual disturbances, including temporary blindness, are common in migraine. Commonest in, but not confined to, the young and middle-aged.
* Shimmering lights in the eyes.
* Nausea.
* One-sided blindness.
* Possibly slurred speech, loss of use of one hand.
* As symptoms fade, a severe headache begins.

The first time this happens, it may seem like a stroke. Many doctors recommend further tests, since occasionally there is a cause for the migraine within the brain.

■ OPTIC NEURITIS
Inflammation of the optic nerve, usually in a young adult.
* Sudden loss of vision in one eye.
* Usually, the loss is confined to the central field of vision, so the individual can still see 'at the edges of vision'.
* The eye may ache.

Recovery after a few days. Optic neuritis can be a warning sign of multiple sclerosis. Other underlying causes may be syphilis, diabetes, and lack of B vitamins.

■ VITREOUS HAEMORRHAGE
Bleeding into the fluid within the eyeball. Associated with diabetes, and with general arterial disease.
* Mild cases give rise to multiple floaters — *see page 42*.
* Otherwise painless partial loss of vision in one eye.

The condition is confirmed by looking at the interior of the eye with an opthalmoscope. There is rarely any treatment. The outcome depends on the size of the bleed and any underlying disease.

■ ACUTE GLAUCOMA
See page 45. Suggested by the sudden onset of:
* Excruciating pain in one eye.
* Red eye.
* Glazed appearance of the eye.

Requires emergency treatment.

RARE

■ METHYL ALCOHOL
Drinkers of methylated spirits are at risk of sudden blindness in one or both eyes. It may be total.

■ INJURY
A head injury can cause sudden blindness by damaging the part of the brain involved in vision, or by causing retinal detachment — see above.

■ HYSTERIA
Blindness of psychological origin is suspected if the back of the eye appears normal and if electrical tests show that visual stimuli are reaching the brain. The individual has usually exhibited other odd physical symptoms, such as:
* Unexplained paralysis.
* Loss of speech.
* Abnormal gait.
* Does not show the expected

emotional reaction to blindness, when for most people it is a devastating event.

There is often previous psychotic history.

BLIND SPOTS

You may become aware of an area of your field of vision where the vision is dim or absent altogether. Wherever you look, that patch remains fixed in relation to the rest of your visual field. This is known as a scotoma. A scotoma that suddenly appears draws attention to itself, whereas a slowly enlarging scotoma can be entirely overlooked until it is a considerable size — you are aware only of unspecific blurring of vision.

Scotomas in both eyes are due to damage to the optic nerves somewhere in the brain. A scotoma in one eye is nearly always due to a cause within that eye.

A scotoma should not be confused with the blind spot which every one has: an area of dim vision which might possibly be noticed if one eye is covered and an object slowly moved to the side. There is a point at which the object briefly disappears from vision. This corresponds with the part of the retina where the optic nerve leaves the eye and where, therefore, there are no visual receptors.

PROBABLE
MACULAR DEGENERATION
STROKE
INJURY

POSSIBLE
PITUITARY TUMOUR

RARE
POISONING
CAROTID ANEURYSM
HEREDITARY

PROBABLE

■ MACULAR DEGENERATION
Age-related deterioration of the eye causing a fixed area of dim or absent vision. *See page 44.*
* One eye affected more than the other.
* A loss of vision in the centre of the field.
* The area of loss may increase very slowly.

■ STROKE
A stroke affecting the back of the brain causes:
* Loss of part of the field of vision.
* Both eyes are affected.
* Other features of a stroke, such as paralysis, confusion.

See also page 47.

■ INJURY
A blow to the head severe enough to damage the eye or the brain

may cause loss of vision.
* Usually both eyes are affected.

POSSIBLE

■ PITUITARY TUMOUR
The pituitary gland is a structure in the brain which lies close to the nerves coming from the eyes. Any tumour in the gland presses on those nerves, producing a characteristic blind spot.
* Painless.
* Loss of the outer field of vision.
* Both eyes affected.
* Mild headache.

There may be other symptoms as a result of abnormal hormone production: for example, excessive height, absent periods, breasts constantly leaking milk.

RARE

■ POISONING
Tobacco, ethyl alcohol and lead are some of the many poisons that may affect the optic nerve.
* Gradual loss of the central field of vision.
* Vision is generally dimmed.
* Loss of vision may be abrupt after a binge.

Recovery depends on how long-standing the damage is.

■ CAROTID ANEURYSM
Caused by the effect of pressure from a swollen carotid artery within the brain, which presses on the optic nerve.
* A blind area in the outer field of vision.
* Affects one eye at first.
* Gradually involves both eyes.

■ HEREDITARY
Rare, inherited conditions might be considered in young adults who develop a scotoma.

NIGHT BLINDNESS

PROBABLE
RETINITIS PIGMENTOSA

POSSIBLE
SEVERE SHORT-SIGHTEDNESS
CONGENITAL

RARE
VITAMIN A DEFICIENCY

PROBABLE

■ RETINITIS PIGMENTOSA
See page 46. Suspected in a young adult with:
* Night blindness.
* Tunnel vision.

POSSIBLE

■ SEVERE SHORT-SIGHTEDNESS
* Difficulty seeing when the light is poor.
* Blurred vision, helped by glasses.

■ CONGENITAL
Occasionally, poor night vision is present from birth.

RARE

■ VITAMIN A DEFICIENCY
Vitamin A is required for vision, this being the basis for the parental wisdom that eating carrots, a rich source of Vitamin A, will help night vision. It is a fair bet that this explanation will leave children unimpressed and carrots uneaten, but children should, at least, be aware that lack of this vitamin is a major cause of blindness in the Third World.
* Night blindness is an early symptom.
* The eyes appear leathery, the lenses clouded.

Given soon enough, high doses of Vitamin A save sight.

COLOUR BLINDNESS

A condition affecting about one in 12 males and about one in 200 females. In the commonest form, red–green vision is partly or completely absent; less commonly, blue–green vision is affected. Total absence of any colour vision is very rare. So adaptable is the brain that it is possible to reach adult life without any suspicion of a problem. The individual appears to distinguish colours by noting subtle differences in brightness and greyness; context also helps — for example the lowest traffic light is green because that is what everyone else calls it. The writer has even known a successful colour-blind interior designer. Normal colour vision is needed in certain occupations — typically pilots and train drivers — where it is essential to see colour absolutely correctly.

Occasionally, someone with previously normal colour vision finds it deteriorating for one of the following reasons:

PROBABLE
CATARACT
DAMAGE TO THE RETINA

POSSIBLE
MALNUTRITION

RARE
TOXIC DRUGS

PROBABLE

■ CATARACT
This common problem, typically experienced as haziness in the lens, does not really destroy colour vision but makes colours less easy to distinguish. *See page 25.*

■ DAMAGE TO RETINA
Many retinal diseases can affect colour vision by damaging the receptors responsible for seeing colour. Other symptoms, considered fully elsewhere in this section, can include:
* Gradual loss of vision.

THE EYES

* Sudden loss of vision.
* Blind spots.

It is not possible to be more specific without medical assessment of the eye, optic nerve and the parts of the brain responsible for vision.

POSSIBLE

■ MALNUTRITION
Lack of vitamins and protein needed for the visual receptors can cause colour vision to deteriorate. It is a possibility among the very poor, alcoholics, those with wasting diseases or the mentally disturbed.

There is likely to be also:
* Night blindness. *See page 000*.
* In children, failure to grow.
* Hair loss, loss of skin colour.
* Swollen ankles.

RARE

■ TOXIC DRUGS
This includes massive over-use of tobacco, and alcoholism.

Overdosage of digoxin, as used in heart disease, can make the world look yellow or green.

SQUINTS

A squint is the result of the eyes being out of alignment: they appear to point in different directions. Often a squint is suspected as an impression rather than definitely seen: you may have the feeling on looking at someone that their eyes are not quite in line. If that someone is a child, please do not ignore your feeling, for squint is an important symptom and should never be ignored.

Forget the old wive's tale of children growing out of a squint; it does not happen. What does happen is that the child experiences double vision and gradually its brain learns to ignore the vision from one eye in an effort to overcome the defect. If unrecognized, this leads to permanently damaged vision in one eye. Symptoms which suggest a squint are:
* Obvious deviation of one or both eyes.
* Head held in an unusual posture, to compensate.
* Squint noticed if child is tired.

The assessment and treatment of squint is a complex area. In most cases the cause is either muscle imbalance or different strengths of lens of each eye. Both causes are treated by surgery or by glasses.

PROBABLE
MUSCLE IMBALANCE OR INEQUALITIES OF VISION

POSSIBLE
PROMINENT SKIN FOLDS

RARE
NERVE PALSIES
TUMOURS OF EYE OR SOCKET

PROBABLE

■ <u>MUSCLE IMBALANCE OR INEQUALITIES OF VISION</u>
If the head is held at an unusual angle, it suggests the likelihood of muscle imbalance underlying the squint. You may also notice that one eye cannot turn beyond a certain point. Otherwise it is likely that one eye is long-sighted or, less commonly, short-sighted compared to the other. Usually, however, it is a matter of specialist assessment to differentiate these possibilities.

POSSIBLE

■ <u>PROMINENT SKIN FOLDS</u>
In children, the folds of skin by the bridge of the nose may be unusually wide, giving the impression that the eyes turn in. Even if this happens to be the case, the child should still be checked.

RARE

■ <u>NERVE PALSIES</u>
It has been mentioned (*see PARALYSIS OF THE EYE MUSCLES page 40*) that six muscles control movements of the eyes. Each muscle is subject to paralysis for a variety of reasons. Nerve palsy is probably the cause if there is:
* Sudden onset of a previously unnoticed squint.
* A drooping eyelid.
* Changes in size of the pupil; *see page 19.*

Nerve palsies have a variety of causes, which themselves need further investigation.

■ <u>TUMOURS OF EYE OR SOCKET</u>
These can occur at all ages, producing a squint by pressure on one eyeball. So don't ignore a newly appeared sqint, especially in children.
* The eye protrudes more and more.
* There is a pain behind the eye.
* The pupil may appear white if the tumour is inside the eye.

THE NOSE

NOSE AN ODD SHAPE

There is, of course, no such thing as a 'normal' shape for a nose. The 'one-off' factors that can deform it are considered here.

PROBABLE
INJURY

POSSIBLE
RHINOPHYMA

RARE
NASAL SEPTAL NECROSIS
LEPROSY
MALIGNANT TUMOUR

PROBABLE

■ INJURY
Typically, the nose is flattened or made crooked (you may hear doctors describe the latter as 'deviation'). This is likely to be accompanied by fracture of the nose bone, swelling and bleeding.

It is normal to wait for a week to allow swelling to go down before deciding whether the nose needs straightening by surgery.
* Nasal bone fracture.
* Flattening of the nose.
* Deviation of the nose.
* Swelling.
* Bleeding.

POSSIBLE

■ RHINOPHYMA
Also known as 'potato nose' or 'bottle-nose'. Caused by over-activity of the sebaceous gland of the nose. It takes some years to develop.
* Large, bulbous nose.
* Purplishred in colour.
* Irregular 'pitted' surface: the pits mark the entrances to the glands.
Can be treated easily by surgery.

RARE

■ NASAL SEPTAL NECROSIS
A blow to the nose may not break the nasal bones, but instead damage the nasal septum (a thin layer of cartilage separating the two sides of the nose). Pressure from a blood clot under its mucous membrane covering causes:
* Headache.
* Local pain at the tip of the nose.
* Apparent widening of the tip of the nose.
* Loss of sensation over the skin of the nose.
* Destruction of septal cartilage over a matter of weeks, causing the nose to dip at the bridge.

■ LEPROSY
Causes collapse of the nose due to septal ulceration.

This is one of several obvious symptoms which will be apparent.

■ CANCER OF THE NOSE
Any irregular sore on the nose that enlarges over months or years,

that bleeds, ulcerates or is painful could be malignant. Enlargement of local lymph nodes suggests malignancy.

REDDENED NOSE

PROBABLE
STAPHYLOCOCCAL INFECTION

POSSIBLE
ACNE ROSACEA
ERYSIPELAS
RHINOPHYMA

PROBABLE

■ STAPHYLOCOCCAL INFECTION
An infection of the skin follicles in a part of the nose.
* Local swelling.
* Local redness
* Local pain.
* Local heat.

May require antibiotics.

POSSIBLE

■ ACNE ROSACEA
A rash caused by over-activity of the sebaceous glands.
* Associated with facial flushing.
* Redness from small blood vessels.
* Rash covers nose, brow, face and chin.
* Small pustules may be evident.
* May persist for years.

Treatment is available, but can be difficult.

■ ERYSIPELAS
A bacterial skin infection.
* Associated with a break in the skin.
* Often near eye, nose or mouth.
* Fever.
* Malaise.
* Hot, reddened swelling all over affected area.
* Painful.
* Blisters may appear.

Antibiotics will treat this effectively if given at an early stage.

■ RHINOPHYMA
See page 54.

STREAMING NOSE

PROBABLE
COMMON COLD
VASOMOTOR RHINITIS
ALLERGIC RHINITIS

POSSIBLE
SINUSITIS
FOREIGN BODY
NASAL POLYP
DRUG WITHDRAWAL

RARE
CANCER OF THE NOSE

The Nose

PROBABLE

■ COMMON COLD
See page 454. There are many different types of common cold virus. As you throw off each new one, you develop a natural immunity to it. Children often have a 'perpetual runny nose'. This is because they are being exposed to new viruses every day at school. The elderly rarely get colds for they have built up immunity to so many of the viruses.

■ VASOMOTOR RHINITIS
See also page 129. Some individuals suffer from over-reaction of the nasal lining. This leads to an excess of the usually small amounts of 'normal' nasal discharge. Some drug treatments taken as nasal sprays may help this condition. Its features are similar to those of allergic rhinitis.

■ ALLERGIC RHINITIS
See also page 129. In the same way that hay fever is caused by pollen, many allergens can cause a running nose. Locally applied steroid nasal sprays can be effective in preventing the reaction.

POSSIBLE

■ SINUSITIS
See page 129. Nasal discharge will often be yellow or green, sometimes thick. There may be an associated headache.

■ FOREIGN BODIES
See page 57. Discharge is foul-smelling and on one side only.
Antibiotics may help.

■ NASAL POLYP
Polyps — which are benign, fleshy growths — can appear inside the nose. As well as obstructing the nasal passages and blocking the nose, they can cause an increase in the volume of secretions, which will appear as a runny nose.
Treatment is surgical removal of the polyps.

■ DRUG WITHDRAWAL
A clear, runny discharge is a common symptom when withdrawing from a `hard' drug such as heroin, or its substitute, methadone. Other signs include:
* Running eyes.
* Sweating.
* 'Goose flesh'.
* Yawning.
* Stomach cramps.
* Diarrhoea.

RARE

■ CANCER OF THE NOSE
See page 59. Any tumour of the nose or in the spaces around the nose may cause a nasal discharge. Recurrent nosebleeds or bloody streaks in the discharge may be a feature.

NOSEBLEEDS

Also known as epistaxis. A particularly common problem in children, although most adults have episodes of bleeding from the nose at some time. There are many causes, some due to local disease and some indicative of systemic, or 'whole body', disease. Most nosebleeds can be treated by continuous, firm pressure across the fleshy part of the nose just below the bridge. Pressure should be maintained for as long as ten minutes in severe cases. Sit forward with the head supported and breathe through your mouth. Local application of ice may also help. Only in rare cases is medical or surgical intervention required. But see your doctor or local hospital emergency department about any profuse or prolonged bleeding.

PROBABLE
MINOR INFECTION
NOSE-PICKING
INJURY
COMMON COLD

POSSIBLE
FOREIGN BODY
CHRONIC SINUSITIS
DRUG-INDUCED
BENIGN TUMOURS, INCLUDING NASAL POLYPS

RARE
HEREDITARY HAEMORRHAGIC TELANGIECTASIA
DISORDERS OF BLOOD CLOTTING
HIGH BLOOD PRESSURE
CANCER OF THE NOSE

THE NOSE

PROBABLE

■ MINOR INFECTION
The commonest cause of persistent and recurrent nosebleeds is a minor nasal infection. This brings blood vessels very close to the surface on the inside of the nose. The slightest disturbance will then set off a nosebleed. Antibiotic ointment used inside the nose over a few days can have dramatic results.

■ NOSE-PICKING
Probably the commonest cause in children. The finger, or the fingernail, damage an area of skin, known as Little's area, situated at the entrance to the nose.
* Occasionally, profuse bleeding.
* Often occurs at night.
* Almost always cures itself after applying pressure.
* May be recurrent.

■ INJURY
If the nose is clearly deformed or misaligned as a result of a blow, see a doctor. There could be an underlying fracture.

■ COMMON COLD
Nosebleeds are a surprisingly frequent symptom of common colds. The inflammation compromises the fine blood vessels.

Repeated nose-blowing to clear mucus may also bring on bleeding.

POSSIBLE

■ FOREIGN BODY
A toddler or young child pushes a

The Nose

bead or some other small object into a nostril, which remains unrecognized for days, weeks or months. Inflammation develops, causing:
* Discharge from one nostril; it may be
* Purulent — yellow-green.
* Possibly bloodstained and smelly.

Removal may require a general anaesthetic.

■ CHRONIC SINUSITIS
The linings of the bony sinuses become chronically infected.
* Profuse discharge back into throat, rather than out through the nostrils.
* Obstruction of the nose.
* Head pain, particularly in the forehead or under the eyes.
* Loss of sense of smell.
* Nosebleeds, often with excessive noseblowing.

■ DRUG-INDUCED
A number of drugs, typically warfarin, which thins the blood, and some drugs used to treat arthritis may cause nosebleeds.

If nosebleeds occur while you are taking warfarin they may indicate that you are taking too much.

■ BENIGN TUMOURS, INCLUDING NASAL POLYPS
These can bleed from time to time, particularly after nose-picking or blowing.
* Obstruction of the nose.
* Associated sinusitis.
* Discharge of mucus.
* Loss of sense of smell.

The sinuses

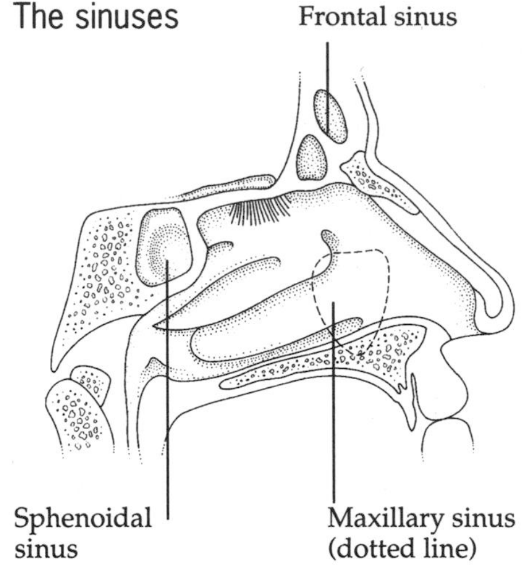

RARE

■ HEREDITARY HAEMORRHAGIC TELANGIECTASIA
See page 86.

■ DISORDERS OF BLOOD CLOTTING
The commonest are Factor 8 deficiency (true haemophilia) Christmas disease and von Willebrand's disease. Common features include:
* Persistent bleeding after minor cuts and abrasions.
* Marked bruising.
* Bleeding after extraction of teeth.
* Bleeding into joints, causing eventual degeneration.
* Spontaneous bleeding, nosebleeds.

Simple blood tests will determine whether there is any abnormality of clotting. It is particularly important to know if you have a disorder before dental treatment If in doubt, check.

■ HIGH BLOOD PRESSURE
In the middle-aged and elderly. An otherwise fit individual who suddenly gets recurrent nose-bleeds must have blood pressure measurements and tests to check clotting ability.

■ CANCER OF THE NOSE
There are several potential symptoms:
* Obstruction of the nose.
* Discharge from the nose.
* Pain in the teeth.
* Loosening of the teeth.
* Ill-fitting dentures.
* Associated sinusitis.
* Nose-bleeds.
* Protruding eyes.
* Visual disturbance.
* Sensory changes in face, nose and mouth.
* The skin may be involved.
* Lymph nodes may enlarge.

It is *very* rare for anyone to present nosebleeds to their doctor as a symptom of cancer of the nose.

NASAL-SOUNDING SPEECH

Any disease or injury that blocks the nose or distorts the naso-pharynx will alter the quality of the sound produced. Commonest of the causes are the common cold; septal deviation *(page 61)* ; 'adenoids' *(page 60)*; and injury. Less common, but worth considering, are: cleft palate *(page 87)*; a foreign body *(page 57)*; chronic sinusitis *(page 58)*; and benign tumours, including polyps *(page 58)*.

The naso-pharynx

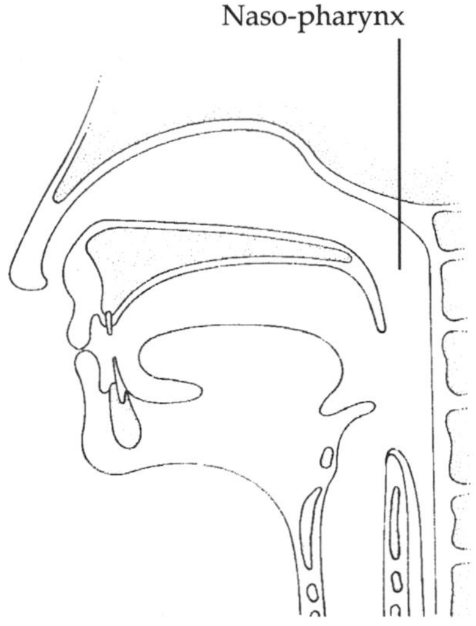

SNORING

An all-too-common problem, rarely reported to doctors by snorers.

It happens when the tongue obstructs air flow, setting up vibrations of structures in the mouth, particularly the uvula (the fleshy, wriggly bit that hangs down between your tonsils), soft palate and tongue. Most common in drinkers, the obese, the over-40's and males, and those with nasal obstruction or misshapen noses. Sleeping on the side, rather than the back, will probably help. If you find your partner's snoring is making you seriously dissatisfied with him (or her), you will not want a doctor to tell you to be understanding because snorers cannot help it. However, you should be interested in the fact that some snoring, some of the time, is inevitable.

Exceptionally severe, persistent snoring justifies surgery. A modern operation known as a uvuloplasty, which reshapes the soft palate at the back of the mouth, can transform the lives of severe snorers.

For less severe cases, one trick that is said to work is to sew a hairbrush inside the back of your pyjama jacket. This wakes you when you roll on to your back — the snoring position. Also try adjusting pillows and bedding, changing the ventilation in your bedroom and eating bedtime snacks — all of which are said to have made a difference to some people's snoring.

BREATHING THROUGH THE MOUTH: A BLOCKED NOSE

The effects of an obstructed nose depend somewhat on the cause, but may include:
* Pain in the nose.
* Discharge from the nose.
* No sense of smell.
* Breathing through the mouth.
* Snoring.
* Dry mouth.
* Bad breath.

For details, see the sections concerning those symptoms. Causes of obstruction include:

PROBABLE
'ADENOIDS'
SEPTAL DEVIATION
INJURY
COMMON COLD
VASOMOTOR RHINITIS
ALLERGIC RHINITIS

POSSIBLE
FOREIGN BODY
CHRONIC SINUSITIS
BENIGN TUMOURS, INCLUDING NASAL POLYPS

PROBABLE

■ 'ADENOIDS'
Perhaps the commonest reason for 'mouth breathing'. The adenoids are lymph tissue lying at the back of the nose and pharynx near the soft palate. They are prone to acute or chronic infection. **Acute infection gives:**
* Pain behind nose.
* Catarrh.
* Nasal obstruction (due to enlargement).
* Enlarged neck lymph nodes.

Chronic infection gives:
* Enlarged adenoids.
* Chronic catarrh.
* Persistent cough.
* Breathing through the mouth.
* Ear infection, possibly leading to impaired hearing.

Both types of 'adenoiditis' cause alteration in the quality of speech. As the adenoids perform no essential function, removing them is a common and usually very helpful operation: common, of course, in childhood.

This operation used to be carried out frequently. Current understanding of how both the adenoids and the tonsils develop is that there is a natural shrinkage of these tissues as a child reaches his or her tenth birthday. An operation can be avoided if symptoms are not too troublesome.

■ SEPTAL DEVIATION
The septum is the thin layer of cartilage separating the tow sides of the nose. 'Deviation' may occur during birth (one to two per cent of babies have permanently deviated septa). It may also occur as the result of injury at a later age. The result is obstruction of one or other of the nostrils, either partially or completely. *See NOSE AN ODD SHAPE, page 54.*

■ INJURY AND COMMON COLD
See page 54; and page 454.

■ VASOMOTOR RHINITIS and ALLERGIC RHINITIS
See page 129.

POSSIBLE

■ FOREIGN BODY, CHRONIC SINUSITIS AND BENIGN TUMOURS INCLUDING NASAL POLYPS: *see pages 57 and 58.*

PAINFUL NOSE

This is such a general symptom that analysing it in its own right is not helpful. There will always be some other accompanying factor(s) to pin it down. Is there nasal discharge or bleeding? Is the speech affected? Is the nose misshapen? Does the nose itch? Has the sense of smell gone? These are all covered in detail in neighbouring pages and will give proper insight into 'pain in the nose'.

TINGLING NOSE; SNEEZING

Look for an outside cause first: is it the smell of a houseplant, or an animal? Or a chemical? Or chili powder or pepper? Some people sneeze in bright sunlight. There are many different causes, a large number unique to individuals. Failing these, consider vasomotor rhinitis, or allergic rhinitis, *page 129.*

NO SENSE OF SMELL

Any progressive loss of the sense of smell suggests an underlying disorder and needs proper medical attention.

THE NOSE

PROBABLE
SMOKING
COMMON COLD
VASOMOTOR RHINITIS
ALLERGIC RHINITIS

POSSIBLE
OBSTRUCTIVE LESIONS OF NOSE
BREATHING THROUGH THE MOUTH
SINUSITIS

RARE
HEAD INJURY
MENINGIOMA
FRONTAL LOBE TUMOUR

PROBABLE

These diagnoses are either self-evident or covered in detail elsewhere: *see pages 454 and 129.* With a common cold, the loss is transient; vasomotor rhinitis and allergic rhinitis cause intermittent loss, which may become long-term.

POSSIBLE

■ OBSTRUCTIVE LESIONS OF THE NOSE
See BREATHING THROUGH THE MOUTH etc, page 60.

■ BREATHING THROUGH THE MOUTH
See page 60.

■ SINUSITIS
See page 129. Acute sinusitis may lead to transient loss and chronic sinusitis to long-term loss.

RARE

■ HEAD INJURY
A blow to the head may sever the filaments of the cranial nerve in the roof of the nose. As the nose is pushed in, or the forehead struck, there is a bony displacement which can cut the nerve responsible for sensing smell.
Permanent loss.

■ MENINGIOMA
A tumour of the sheath covering the brain. It can press on the olfactory nerve, causing progressive loss of smell and other symptoms, such as headache.

■ FRONTAL LOBE TUMOUR
This can cause pressure on brain tissue involved in sensing smell, and it can damage the pathways conducting sense of smell. Loss is progressive and other symptoms will be apparent.

THE EAR

This organ has something in common with an iceberg: there is so much more to it than you see. The visible ear is cartilage, covered with skin, and it is subject to any of the problems that affect skin elsewhere: bruising, infections and eczema.

Hidden from view is the eardrum, which guards the inner ear, a beautifully intricate structure that turns sound waves into the electrical impulses for transmission to the brain.

The inner ear also contains the fluid-filled semi-circular canals which give you your sense of balance and orientation. Then there are the passages connecting the inner ear to the back of the throat: they allow equalization of air pressure on both sides of the eardrum, without which you experience pressure or 'popping' in the ears. Skin, nerves, bones, fluid: little wonder that there are many minor diseases which can afflict the ear, and a few serious ones.

BLEEDING EAR

Blood from the ear, usually mixed with pus, is a common symptom, not often due to a serious cause.

PROBABLE
MIDDLE EAR INFECTION

POSSIBLE
BOIL
POLYP
INJURY

RARE
CANCER

PROBABLE

■ MIDDLE EAR INFECTION
This problem is inescapable in childhood, occasional in adults and usually accompanies a common cold. The eardrum becomes red and bulges. If the drum bursts, pus and blood ooze from the ear for a few days.
* Pain in the ear for a day or two.
* Then, suddenly, a smelly, blood-stained discharge.
* The pain goes.
* The discharge lessens over a few days.

The eardrum nearly always heals, but your doctor will want to watch progress in order to be certain.

POSSIBLE

■ BOIL
Just like a pimple elsewhere, a boil in the canal of the ear may burst, discharging a few specks of blood.
* An extremely tender spot, just inside the ear canal.
* Bursts after a day or two.
* Symptoms then rapidly vanish.

THE EARS

■ POLYP
These fleshy lumps can form deep inside the ear if there is recurrent infection. They are painless, but may ooze or bleed and can be seen through an instrument for seeing inside the nose.

■ INJURY
A severe blow to the head may rupture the eardrum and cause bleeding.

RARE

■ CANCER
Growths within the ear canal or within the inner ear are unusual.
* Intense, persistent pain in the ear.
* Constant discharge of pus mixed with blood.
* Partial paralysis of one side of the face.

BOIL IN THE EAR

PROBABLE
BOIL

POSSIBLE
HERPES SIMPLEX
RAMSAY-HUNT SYNDROME

PROBABLE

■ BOIL
Boils form at the root of the tiny hairs lining the ear canal. They cause pain out of all proportion to their tiny size because the skin of the ear canal is unable to stretch much without intense pain.
* Localized, throbbing pain.
* You may be able to feel a tender lump.
* Reaches a peak after a day or two.
* Discharges small amounts of blood and pus for a couple of days.

Will usually clear by itself, but antibiotic drops help.

POSSIBLE

■ HERPES SIMPLEX
A cold sore in the ear canal will give symptoms similar to a boil, but:
* The pain is more prolonged and recurrent.
* The sore is filled with clear fluid, rather than pus.

■ RAMSAY-HUNT SYNDROME
See page 69.

LUMPS AND BUMPS ON THE EAR

PROBABLE
RESOLVED BOIL
CAULIFLOWER EAR

POSSIBLE
AURICULAR APPENDAGE
WART

RARE
GOUT
TUMOURS

PROBABLE

■ RESOLVED BOIL
Meaning the aftermath of a boil.
* Initially, pain and redness from the boil.
* May discharge pus.
* Becomes smaller over a few days.
* Firm lump left at the site.

Usually the lump disappears, but this can take months.

■ CAULIFLOWER EAR
This is the permanently enlarged, fleshy, misshapen ear left after injury. It results from permanent scarring of the cartilage that makes up the external ear and is an occupational hazard of boxers and rugby players.

POSSIBLE

■ AURICULAR APPENDAGE
A small, painless outgrowth between the ear canal and the cheek. It is present from birth, harmless and removable.

■ WART
Can occur on the ear as on other parts of the skin.
* Appears rapidly, then stops growing at about 2/10 in/5 mm in length.
* The end is rough, with black spots.

Removable.

RARE

■ GOUT
A disorder of body chemistry leading to the appearance of crystals of uric acid in many parts of the body, especially the joints.
* Firm, irregular lumps called tophi in the outer ear.
* These become extremely painful.
* Pain in other joints, classically the big toe.

■ TUMOURS
A slow-growing skin cancer can involve the ear.
* Begins as a small, crusted spot.
* Develops a rolled edge.
* May bleed.
* Does not heal.
* Gradually enlarges.

This is a benign form of cancer, treated by freezing or by radiotherapy.

DISCHARGING EAR

PROBABLE
EAR INFECTION
OTITIS EXTERNA

POSSIBLE
CHRONIC OTITIS MEDIA

RARE
CHOLESTEATOMA
POLYP
RUPTURE OF EARDRUM

The Ears

PROBABLE

■ EAR INFECTION
See page 63.
Gives pain, pus and blood for a few days.

■ OTITIS EXTERNA
Meaning eczema of the skin lining the ear canal. The skin of the ear canal is as prone to eczema as is skin elsewhere in the body.

Aggravating factors include swimming-pool chemicals, poking about in the ear with pencils or earbuds, and even medicated ear drops. Frequently, bacteria or fungi invade the eczema, giving a mixed picture of infection and irritation which it is difficult to cure.
* Intensely itching ear canals.
* Persistent, thin, watery discharge.
* Discharge thicker if infection occurs.

Treatment is with anti-fungal, anti-inflammatory ear drops and often needs to continue for many weeks.

POSSIBLE

■ CHRONIC OTITIS MEDIA
Literally, chronic infection of the inner ear, with pus discharging for weeks on end through a hole in the eardrum. There is usually a previous history of repeated ear infection.
* Yellowish discharge.
* Quantity varies from day to day.

Treatment involves eradicating infection, getting air into the ear and, eventually, repairing the hole in the eardrum.

RARE

■ CHOLESTEATOMA
This is a mass of abnormal cells which forms usually as a result recurrent ear infections. The cells destroy surrounding tissues, so causing symptoms of:
* Deafness.
* Discharge.
* Vertigo.

Treatment consists of surgically removing the cholesteatoma and refashioning the inner ear. This is a complex operation.

■ POLYP
A fleshy, non-cancerous growth arising from a cholesteatoma and causing discharge, sometimes bloodstained.

■ RUPTURE OF EAR DRUM
Caused by injury and resulting in:
* Deafness, which may be partial or total.
* Ringing in ears.
* Bloody discharge.

An injury serious enough to fracture the skull near the ear means that the fluid which surrounds the brain may leak out of the ear. This significant condition causes the above symptoms plus:
* Painless, persistent leakage of clear fluid.

EARACHE

Pain in the ear is usually caused by a relatively minor problem within the ear. It nonetheless keeps doctors on their toes because it can be a symptom of disease elsewhere.

PROBABLE
INFECTION
EUSTACHIAN CATARRH
WAX
BOIL

POSSIBLE
THROAT INFECTION
TEETH PROBLEMS
MASTOIDITIS
PERICHONDRITIS

RARE
RODENT ULCER
TIC DOULOUREUX
RAMSAY-HUNT SYNDROME
CANCER OF EAR
CANCER OF TONSIL
CANCER OF TONGUE

PROBABLE

■ EAR INFECTION

See page 63.

Pain, pus and discharge arising over a few hours or days. A routine symptom in children with common colds.

■ EUSTACHIAN CATARRH

This condition may be described by your doctor as Eustachian tube dysfunction.

If fluid builds up inside the inner ear, it muffles hearing. This condition is common for a few days or weeks after a common cold. Chronic catarrh is also familiar to those who suffer from hay fever or sinusitus. It is particularly important to pick up in childhood since it can cause deafness severe enough to interfere with speech and to hinder progress in school.

* Hearing is muffled.
* A feeling of pressure inside the ear.
* Yawning relieves pressure temporarily.
* In children, delay in learning to speak.

Adults rarely need any treatment other than decongestants; children suffering deafness may need surgery to drain the fluid.

The Eustachian tube is a ventilation pipe which goes from the back of the throat to the inner ear. Air passes through the tube to equalize the pressure on either side of the eardrum. This is why swallowing relieves popping ears. The tube is narrowest in childhood and it is then that most problems occur.

■ WAX

A block of hard wax may eventually become painful and give rise to muffled hearing. People vary enormously in how much ear wax they produce and often recognize

The Ears

for themselves when so much has built up that they need their ears cleared by syringing. If possible, however, leave your ears alone.

The ear is a self-cleaning organ. It is rarely necessary to have ears syringed. Small hairs move the wax to the outer ear where it can be wiped away.

Avoid cleaning your ears with cotton buds — it causes more problems than it cures. Ear syringing, once it has been started, tends to need repeating. This is thought to be due to damage to the hairs in the ear canal. Always try simple earwax softening drops first, and try to allow the ear to clear naturally.

■ BOIL
See page 64. A pimple in the ear canal, causing a remarkable amount of pain for such a small object.

POSSIBLE

■ THROAT INFECTION
A throat infection (including tonsillitis) may seem obvious and recognizable, but often the throat symptoms are overshadowed by earache. Especially common in young children.
* Sore throat.
* Pain on swallowing.
* If tonsillitis, white patches may be present on tonsils.

■ TEETH PROBLEMS
The large molar teeth, if decayed, may cause aching which appears to radiate into the ear. In children, eruption of the back teeth can cause a combination of symptoms easily taken for an ear infection:
* Feverish, unhappy child.
* Rubbing ear.
* Dribbling.

■ MASTOIDITIS
The mastoid bone is the prominent swelling behind the ears and it was once common for ear infection to spread into that area. With the routine use of antibiotics, this is now unlikely.
* Pain behind the ear.
* Tender, red swelling of the mastoid bone.
* Fever and malaise.
* Heavy yellow discharge from the ear.

The condition urgently needs surgical drainage of the mastoid bone.

■ PERICHONDRITIS
Occasionally, the outer ear, which is made up of cartilage, becomes inflamed, typically after a knock, or in cold weather.
* Throbbing pain over part of the outer ear.
* Skin is reddened.

Symptoms settle of their own accord over a few days, just occasionally needing antibiotic treatment.

RARE

■ RODENT ULCER
A form of skin cancer that can occur anywhere on the ear or in the ear canal.
* Starts by looking like a small sore

that does not heal.
* Grows very slowly.
* May bleed and cause pain.

Cured by treatment given at an early stage.

■ TIC DOULOUREUX

The medical term for this is trigeminal neuralgia.

An unpleasant condition arising from irritation of the nerve which supplies feeling to much of the face and the ear. The cause is unknown. Commonest in the late middle-aged and elderly.
* Sudden, severe shooting pains across ear, face, nose.
* Pains set off by eating, the cold or other triggers.

There are several drug treatments for this miserable, though harmless illness.

■ RAMSAY-HUNT SYNDROME

This is a form of shingles which can be a puzzling cause of pain.
* Pain in one side of throat and the ear on that side.
* Hearing may seem hyper–sensitive.
* Loss of taste on that side of the tongue.
* Small, crusting spots appear on throat and ear after a week or two.

■ CANCER OF THE EAR

Cancer of the ear canal or inner ear is unusual.
* Intense, prolonged pain.
* Bloody discharge.

■ CANCER OF THE TONGUE

It is important to check the back of the tongue in cases of persistent earache where there appears to be no cause within the ear itself.
* A persistent, shallow ulcer on the back of the tongue.
* Commonest in smokers.
* Gradually enlarges, with pain and bleeding.

■ CANCER OF TONSIL

Another unusual cancer, most common in old age.
* One tonsil is enlarged.
* Earache.
* Pain on swallowing.

EAR FEELS 'FULL'

A familiar sensation, variously described as fullness, cotton wool between the ears, pressure in the ears, muzziness in the head. The basic features are slight deafness and muffled hearing due to some physical obstruction to hearing. The causes are often obvious and readily treatable.

PROBABLE

EUSTACHIAN CATARRH
WAX
INFECTION

POSSIBLE

HAY FEVER

RARE

CHRONIC OTITIS EXTERNA

THE EARS

PROBABLE

■ EUSTACHIAN CATARRH
See EARACHE, page 67. Caused by build-up of fluid within the inner ear as after a common cold; treatment, if needed, consists of decongestants and aromatic inhalations

■ WAX
Probably the commonest cause of a slight feeling of fullness, often accompanied by dizziness, discomfort, mild earache *(see page 67)*.

Simple earwax softening drops often allow the ear to clear naturally.

■ INFECTION
Rather than causing the painful picture described elsewhere (*see, for example, EARACHE, page 67*, infections sometimes run a less obvious course with:

* Vague mild discomfort.
* Fluctuating, mild deafness.
* Feeling of pressure in ear.

The diagnosis has to be made by a doctor or nurse who can see the eardrum.

POSSIBLE

■ HAY FEVER
Causes fullness as a result of swelling of the lining of the nose and ears.

* Seasonal sneeezing, sore eyes.
* Persistent runny nose during the pollen season.
* Often associated with eczema, asthma.

Treatments include anti-histamine tablets and nose sprays.

RARE

■ CHRONIC OTITIS EXTERNA
Severe cases give rise to chronic swelling of the ear canal, which also becomes blocked up with debris. Cleansing is needed for a long time. *See page 66.*

DEAFNESS OR HEARING DIFFICULTIES IN ADULTS

Adult deafness or loss of hearing is, to a large extent, a normal part of the ageing process. The hearing loss can gradually worsen, unnoticed, until it interferes with work or social relationships, at which point it is suddenly seen as a 'new' problem. Special attention should always be given to sudden deafness, deafness affecting one ear only or when it is associated with pain, giddiness (vertigo), or ringing in the ears (tinnitus).

PROBABLE
WAX
CHRONIC OTITIS MEDIA
OTOSCLEROSIS
PRESBYACUSIS

POSSIBLE
MENIERE'S DISEASE
ACOUSTIC TRAUMA
ARTERIOSCLEROSIS

RARE

INFECTION
ACOUSTIC NEUROMA
SKULL FRACTURE
DRUGS
PAGET'S DISEASE

PROBABLE

■ WAX
An extremely common cause for a mild degree of hearing loss.
* Often causes sudden, partial hearing loss.
* 'Blocked' feeling in ears.

■ CHRONIC OTITIS MEDIA
Long-term infection within the ear leads to:
* Deafness.
* Persistent discharge of pus-like material.
* Sometimes pain and vertigo.

Treatment is meticulous cleansing of the ear in a specialist clinic. The sudden appearance of pain and vertigo calls for urgent specialist assessment: this could indicate a deterioration of the condition. Normally, continuous cleansing of the ear will allow healing. Occasionally, when the infection has cleared, skin grafting to the ear drum is necessary to allow complete healing.

■ OTOSCLEROSIS
A condition causing increasing stiffness of one of the bones that transmits sound waves from the eardrum.
* Often runs in families.
* Commonest in women, and gets worse in pregnancy.
* Progressive deafness, starting in early adulthood.
* Ringing in the ears — tinnitus — is common.

Surgery can help, but usually a hearing aid is the simplest treatment.

■ PRESBYACUSIS
This is the familiar hearing loss that comes with age, caused by degeneration of the pathway that turns sound waves into electrical impulses for transmission to the brain.
* Typically noticed in late 60s.
* Both ears affected.
* Pain-free.

POSSIBLE

■ MENIERE'S DISEASE
Suggested by repeated attacks of deafness along with vertigo and ringing in the ears — tinnitus.

■ ACOUSTIC TRAUMA
Repeated loud noise damages hearing. It is said, however, that five years of exposure is needed for any significant damage to occur, by which time the most dedicated disco-goer may well have moved on to embroidery.

Actually, discotheque deafness is usually temporary; but prolonged and repeated exposure to loud noise can result in some loss of hearing. Ringing in the ears is common after hearing loud noises. Workers exposed to loud noise should wear ear protection and have regular hearing checks.

THE EARS

Prolonged use of personal stereos at high volume damages ears. The direct application of earphones, delivering high volume sound, has been shown significantly to affect young people's hearing. If others around you can hear it — it is too loud.

■ ARTERIOSCLEROSIS
Poor blood flow to the arteries supplying blood to the ear can cause a range of symptoms, usually confined to the elderly.
* Fluctuating deafness, giddiness, ringing in the ears.
* Symptoms may vary, depending on the position of the neck.
There is no specific treatment.

RARE

■ INFECTION
Deafness is a rare and unpredictable complication of certain infectious illnesses, notably measles and mumps. It is also a possible consequence of meningitis and syphilis.

Children who have recurrent ear infections may have decreased hearing. *See also HEARING DIFFICULTIES IN CHILDREN, this page.*

■ ACOUSTIC NEUROMA
A slow-growing tumour on the nerve of hearing. Though rare, it is suspected frequently on the basis of the following suggestive symptoms:
* One-sided progressive deafness.
* One-sided tinnitus.
* Vertigo.
* Later numbness of face, unsteadiness.

A brain scan allows for quite precise localization, improving the chances of successful removal by surgery.

■ SKULL FRACTURE
Could damage the nerve of hearing and disrupts the delicate bones that transmit sounds, causing sudden loss of hearing.

■ DRUGS
The nerve of hearing is sensitive to several drugs. The commonest among adults is aspirin, taken in overdose.
* Tinnitus is an early warning sign.
* Giddiness.

■ PAGET'S DISEASE
A not uncommon condition of later life in which:
* Bones become tender.
* Bowing of the legs.
* Enlargement of the head.
* Gradual deafness.

The deafness is caused by a squeezing of the nerve of hearing by enlarged bone. This disease is frequently unrecognized until characteristic signs are noticed on an X-ray.

DEAFNESS OR HEARING DIFFICULTIES IN CHILDREN

Hearing difficulties in childhood are difficult to detect, but every effort must be made to do so. In a baby, suspect a hearing problem if there is no startled reaction to sudden, loud noises, or if, as he or she develops, the baby does not turn to a sound. Later, delay in starting to speak should arouse suspicion. Later again, a schoolchild's performance may deteriorate for no obvious cause; once more, consider the possibility of loss of hearing. You cannot be too careful.

PROBABLE
WAX
SEROUS OTITIS MEDIA

POSSIBLE
CONGENITAL

RARE
CONGENITAL RUBELLA
INFECTIONS
NEO-NATAL JAUNDICE
DRUGS
HYPOTHYROIDISM

PROBABLE

■ WAX
Simple to detect, and simple to remedy with drops to soften the earwax. Most ENT specialists would advise against syringing ears. The wax will clear naturally.

■ SEROUS OTITIS MEDIA
A common reason for hearing loss in children who have recurrent ear infections leading to a build-up of fluid within the inner ear. The condition is also known as glue ear because the fluid can be thick and sticky. The condition often cures itself over a few months, but frequently other treatment is needed. The symptoms are:
* Deafness, which may be partial or total.
* Occasional pain in ear.

Certain typical changes in the appearance of the eardrum will alert a doctor to the condition. As a remedy, grommets may be inserted.

POSSIBLE

■ CONGENITAL
Always to be considered in children born deaf, in whom there may have been a failure of development of the organs of hearing. Sometimes deafness runs in the family; sometimes the mother has been exposed to drugs which damage the ear (*see below*) or has had German measles — Rubella.

There are also many syndromes in which deafness is one of several abnormalities, but this is a matter for specialist assessment. In most cases of congenital deafness, however, no cause can be found.

RARE

■ CONGENITAL RUBELLA — GERMAN MEASLES
A rarity since vaccination has become generally available. Rubella contracted in the first four months of pregnancy wreaks havoc on the developing child. As

well as deafness, it can cause:
* Poor development of the brain and mental retardation.
* Cataracts.
* Heart defects.

This tragic outcome is becoming much less frequent as national immunization programmes against Rubella improve. Check on your Rubella immunity before you get pregnant.

■ INFECTION
Deafness is an unusual and unpredictable complication of certain infectious illnesses, notably measles and mumps, both of which are increasingly rare, thanks to immunization. It may also be a consequence of meningitis.

■ NEONATAL JAUNDICE
Severe jaundice in the days after birth can cause brain damage, including deafness. Hence the vigorous treatment given to babies who develop the condition.

■ DRUGS
The nerve of hearing is sensitive to several drugs, the commonest of which is aspirin taken in overdose. Another is gentamicin, now reserved for life-threatening disease such as meningitis, where the risk of damage to hearing is outweighed by the risk to life.
* Tinnitus (ringing in the ears) is an early warning sign.
* Giddiness.

If a potentially harmful drug has to be used, blood levels will be monitored to avoid damage.

■ CONGENITAL HYPOTHYROIDISM
An under-active thyroid gland, giving a child with:
* Coarse features.
* A gruff cry.
* Enlarged tongue.

In many countries there are screening programmes to detect this curable illness as early as possible in new-born babies.

ITCHING EAR

PROBABLE
OTITIS EXTERNA

POSSIBLE
FUNGAL INFECTION

PROBABLE

■ OTITIS EXTERNA
A form of eczema affecting the skin of the ear canal. Common in adult life, typically in those with eczema elsewhere.
* Intense itching.
* Skin of ear canal and ear itself is flaking, crusting, swollen.
* Ear feels wet, with a thin, clear discharge.

Like any other skin, that of the ear can become sensitised to chemicals. Common among these are chlorine in swimming pools, hair spray and the antibiotics in the very drops used to treat otitis externa.

POSSIBLE

■ FUNGAL INFECTION
Organisms known as fungi can invade skin which is already broken down by otitis externa.
* Symptoms of otitis externa.
* Black spores may be visible in the discharge.
Treatment is with anti-fungal drops.

NOISES IN THE EAR

Noises other than ringing in the ear are very common and very rarely due to worrying underlying causes. They nearly always pass within a fortnight. Many cases remain unexplained, the symptoms going as mysteriously as they came. If noises occur in a particular location, check for a cause as simple as the hum from central heating, power lines or similar noise source. *See also RINGING IN THE EAR, page 76.*

PROBABLE
EUSTACHIAN CATARRH
ACUTE INNER EAR INFECTION

RARE
HEART MURMUR
ANAEMIA

PROBABLE

■ EUSTACHIAN CATARRH
Blockage caused by fluid building up inside the ear, often experienced with a common cold.
* Muffled hearing.
* Popping or crackling inside the ears.
* Slight discomfort from a feeling of pressure in the ears.
* Swallowing gives temporary relief.

■ ACUTE INNER EAR INFECTION
Causes noises for similar reasons as does acoustic catarrh (*see above*).
* Rapid onset of pain.
* Deafness.
* Crackling inside ears.
Antibiotics are usually given for this condition.

RARE

■ HEART MURMUR
The sound arising from a diseased valve in the heart may be heard inside the head when there is no competing noise.
* A whooshing noise.
* In time with heart beat.
Needs to be assessed by a doctor.

■ ANAEMIA
If extreme, anaemia is said to cause noises in the ear. This symptom is likely to be over–shadowed by other features of anaemia such as:
* Pallor.
* Tiredeness.
* Sore tongue.

* Dizziness on standing.
A blood test will quickly confirm the diagnosis.

TENDERNESS BEHIND THE EAR

Immediately behind the ear is a bone known as the mastoid, felt as a prominent swelling. Pain and swelling in this area is always to be taken seriously.

PROBABLE
ACUTE EAR INFECTION

POSSIBLE
MASTOIDITIS

PROBABLE

■ ACUTE EAR INFECTION
Although the infection is confined to the middle ear, occasionally there is a mild degree of tenderness over the mastoid bone. Middle ear infections are usually treated with an antibiotic, which should prevent further spread.

POSSIBLE

■ MASTOIDITIS
Though now uncommon, this was once a feared consequence of ear infections, since infection can spread from the mastoid region into the brain.
* Begins with an ear infection.
* Redness, swelling over mastoid bone.
* Yellow/green discharge from ear.
* Fever, pain, malaise.
Urgent surgical treatment is needed.

RINGING IN THE EAR — TINNITUS

Of all ear diseases, this causes most misery — because of its persistence. It is usually described as a ringing noise, but sometimes it is lower-pitched than that, more of a hum. As an occasional symptom it is quite common, no more than a nuisance.

Chronic tinnitus is another matter. Treatments vary from drugs to devices that mask the sound, but there is no real cure. Brief episodes of tinnitus may be caused by a blow to the head, wax in the ears, a foreign body, infection or sudden changes in air pressure. Prolonged cases may be due to the following:

PROBABLE
OTOSCLEROSIS
MENIERE'S DISEASE
PRESBYACUSIS

POSSIBLE
ARTERIOSCLEROSIS
DRUGS
PSYCHOLOGICAL

RARE
PAGET'S DISEASE

PROBABLE

■ OTOSCLEROSIS
This is a common cause of deafness. *See page 71.* Tinnitus tends to be the earliest symptom of the condition, which is due to increasing stiffness of one of the bones that transmit sound.

■ MENIERE'S DISEASE
The classic symptoms of this disease are varying combinations of:
* Tinnitus.
* Vertigo.
* Deafness.

■ PRESBYACUSIS
Hearing loss as part of the ageing process is frequently accompanied by tinnitus. *See page 71.*

POSSIBLE

■ ARTERIOSCLEROSIS
The blood supply to the brain and ear arrives via major arteries in the neck which, with age, can get furred up. This is thought to underlie cases of tinnitus in the elderly associated with:
* Giddiness on standing up.
* Giddiness set off by head movements, especially looking up.
* Deafness.

It helps to take your time when getting up and to avoid sudden, extreme movements of the neck.

■ DRUGS
Common drugs which can cause tinnitus include aspirin, quinine and streptomycin.

■ PSYCHOLOGICAL
Occasionally, tinnitus or other noises in the ears are actually hallucinations in someone suffering from serious mental disease. Suspicion aroused by reports of:
* Bizarre noises.
* Voices commenting on the individual's activities.

The individual may also appear:
* Unusually suspicious.
* Moody to an exaggerated degree.

This situation needs sensitive, expert assessment.

RARE

■ PAGET'S DISEASE
A disease of bone which can squeeze the nerve of hearing, resulting in:
* Deafness.
* Tinnitus.

See also page 72.

The Ears

VERTIGO

Vertigo means a sense of rotation. Giddiness is a mild form of the same symptom. They are frequently caused by disorders of the ear, although the connection may not be obvious since there may be no other features of ear trouble such as pain, discharge or tinnitus. For that reason, vertigo/giddiness is covered in detail elsewhere in this book. *See THE BRAIN AND NERVOUS SYSTEM*. The following conditions are, however, relevant to the ear.

PROBABLE
CATARRH
VESTIBULITIS
MENIERE'S DISEASE

POSSIBLE
CHRONIC OTITIS MEDIA
OTOSCLEROSIS
WAX

RARE
ACOUSTIC NEUROMA

PROBABLE

■ CATARRH
The congestion which accompanies a cold often also causes mild giddiness for a few days.
* Nasal congestion.

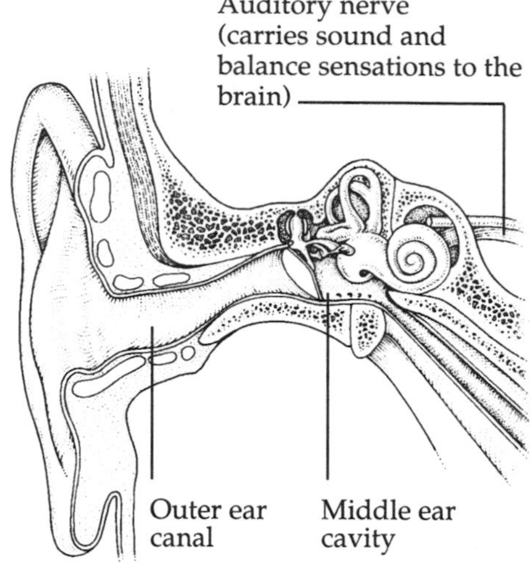

* Slight pressure in ears.
* Mild deafness and ringing in the ears — tinnitus.

■ VESTIBULITIS
A common, alarming, but harmless condition, occurring in mini-epidemics. It is a viral infection of the balance organ which is sited in the ear. The nerve endings that normally transmit messages telling us how we are balanced become inflamed and send off inaccurate and confusing messages. This causes acute loss of balance and intense true vertigo, with the room spinning round.
* Abrupt, disabling vertigo: you may even find it impossible to stand up.
* Usually noticed on attempting to get up in the morning.
* Nausea or vomiting are common.
* Vertigo returns each time you move your head.

This is a panic-inducing illness: but be reassurred that the symptoms will fade over two or three weeks. Minor recurrences are

Ear syringing

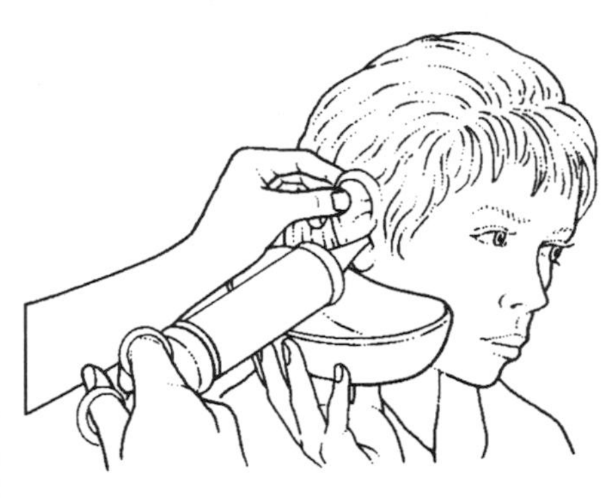

Ear examination

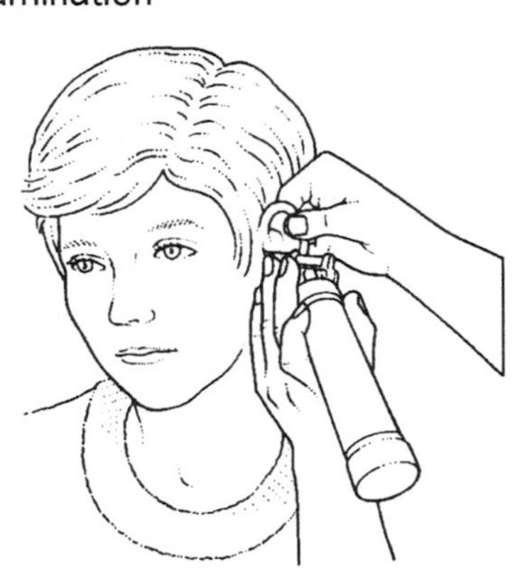

possible for several months afterwards.

■ MENIERE'S DISEASE
Vertigo can be an early symptom of this condition. Later there is:
* Ringing in the ears — tinnitus.
* Deafness.

POSSIBLE

■ CHRONIC OTITIS MEDIA
See page 71. Persistent yellow or green discharge from one ear, together with:
* Discomfort.
* Deafness.

Needs specialized treatment to clean the ear and to eradicate infection.

■ OTOSCLEROSIS
A cause of deafness in middle life, but as early features there can be:
* Tinnitus.
* Vertigo.

■ WAX
A convenient scapegoat for many ear problems, perhaps too convenient. However, if there is just mild giddiness, with no other symptoms except that the ears are full of hard wax, it is reasonable for a doctor to suggest clearing the wax with drops to soften it, or, if necessary, syringing the ears, to exclude wax as a cause of vertigo.

RARE

■ ACOUSTIC NEUROMA
See page 72. This growth on the nerve of hearing is suspected if, as well as vertigo, there is progressive:
* One-sided deafness.
* One-sided vertigo.
* One-sided tinnitus.

THE MOUTH, FACE, HEAD, THROAT AND NECK

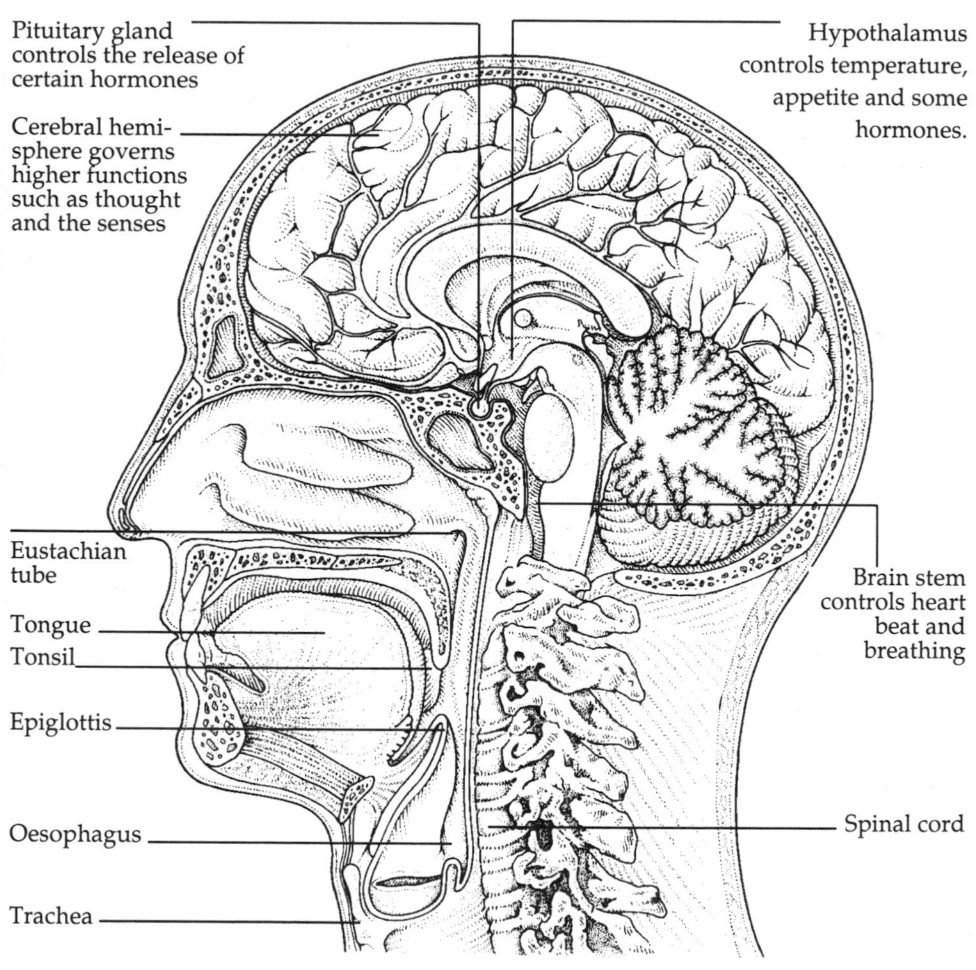

BLUISH-PURPLE LIPS

A feature of cyanosis, covered in detail on *page 424.* It can be caused by low body temperature. But long-term cyanosis suggests that blood oxygen levels are low. Similar discolouration may be noticed in the ear lobes, all the mucous membranes, the tongue and anywhere that blood flows close to the surface of the skin, such as the beds of the fingernails. In general, cyanosis suggests either heart or lung disease.

PROBABLE
LOW TEMPERATURE
CHRONIC BRONCHITIS
EMPHYSEMA
PULMONARY OEDEMA

POSSIBLE
SHOCK
PNEUMONIA

RARE
PULMONARY EMBOLUS
CONGENITAL HEART DISEASE
AIRWAYS OBSTRUCTED BY A FOREIGN BODY
LARYNGEAL OEDEMA
FIBROSING ALVEOLITIS
PNEUMOCONIOSIS
EXTRINSIC ALLERGIC ALVEOLITIS

PROBABLE

■ LOW TEMPERATURE
Commonly seen in shivering children on the beach. It may, however, accompany low temperature in the elderly. Consider hypothermia if there are other symptoms, such as:
* Confusion.
* Slowness of thought.
* Decreased movement

The individual should be warmed gradually: layers of blankets are best. Hot drinks, such as tea, may be given. Avoid alcohol, which increases heat loss. In all cases, seek medical help urgently — hypothermia must be dealt with in hospital.

■ CHRONIC BRONCHITIS
See page 222.

■ EMPHYSEMA
Described in detail on *page 222.*
* Shortness of breath which gets progressively worse.
* The chest becomes expanded, as though permanently inhaling.
* May accompany chronic bronchitis.
* Respiratory infections.
* Cyanosis.
* Respiratory failure.

■ PULMONARY OEDEMA
Retention of fluid in the lungs as a result of failure of the heart to pump effectively. Heart failure may have occurred because of either poor blood supply to the heart, or because of structural abnormality such as disease of the heart's valves. Symptoms include:

MOUTH

* Shortness of breath on exertion.
* Shortness of breath when lying down flat.
* Night-time shortness of breath.
* Frothy sputum, sometimes pink with blood.
* Cyanosis.
* Fast or irregular heart rate.
* Swelling of ankles.

POSSIBLE

■ SHOCK
Covered in detail on *page 408.* Cyanosis is just one of several noticeable features. May be an emergency.

■ PNEUMONIA
Actually, 'pneumonias' would be a better term, since there are several types. Cyanosis is a typical feature of all of them. *See page 214.*

Some types of pneumonia may still be fatal, particularly in the very young or the elderly: see a doctor without delay.

RARE

■ PULMONARY EMBOLUS
Covered in detail on *page 218.* Bluish lips are just one of several more dramatic features, such as sudden shortness of breath, chest pain, bloody sputum and collapse.

■ CONGENITAL HEART DISEASE
Cyanosis is a typical and obvious feature of new-born babies with heart abnormalities. Fallot's tetralogy and transposition of the great arteries are probably the most well known. Heart defects may also accompany abnormalities such as Down's Syndrome, or those caused by the mother having Rubella during pregnancy. In addition to cyanosis:
* Shortness of breath.
* Finger clubbing.
* Toe clubbing.
* Polycythemia: excess haemoglobin to compensate for poor oxygenation.
* Malaise.
* Poor growth.

■ AIRWAYS OBSTRUCTED BY A FOREIGN BODY
Any object that obstructs the free passage of air in an out of the lungs may result in cyanosis. The sudden onset of blueness, choking in someone eating, or in a child, must be considered as being possibly due to inhalation of a foreign body, perhaps a peanut, or a piece of a toy. This is a life-threatening emergency. *See HEIMLICH'S MANOEVRE, page 204.*

■ LARYNGEAL OEDEMA
An infection (typically diphtheria, epiglottitis) or a severe allergic reaction may cause swelling of the soft tissues of the larynx, preventing air getting into the lungs.
* Blue lips.
* Stridor: a harsh and frightening noise heard as air is forced past a blockage in the airways.
* Distress.

If caused by an infection of the upper airway, all the usual features will also be noticed. Laryngeal oedema is an emergency: get help quickly.

■ FIBROSING ALVEOLITIS
Tends to develop in middle age and progresses gradually.
* Increasing shortness of breath.
* Dry cough.
* Clubbing.
* Cyanosis.

■ PNEUMOCONIOSIS
A term used for a number of occupationally related chest diseases, typically associated with work in dusty environments.
* Slow onset.
* Increasing shortness of breath on exertion, and then at rest.
* Intermittent cough.
* Onset of bronchitis.
* Cyanosis.
* Respiratory failure.
* Heart failure.

■ EXTRINSIC ALLERGIC ALVEOLITIS
A disease that develops because of recurrent allergic reactions to dusts from animals or plants. Quite common in farm workers.
* Recurrent brief attacks, up to a couple of days, of shortness of breath, malaise, fever and cough, when exposed to the dust.

After repeated exposure over the years a chronic condition develops, with:
* Shortness of breath.
* Finger and toe clubbing.
* Cyanosis.
* Respiratory failure.
* Heart failure.

CRACKING AT CORNERS OF MOUTH

The medical terms are angular stomatitis or cheilosis. In isolation, this is normally of no great significance.

PROBABLE
CHILDHOOD CRACKING
AGE

POSSIBLE
BRAIN INJURY

RARE
SCURVY
ZINC DEFICIENCY
RIBOFLAVIN DEFICIENCY

PROBABLE

■ CHILDHOOD CRACKING
If the corners of your child's mouth are constantly wet, they will be at increased risk of cracking. Children taking bottles or who suck their thumbs may develop inflammation at the corner(s) of the mouth. This may also occur in older children, with no very obvious cause.
* Redness.
* Cracking.
* Pain.
* Clears up ot its own accord.
* May develop on one side only.

MOUTH

■ AGE
As individuals age, they can develop a crease running downwards from the angle of the mouth, along which saliva flows, causing skin irritation and:
* Redness.
* Cracking.
* Pain.
* May be on one or both sides. Clears up of its own accord.

POSSIBLE

■ BRAIN INJURY
Anyone who has suffered brain injury (stroke, accident) or with chronic neurological disease may have facial weakness or swallowing problems that allow saliva to pool in the mouth and dribble out.
* Redness.
* Cracking.
* Pain.
* Clears up of its own accord.
* May be on one side only (after stroke) or on both sides if there is a swallowing problem.

RARE

■ SCURVYAND ZINC DEFICIENCY: *see pages 426 and 86 respectively.* RIBOFLAVINE is a water-soluble vitamin present in many foods. Deficiency is likely to be a feature only of severe, general malnutrition. Glossitis, *page 125,* may be present.

HARE LIP

Colloquial term for cleft lip. *See CLEFT LIP AND PALATE, page 87.*

LIPS — CRACKED, SORES OR PATCHES

Sore, inflamed lips are common in adults and children: the lips look red and are often cracked. The usual cause is intermittent exposure to heat and cold. The skin of the lips loses its natural oil, becoming dry and uncomfortable or 'chapped'.

Other common causes are lip-licking and lip-chewing. The first is typical of children with colds who develop running noses and continually lick or wipe their upper lips, causing inflammation. The second is a comfort habit adopted at times of stress.

The lips and the surrounding skin are possible sites of sores or lesions for many diseases. Some are local and some are general; some are permanent and some temporary, some need treatment and some don't. The following list cannot be exhaustive, but it does highlight examples of all these types.

PROBABLE
APHTHOUS ULCER
HERPES SIMPLEX
MUCOCOELE OR RETENTION CYST
BURN
IMPETIGO

MOUTH

POSSIBLE
CANDIDIASIS
LEUKOPLAKIA

RARE
ZINC DEFICIENCY
HEREDITARY HAEMORRHAGIC TELANGIECTASIA
CHANCRE
DERMATITIS
BEHCET'S SYNDROME
ERYTHEMA MULTIFORME
CANCER
LICHEN PLANUS
DRUGS

PROBABLE

■ APHTHOUS ULCER
May develop after injury, when the individual is run-down (physically or mentally) or more commonly for no clear reason.
* Exquisitely painful.
* After 24 hours mucous membrane breaks down to form an ulcer.
* Often a greyish/white appearance.
* Ulcer is normally about 3-4 mm in diameter and oval shaped.
* Pain can make, eating, talking or brushing teeth difficult.
* May be multiple.
* Tend to be on inner aspect of lips.
* Healing occurs between five days and two weeks.

■ HERPES SIMPLEX
Also known as a cold sore. A virus which infects the skin.
* Often precipitated by upper respiratory tract infection when the individual is run down.
* Also precipitated by weather extremes (heat or cold).
* Initially a slightly irritating itchy patch on the lip or local skin.
* Little fluid filled vesicles develop.
* These become crusted and a scab develops.
* The disease runs its course in ten to 14 days.

If severe, and recognized at an early stage, can be helped by antiviral medication.

■ MUCOCOELE OR RETENTION CYST
Blockage of one of the small glands on the inner aspect of the lips causes:
* Sudden appearance of a lump, a few millimetres in diameter.
* Painless.
* Translucent/bluish colour.
* Suddenly empties.
* Rarely lasts for more than a couple of days.

■ BURN
Local areas of pain and ulceration on one lip (particularly in the middle of the lower lip) are often caused by smokers under the influence of alcohol placing the cigarette the wrong way round in their mouth. Often, the individual cannot recall the incident. The patch will heal in about five days.

■ IMPETIGO
A nasty and highly infectious skin

MOUTH

infection, which can occur anywhere, but commonly on the face and lips and other exposed parts. Commonest in children.
* Starts with redness.
* Vesicles and bullae (fluid filled sacs) develop on the skin surface.
* These burst and crusting occurs.
* May spread over a large area of the face.
* Asymmetrical: does not spread evenly over both sides of face.

Needs antibiotic treatment.

POSSIBLE

■ CANDIDIASIS
A 'thrush' infection of the lips, typical of the elderly, those with dentures, those who are 'run-down' or with diets deficient in vitamins or iron. Treatment is anti-fungal creams or lozenges.
* Redness.
* Soreness.
* Slight swelling.
* Occasional cracking and bleeding.
* White plaques or patches may be seen.

■ LEUKOPLAKIA
* White patches on the tongue or lining of the mouth.
* Cannot be scraped off.
* Occasionally disappear leaving a red base.
* Localized hardening under the patch may occur.

It is associated with smoking, spirits, spices, sepsis, sharp teeth, and syphilis.

Leukoplakia may also be an early warning sign of cancer, so long-standing firm white patches on the tongue or in the mouth must not be ignored.

RARE

■ ZINC DEFICIENCY
Any elderly person on a poor diet or with malabsorption or malnutrition problems who develops intermittent sores on around the mouth may be zinc-deficient. A bloodtest may be needed to confirm this, and zinc supplements can be given.

■ CANCER
Any long-standing ulcer or growth on the lip, particularly in elderly smokers with poor oral hygiene, may be cancerous.
* Persistent ulcer or irregular lump.
* Persistent painless, but enlarged lymph nodes.
* Bleeding from lesion.
* Loss of weight.
* Malaise.

■ HEREDITARY HAEMORRHAGIC TELANGIECTASIA
Also known as Osler-Weber-Rendu Disease. Hereditary.
* Small red vascular lesions on lips and in mouth.
* Similar lesions throughout gastro-intestinal tract.
* The gastro-intestinal lesions may cause internal bleeding.
* Rarely seen before the age of 40.

■ CHANCRE
The first sign of infection with syphilis. May occur on the lips or in the mouth after oral sex.
* Appears three to four weeks after contact.

* Initially, a hardened, elevated solitary lesion.
* Becomes a shallow ulcer.
* Painless.
* Does not bleed.
* Raised, red edges.
* Local, painless lymph node enlargement.

If suspected must be seen and treated by a doctor.

■ DERMATITIS

Any area of skin may develop sensitivity to some irritant. Habitual sucking or chewing of pens or application of some lipsticks or lip balms are examples of agents to which some may react.
* Redness.
* Itchiness.
* Soreness.
* Sometime crusting and weeping.
* Normal lips when the irritant is not being used

■ BEHCET'S SYNDROME

Commonest in men from the teens to the early thirties.
* Painful ulceration of the mouth.
* Genital ulceration a few weeks after the oral lesions.
* Eye inflammation (uveitis) with the genital ulceration.

The condition repeats and relapses. Treatment is aimed at relieving the symptoms. This condition is commonest in the Middle East.

■ ERYTHEMA MULTIFORME

Associated with reaction to drugs or infection. Commonest in young males.
* Extensive painful ulcers inside the mouth.
* Gum inflammation.
* Crusting, bloodstained lesions on lips.

Treatment consists of identifying and removing or treating the cause.

■ LICHEN PLANUS

In the over-30s.
* Multiple, fine white lines on lips. tongue and the cheek
* Tiny white spots in the same region.
* Sometimes ulcers between the spots and lines.
* Occasionally fluid-filled sacs form which then burst, causing painful ulcers.

■ DRUGS

A number of drugs, such as arsenic, bismuth, lead and mercury, will cause pigmentation of the mouth and lips, in addition to their other symptoms and signs. In the absence of other definite causes for mouth pigmentation, accidental or deliberate taking of such drugs should be considered.

CHAPPED LIPS

Essentially the same as *SORE LIPS, page 84*.

CLEFT LIP AND PALATE

These terms cover a fairly wide range of abnormalities that occur during development in the womb. They are quite common — one in 750 births. For some reason, generally unknown, areas of tissue fail

to 'join', and the resulting gap is seen at birth, sometimes on one side, or in severe cases as a cleft lip and palate on both sides beneath the nose.
* Distortion of the nostril on the affected side.
* In more than half the cases, there is also a defect in the hard palate.
* Speech problems, typically nasal speech, will develop if left untreated.

The trend at present is to repair these deformities by plastic surgery as soon as reasonable after birth so that breast feeding and speech development are affected as little as possible.

SKIN AROUND MOUTH LOOKS PALE

This is a very specific symptom, otherwise known as circumoral pallor, associated with scarlet fever. It should not be confused with more general pallor of skin, mucous membranes and nails associated with anaemia or blood loss. *See pages 417-24.* The symptoms of scarlet fever are:
* Tonsillitis and pharyngitis.
* Red rash, predominantly on trunk.
* Sore and coated tongue.
* Circumoral pallor.
* Otitis media may develop; *see page 66.*

BLEEDING GUMS

This is almost always due to over-vigorous brushing of the teeth, and can be a normal daily occurrence for some people. If bleeding is persistent, or the gums are painful, some degree of *GUM DISEASE* (also known as gingivitis or periodontal disease) may be present; *see page 90.* This may settle without treatment but if there is infection too, antibiotics may be necessary. The care of a dental hygienist may be beneficial. A very rare cause of bleeding gums is scurvy, caused by Vitamin C deficiency.

FOUL-SMELLING BREATH

Halitosis. Most dentists and doctors would attribute bad breath to poor oral hygiene. This is by far the commonest cause of bad breath. There are, however, other causes, related to a variety of abnormalities of the mouth, the sinuses, and the lungs, as well as disease elsewhere in the body.

PROBABLE

POOR ORAL HYGIENE
FOOD OR DRINK
SMOKING
DENTAL CARIES
MOUTH BREATHING
MOUTH OR THROAT INFECTION
GUM DISEASE
DENTURES
POST NASAL DRIP

POSSIBLE
SINUSITIS
CATARRH
CHRONIC LUNG CONDITIONS
PYORRHOEA ALVEOLARIS
DIABETIC KETOACIDOSIS

RARE
VINCENT'S ANGINA
CANCERS OF THE MOUTH, UPPER RESPIRATORY TRACT AND LARYNX
RENAL FAILURE – URAEMIA
LIVER FAILURE
DRUGS AND POISONING

PROBABLE

■ POOR ORAL HYGIENE
The surest way to develop bad breath is to fail to clean your teeth. Even regular tooth brushing may not be enough to prevent the accumulation of food debris, which collects in the cracks between teeth and generates generates odours as it decays. Dental flossing (passing a special thread between teeth) clears these crevices and helps prevent bad breath.
* Staining between teeth.
* Irregular colour to teeth.
* Breath worse in the morning, on waking.

In addition to brushing and flossing your teeth, regular descaling by a dentist or an oral hygienist can help prevent bad breath.

■ FOOD AND DRINK
* Individual has recently eaten spiced foods or drunk alcohol.
* No other evidence of disease in mouth or elsewhere.
* Not present if diet is confined to non-spicy food, or if alcoholic drink is stopped.

■ SMOKING
* Halitosis.
* Stained teeth.

■ DENTAL CARIES
Caries means tooth decay. The enamel covering of the tooth is damaged by bacteria. Regular brushing and avoidance of sugary foods may help, as may fluoride — ask your dentist's advice.
* 'Sensitive teeth'.
* Painful tooth or teeth.
* Halitosis.
* Worse on drinking and eating very hot or cold foods and drinks.

■ MOUTH BREATHING
Any condition which makes you breath through your mouth rather than your nose may result in halitosis because of drying up of the salivary secretions which act as a rinsing agent. Thus nasal polyps, a broken nose, hay fever or even snoring may cause halitosis, because they make it difficult to breathe through the nose.

■ MOUTH OR THROAT INFECTION
Any mouth or throat infection may cause bad breath; all may be associated with:
* Pain.
* Fever.
* Malaise.

MOUTH

* Halitosis.
* Unpleasant taste in the mouth.

■ GUM DISEASE
Disease of the gums and tooth sockets, with inflammation of the gums (also known as gingivitis). Caused mainly by poor oral hygiene.
* Bleeding gums particularly after brushing teeth.
* Sensitive gums.
* Halitosis.
* Often associated with dental caries.

■ DENTURES
If not cleaned regularly and adequately, food debris or saliva may accumulate on dentures, giving off an offensive smell, even when in the mouth.

■ POST NASAL DRIP
* May be present for some weeks after flu/colds.
* Mucus drips back into throat causing reflex coughing.
* Worse at night.
* General health otherwise good.
* Halitosis may be present.

See also PHLEGM IN THE THROAT, page 128.

POSSIBLE

■ SINUSITIS
Infection of any of the sinuses may cause:
* Persistent nasal discharge (out through the nose or back into the throat).
* May be green or yellow.
* Possibly headache.
* Occasionally pyrexia.

The sinuses

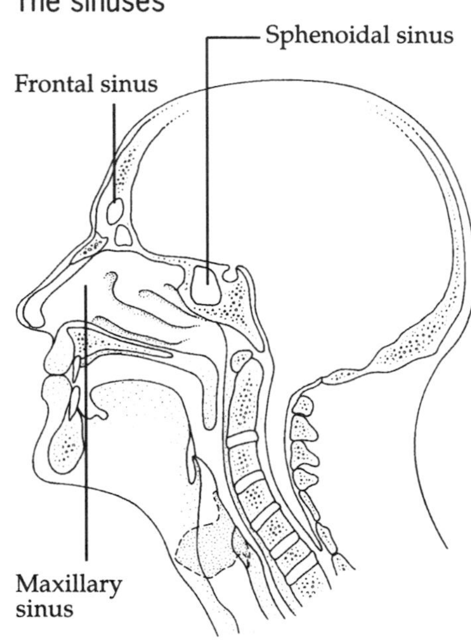

* Malaise.
* Halitosis.

■ CATARRH
A term with many different meanings: some use it to describe a blocked nose (because of nasal inflammation); some use it for large amounts of infected mucus. It often results in bad breath, either because of accompanying infection in the mouth or nose, or because a blocked nose is making you breath through your mouth.

■ CHRONIC LUNG CONDITIONS
See also FOUL-SMELLING BREATH AND COUGH, page 92.

Any lung condition that causes persistent production of mucus, or where the lung has a long-standing focus of infection may cause halitosis. Patients with chronic bronchitis, tuberculosis, cystic fibrosis, bronchiectasis,

emphysema and other diseases may well complain of halitosis. The main symptoms of the underlying disease usually include:
* Purulent (green/yellow) mucus.
* Cough.
* Fever.
* Malaise.

■ PYORRHOEA ALVEOLARIS
A disease of gums and tooth sockets, actually a severe, advanced form of gum disease (*see above*).
* Gum margins recede.
* Teeth loosen.
* Pus caused by infection of the tooth socket leaks out between gums and teeth.
* Pain.
* Halitosis.

■ DIABETIC KETOACIDOSIS
Diabetics whose blood sugar is not properly controlled can develop an excess of sugar (ketoacidosis). This is characterized by a sweetish smell on the breath (some describe it as sickly).

RARE

■ VINCENT'S ANGINA
Also known as 'trench mouth', this is a bacterial disease of the tonsils which spreads to the gums. Associated with poor hygiene.
* Fever.
* Sore throat.
* Infected gums.
* Enlarged lymph nodes in the neck.
* Often only one tonsil is affected, with ulceration, and a membrane which may spread to soft and hard palate.

Highly infectious. Responds rapidly to antibiotics.

■ CANCER OF THE MOUTH, UPPER RESPIRATORY TRACT AND LARYNX
Halitosis may be an accompaniment to any site of cancer in the mouth, upper respiratory tract and larynx, particularly if the tumour has become infected and ulcerated. Thus persistent halitosis, in addition to some or any of the following, particularly in elderly smokers, needs close investigation:
* Persistent, painless enlarged lymph nodes.
* Other lumps developing in mouth/tongue or palate.
* Change in voice.
* Loss of weight.
* Feeling unwell.
* Persistent pain in mouth or neck.
* Dentures not fitting.
* Anaemia.

■ RENAL FAILURE
Uraemia is present. Urea is a waste product normally excreted in the urine, produced by the kidneys.
* Browny/yellow appearance of skin.
* Bruising.
* Fast rate of breathing.
* Swollen ankles.
* Heart failure.
* Breath smells of urine/ammonia.
* Altered sensation in limbs.

■ LIVER FAILURE
This may occur as a result of a number of diseases that damage liver tissue, such as hepatitis or

cirrhosis. It may result in a large number of symptoms, including:
* Jaundice.
* Fatigue.
* Mental deterioration.
* Reddened palms ('liver' palms: the fatty parts of the palms are flushed red).
* The appearance of tiny blood vessels in the skin — 'vascular spiders'.
* Fever.
* Halitosis — sweet and faeculent — *foetor hepaticus*.

■ DRUGS AND POISONING
Some drugs have characteristic smells, excreted in air exhaled from the lungs. Examples are paraldehyde, now rarely used, and disulfiram, a drug prescribed for alcoholics.

FOUL-SMELLING BREATH AND COUGH

PROBABLE
CHRONIC BRONCHITIS

POSSIBLE
LUNG CANCER
BRONCHIECTASIS
CYSTIC FIBROSIS

RARE
LUNG ABSCESS
PULMONARY TUBERCULOSIS
(TB OF THE LUNG)

PROBABLE

■ CHRONIC BRONCHITIS
Covered in detail on *page 212*. The typical picture is:
* Smoker's cough, especially in the early morning.
* Cough in winter.
* Wheezing.
* Sputum varying from white to yellow/green.
* Increasing breathlessness over the years.
* Cyanosis.
* Halitosis.

POSSIBLE

■ LUNG CANCER
Covered in detail on *page 224*. Associated symptoms which may be noticeable include:
* Dry cough.
* Bloody sputum.
* Hoarse voice.
* Shortness of breath.
* Chest pain.
* Infection in the lung.
* Malaise.
* Weight loss.
* Superior vena cava obstruction.
* Halitosis.

■ BRONCHIECTASIS
The air passages are widened, preventing oxygen entering the circulation efficiently. Features include:
* History of recurrent chest infections.
* Lots of yellow/green sputum with or without blood.
* Fever.
* Looking unwell.

* Weight loss.
* Malaise.
* Severe halitosis.

■ CYSTIC FIBROSIS
See page 223.
Later in infancy, symptoms may include slow growth, offensive diarrhoea and/or respiratory infections, which may be associated with halitosis.

RARE

■ LUNG ABSCESS
A collection of pus lying within the lung tissue. It may be caused by inhaling infected material, as a complication of pneumonia, or by rare causes such as spread of a liver abscess into the chest. In general, features include:
* A pre-existing infection.
* Fever.
* Shivering.
* Sweats.
* Malaise.
* Pleurisy (pain in the chest on breathing in and out).
* Foul sputum.
* Halitosis.

■ PULMONARY (LUNG) TUBERCULOSIS
Most often in malnourished or immunosuppressed patients. Features may include:
* Malaise.
* Fatigue.
* Weight loss.
* Cough with sputum — sometimes bloody.
* Chest pain.
* Shortness of breath
* Halitosis.

BREATH SMELLS OF URINE

Covered in detail under *RENAL FAILURE* in *FOUL-SMELLING BREATH, page 91.*

BREATH SMELLS SWEET

See *DIABETIC KETOACIDOSIS* and *LIVER FAILURE*, covered in detail under *FOUL-SMELLING BREATH, page 91.*

ABNORMAL TEETH

Including discolouration and deformity. These following diseases and predisposing factors are worth considering:

■ AGE
As is well known, teeth tend to become discoloured with age. Periodontal disease such as gingivitis causes gum loss, making the teeth appear longer than normal: hence the expression 'long in the tooth'.

■ SMOKING
Yellowy-brown staining, even with regular brushing. It also hastens the age-related colour changes of teeth.

■ BETEL-NUT CHEWING
Brownish-red discolouration of all teeth, commonly seen in Asian men and women who are habitual betel nut chewers.

■ TETRACYCLINE STAINING
Some children develop brown transverse staining of teeth which may be caused by the mother taking tetracycline, an antibiotic, during pregnancy.

■ TRANSVERSE RIDGES
Transverse ridges on teeth may be seen in people who had scurvy or rickets while the surface enamel of their teeth was forming.

■ CHONDRO-ECTODERMAL DYSPLASIA
A congenital disorder. Features include:
* Short stature.
* Short fingers.
* Small teeth.
* Dry skin.
* Scanty hair.

■ HUTCHINSON'S TEETH
Rarely seen nowadays; caused by congenital syphilis. The incisor teeth have a notch at the lower edge, are small and taper towards the notched edge. Other signs of congenital syphilis may also be present.

GRATING THE TEETH

This is a symptom of more concern to the partner or parent of the affected person. It is observed commonly at night and may be associated with snoring. Some individuals do it habitually. The noise is caused by the opposing movement of the maxillary and mandibular teeth against each other. The symptom often

Maxillary and mandibular teeth

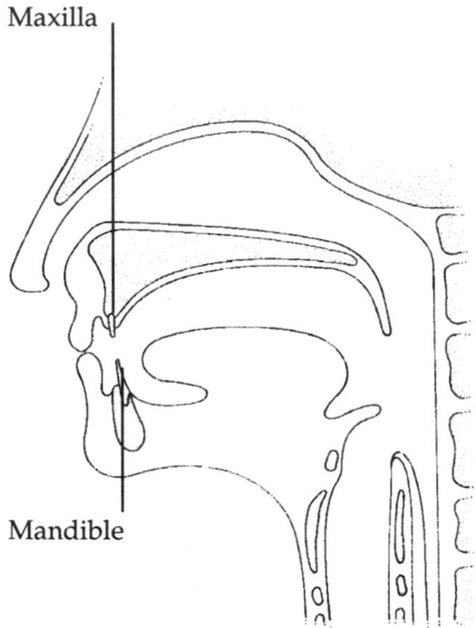

disappears spontaneously. Only rarely does it cause permanent tooth damage. If the symptom persists the advice of a dentist should be sought.

'Made-to-measure' moulds which fit over the teeth can be worn at night to protect the teeth and to prevent grinding.

There is an association between tooth grinding and migraine: many people find that they have both conditions.

DAMAGED TOOTH

If possible, the broken fragment(s) should be kept, and taken with you to a dentist. If the entire tooth and root has been displaced, it may be possible to reimplant it. If there is a possibility that the jaw is fractured, get professional help quickly. The cosmetic problems of a broken or chipped tooth are less important than underlying bone damage. The bones may need to be realigned. *(See UPPER AND LOWER TEETH NOT CLOSING etc, page 100).* Cosmetic repair can be undertaken at a later date, once the bone damage has been treated.

TEETHING PAIN

The first baby teeth, normally the lower central incisors, appear at the age of six to ten months. Teeth continue to appear until about 30 months. Most infants and toddlers will have episodes of crying, fever and salivation which may be attributed (not always convincingly) to teeth erupting or growing.

Fever is not a prominent symptom in a teething child: if your child has a fever, do not attribute it to teething. Pain and discomfort are the major symptoms, leading to irritability and crying. Just as you would take a painkiller for toothache, it is reasonable to use infant paracetamol to soothe a teething child.

It is always important to exclude other obvious sites of infection such as ears or throat.

DRY MOUTH

The PROBABLE causes are, of course, dehydration, mouth breathing and fear or anxiety. The first two are covered on *pages*

Salivary glands

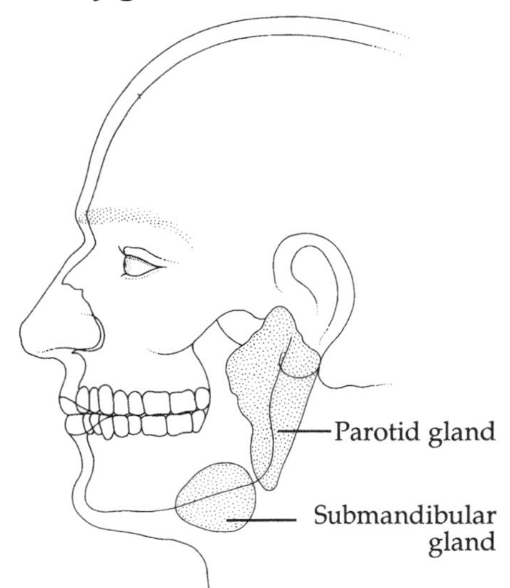

483 and 60, the last on page 377. Remove the cause, and a normal 'wet' mouth returns. If a dry mouth persists, then it might indicate underlying disease.

Anaesthetics and anti-depressants can also cause a dry mouth.

POSSIBLE
SALIVARY GLAND CALCULUS

RARE
SJOGREN'S SYNDROME

POSSIBLE

■ SALIVARY GLAND CALCULUS
Stones can form in the ducts of the major salivary glands, blocking saliva. They are commonest in the

submandibular salivary glands but occasionally occur in the parotids.
* Swelling over the gland on one side.
* Swelling worse at meal times or in the presence of food.
* Swelling is uncomfortable.
* Sensation of dryness on the same side of the mouth.
* Swelling suddenly goes down — you may note saliva trickling into mouth.

Sometimes the stones are passed, sometimes they need surgical removal.

RARE

■ SJOGREN'S SYNDROME
Probably an auto-immune disease, commonest in middle-aged women.
* Dry eyes, causing a painful, gritty feeling.
* Dry mouth, with halitosis.
* Salivary gland swelling.

Other connective tissue disorders may be associated, for example rheumatoid arthritis.

GENERALLY INFECTED MOUTH

Severe generalized infection of the oral cavity, including tongue, plate and gums, is a medical emergency. It is rare, and happens if oral hygiene is extremely poor, or indeed absent.

RARE
VINCENT'S ANGINA AND VINCENT'S ACUTE ULCERATIVE GINGIVITIS
CANCRUM ORIS

RARE

■ VINCENT'S ANGINA AND VINCENT'S ACUTE ULCERATIVE GINGIVITIS
Named after the infecting organisms. Also known as trench mouth. These are bacterial diseases of the mouth which may originate in the gums between the teeth, or the tonsils (Vincent's angina). May spread rapidly to adjacent tissues.

Vincent's angina:
* Pyrexia.
* Local pain.
* Sore throat.
* Enlarged neck lymph nodes.
* Often only one tonsil affected which is ulcerated, with a membrane present.
* The membrane may spread to soft and hard palate.
* Excessive salivation may occur.
* Highly infectious.

Responds rapidly to appropriate antibiotics.

Vincent's acute ulcerative gingivitis: in addition to the preceding symptoms,
* Deep gum ulcers.

■ CANCRUM ORIS
A severe form of the conditions described above which occur in poorly nourished children. Even with treatment, gross scarring of

the cheek can result, also limitation of jaw movement.

DIFFICULT TO OPEN MOUTH

This is usually the result of a disease affecting structures involved in opening the mouth, causing a combination of either pain or swelling. Pain gives the impression that it is difficult to open the jaw. It is, however, rarely a primary symptom. The diseases are listed here in order of **frequency**, not in order of how often they give rise to difficulty in opening the mouth.

PROBABLE
APHTHOUS ULCER
DENTAL CARIES
DENTAL INFECTION
UPPER RESPIRATORY TRACT INFECTION
TONSILLITIS
MUMPS

POSSIBLE
INFECTIOUS MONONUCLEOSIS
PERITONSILLAR ABSCESS
IMPACTION OF WISDOM TOOTH
ARTHRITIS IN TEMPOROMANDIBULAR JOINT

RARE
TETANUS
STRYCHNINE POISONING

PROBABLE

■ APHTHOUS ULCER
See page 85.

■ DENTAL CARIES
See page 89.

■ DENTAL INFECTION
See page 138.

■ UPPER RESPIRATORY TRACT INFECTION
See page 138.

■ TONSILLITIS
See page 138.

■ MUMPS
* Inflammation of the parotid glands, often mistaken for lymph glands.
* Both glands affected and markedly swollen.
* Swelling makes opening the jaw uncomfortable.
* Occasionally, pancreas and testes are affected (after puberty).

POSSIBLE

■ INFECTIOUS MONONUCLEOSIS
See page 138.

■ PERITONSILLAR ABSCESS
See page 139.

MOUTH

■ <u>IMPACTED WISDOM TOOTH</u>
Emerging wisdom teeth, especially if obstructed by existing teeth, may cause such pain, discomfort and infection at the back of the mouth that it is difficult to open your mouth. Dental opinion should be sought if suspected.

■ <u>ARTHRITIS IN TEMPORO-MANDIBULAR JOINT</u>
This joint is where the mandible hinges with the skull. Arthritis can develop with age, or after injury.
* Pain localized just in front of the ear.
* Pain may extend across side of face.
* Pain worse on chewing or moving jaw.
* A grinding sensation over the joint may be noted.
* At first, only on one side.
* May eventually affect both sides.

Temporo-mandibular joint

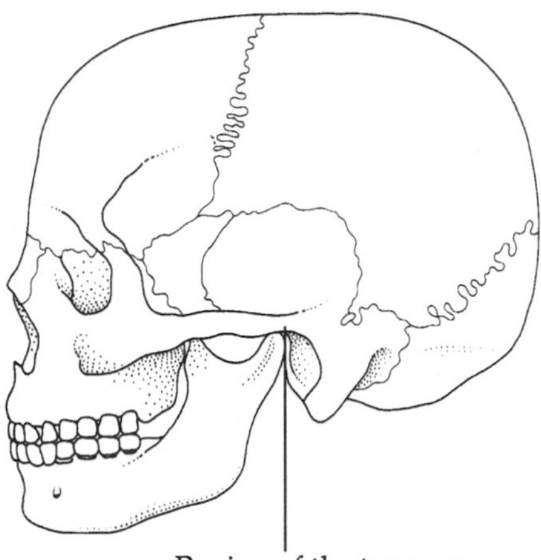

RARE

■ <u>TETANUS</u>
A disease caught by soil penetrating a trivial skin wound and contaminating it with the organism *Clostridium tetani*. It can be fatal.
* Local muscular weakness near the wound.
* Muscular spasms develop.
* Inability to open the mouth, called trismus or 'lockjaw'.
* The spasms and trismus give rise to a grinning appearance, 'risus sardonicus'.
* Fever.

Gradually, spasms are caused by the slightest stimulus. In severe cases, the number and frequency of spasms increases until death occurs. Keeping your tetanus immunization up to date is essential. Choose a birthday as the date for your shot, and have a tetanus shot every tenth year; for example, at 20, 30, 40 years old, and so on.

■ <u>STRYCHNINE POISONING</u>
The symptoms of strychnine poisoning are similar to those of tetanus (*see above*) but without a history of wound contamination.

TOO MUCH SALIVA

In the absence of any other problems, this is rare. Any condition that causes painful swallowing or a sore throat may lead to an apparent excess of saliva, as the pain prevents the usual frequency of clearing of the saliva from mouth to stomach.

However, there are some conditions in which excessive saliva is a notable feature:

PROBABLE
SMOKING
NAUSEA AND VOMITING
TONSILLITIS
PHARYNGITIS

POSSIBLE
INFECTIOUS MONONUCLEOSIS
BRAIN INJURY
NEUROLOGICAL DISEASE
PERITONSILLAR ABSCESS

RARE
CANCER OF THE OESOPHAGUS

PROBABLE

■ SMOKING
Many smokers, especially pipe and cigar smokers, notice that they salivate excessively when smoking, an effect of nicotine. It is unclear why this is not noticed by all smokers.

■ NAUSEA AND VOMITING
Prior to vomiting, the mouth often appears to fill with salty saliva.

■ TONSILLITIS
See page 138. Excessive saliva is a typical feature.

■ PHARYNGITIS
See page 124. There may be an apparent excess of saliva because of pain on swallowing.

POSSIBLE

■ INFECTIOUS MONONUCLEOSIS
See page 138.

■ BRAIN INJURY
See page 84.

■ NEUROLOGICAL DISEASE
See multiple sclerosis, Parkinson's disease, motor neurone disease, pseudobulbar and bulbar palsy, under PROBLEMS WITH SWALLOWING PLUS WEIGHT LOSS, page 122.

■ PERITONSILLAR ABSCESS
See ENLARGED LYMPH GLANDS IN NECK, page 139.

RARE

■ CANCER OF THE OESOPHAGUS
See page 121.

IMPACTED TOOTH

Meaning a tooth that cannot erupt because it is blocked or otherwise prevented from emerging by other teeth. This applies most frequently in adult life to the wisdom teeth. The unerupted tooth may be covered by a flap of gum that can become infected and painful. Extraction of the unerupted tooth is the usual — and effective — treatment. It may have to be done under general anaesthetic.

LOOSE TEETH

See DENTAL CARIES, page 89; GUM DISEASE page 90; PYORRHOEA ALVEOLARIS , page 91. These are associated with, or lead to, loose teeth, decaying teeth and toothache.

UPPER AND LOWER TEETH NOT CLOSING PROPERLY

Medical term, malocclusion. Teeth should snap shut directly opposite each other. Most people have some degree of malocclusion, typically protruding front teeth — overbite), and this needs no further treatment. Some have irregular teeth because as babies their teeth developed too slowly; because of infection, or because of an extra tooth. Dentists can correct deformities to improve function and cosmetic appearance.

Damage to the jaw bones, into which the teeth are bedded, can also give malocclusion. If bone damage is suspected, specialized treatment is essential. Deformity will give rise to pain around the face and ear — *see DIFFICULT TO OPEN MOUTH, page 97.*

Arthritis may develop.

SENSITIVE TEETH

Most people suffer from sensitive teeth at some time, frequently caused by over-vigorous brushing of the teeth, leading to receding gums. This exposes the nerve fibres around the tooth, producing sometimes extreme sensitivity to heat and cold. When a tooth is damaged or infected, again the nerves will be exposed and unusually sensitive.

See DENTAL CARIES, page 89; GUM DISEASE page 90; PYORRHOEA ALVEOLARIS , page 91. Special toothpastes for sensitive teeth coat the nerves and reduce sensitivity. They will not work in cases where there is gum disease, dental caries or infection.

DECAYING TEETH

See DENTAL CARIES, page 89; GUM DISEASE page 90; PYORRHOEA ALVEOLARIS , page 91.

TOOTHACHE

See DENTAL CARIES, page 89; GUM DISEASE page 90; PYORRHOEA ALVEOLARIS , page 91.

THE FACE — INTRODUCTION

Many symptoms of the face can also appear elsewhere on the body. This section concentrates on conditions most likely to be localized to the face.

SWOLLEN OR PUFFY FACE

Generalized swelling or puffiness of the face, as distinct from, say, swelling in the neck, is rather uncommon. Considered here is true, overall facial swelling or puffiness.

For causes of local swelling, see the sections on skin, and on the neck.

PROBABLE
INSECT BITE
DENTAL ABSCESS

POSSIBLE
ANGIONEUROTIC OEDEMA
ERYSIPELAS
CUSHING'S SYNDROME
HYPOTHYROIDISM
ACROMEGALY

RARE
GLOMERULONEPHRITIS
NEPHROTIC SYNDROME

PROBABLE

■ INSECT BITE
* Sudden onset of swelling localized to site of bite.
* Often very itchy.
* Subsides after a day or so.
* Occasionally becomes infected, with swelling becoming red and hot, and fever developing with malaise.

■ DENTAL ABSCESS
* Painful swelling above or below lower or upper jaw.
* Whole cheek may be swollen.
* No obvious dental pain or decay (caries).
* Swelling worsens over two to three days.

A visit to your dentist plus a course of antibiotics should provide rapid relief. Dental treatment may subsequently be required.

POSSIBLE

■ ANGIONEUROTIC OEDEMA
Also known as giant urticaria. Normally caused by allergy, typically to a food or a drug, but often the cause is not identifiable. Symptoms may include:
* Swelling of lips and eyes.
* Marked itching.

■ ERYSIPELAS
An infection of the skin and underlying tissues. Often, germs get in through a cut or graze.
* Red, shiny, hot skin.
* Painful.
* Fever

* Malaise.
Needs antibiotic treatment.

■ CUSHING'S SYNDROME
See page 272.

■ HYPOTHYROIDISM
Weight gain and other changes associated with this condition may give the appearance of a puffy face, although there is no true swelling.
See page 461.

■ ACROMEGALY
Enlargement of the jaw is one of the symptoms of acromegaly and might be mistaken for facial puffiness. *See page 275.*

RARE

■ GLOMERULONEPHRITIS
One of the conditions described by *NEPHRITIS, page 430.*

■ NEPHROTIC SYNDROME
See page 430.

FACIAL NODULES OR BUMPS

A possible cause is gout, covered in detail on *page 279*. A very rare cause is leprosy, *page 318*.

FACIAL BLISTERS OR ULCERATIONS

PROBABLE
COLD SORE
IMPETIGO

POSSIBLE
ECZEMA
SHINGLES

RARE
RODENT ULCER
PEMPHIGUS VULGARIS
DERMATITIS HERPETIFORMIS
PEMPHIGOID
ERYTHEMA MULTIFORME
STEVENS-JOHNSON SYNDROME

PROBABLE

■ COLD SORE
Common, and caused by a herpes virus. They often develop when someone is or has been unwell, or subjected to extremes of weather, either hot or cold, or windblown.
* Initially, irritation noted on skin around mouth.
* Becomes progressively more painful.
* Skin reddens and little vesicles (fluid-filled blisters) appear.
* Vesicles burst and crusts form.
* Clears up in about two weeks.
A similar type of infection may occur in the genital region.

THE FACE

■ IMPETIGO
A bacterial infection of the skin. Very contagious. May occur in children and adults.
* Blisters may develop wherever the infection starts.
* Blisters burst, forming dark scabs.
* Large areas can be infected if untreated.

At some stages, impetigo can be difficult to distinguish from a cold sore.

Antibiotics are required: if the condition is mild, treatment is by ointment; if it is severe, by tablets.

POSSIBLE

■ ECZEMA
Sometimes called dermatitis. On the face, cosmetics are a common cause. Features include:
* Redness (where the cosmetics were applied).
* Red, raised spots.
* Small blisters which weep.
* Crusting and scaling.

It is not uncommon for patches of eczema to appear eventually all over the body.

■ SHINGLES
An infection caused by the virus that also causes chickenpox.
* Red, blistering rash.
* Can be very painful (often preceding the rash).
* May be extensive (typically covering one side of the face).
* Localized to one side of the body's centre line.
* Crusting of the blisters.
* Heals in about two weeks, but in rare cases pain may persist for months or years.

If the eye is affected, seek medical help urgently.

RARE

■ RODENT ULCER
A small cancerous sore, which virtually never spreads to distant parts of the body. Often appears in the elderly around nose, eyes, ears or mouth.
* Starts as a small pink lump.
* After some weeks or months become ulcerated.
* Gradually, if undiagnosed and untreated, it invades underlying tissues, for example the bones of the nose.

Once diagnosed, treatment is straightforward.

■ PEMPHIGUS VULGARIS
See page 240.

■ DERMATITIS HERPETIFORMIS
See page 240.

■ PEMPHIGOID
See page 240.

■ ERYTHEMA MULTIFORME and STEVENS-JOHNSON SYNDROME
The second is a severe form of the first and both are reactions to provocations such as infection or medications. Features include:
* Red rash of different shapes which may be present all over the body.
* Raised red lesions and blisters may occur.
* Each episode may last two to three weeks.

THE FACE

Stevens-Johnson syndrome may also include:
* Fever.
* Malaise.
* Lung inflammation.
* Kidney damage.

REDDENED FACE

The probable causes are, of course, embarassment, heat and alcohol, all of which can make the blood vessels in the skin widen so that they carry more blood than usual. In each case, the redness may well extend across not only face and head but neck and upper trunk. That the blood vessels can respond to a state of mind is proof, if any were needed, that mind and body are indeed not separate but complementary.

POSSIBLE
ACNE ROSACEA
EPILEPSY
MENOPAUSE

RARE
MITRAL VALVE DISEASE
CARCINOID SYNDROME
PHAEOCHROMOCYTOMA
SYSTEMIC LUPUS ERYTHEMATOSIS

POSSIBLE

■ ACNE ROSACEA
Most common in the middle-aged and elderly.
* Facial reddening.
* Some inflamed pustules.
* Skin is shiny.
* May become permanent.

Food, alcohol or embarassment can exacerbate the reddening.

■ EPILEPSY
Epileptics may be aware of facial flushing just before a fit, and observers will often notice it afterwards.

■ MENOPAUSE
Flushing is one of the commonest symptoms women experience as they approach the 'change of life'. Symptoms can persist for years.

RARE

■ MITRAL VALVE DISEASE
* Shortness of breath.
* Lung congestion.
* Coughing blood.
* Bronchitis.
* Heart failure.
* Facial flush, very marked below the eyes.

■ CARCINOID SYNDROME
A tumour that may occur in many parts of the body. Most of its symptoms are caused by chemicals it secretes, and may include:
* Facial flushing, extending over body.
* Diarrhoea, abdominal pain.

* Enlarged liver.
* Wheezy chest.
* Heart problems.

■ PHAEOCHROMOCYTOMA
Another tumour whose symptoms are caused by the chemicals it secretes. It is very rare.
* High blood pressure.
* Diarrhoea.
* Nausea.
* Abdominal pain.
* Facial flushing.

■ SYSTEMIC LUPUS ERYTHEMATOSUS
See page 448.

ADENOIDAL FACE

A term used for individuals who tend to mouth-breathe, rather than breathe through the nose. They tend to walk, move about and even sit with their mouths permanently open. This is because their enlarged adenoids prevent them from breathing through their nose. Their voice may also be affected and is often described as 'adenoidal'. Symptoms may include:
* Breathing through the mouth.
* Snoring.
* Open mouth — the jaw hangs down.
* Nasal speech.

GRINNING

One of the several symptoms of tetanus *(see page 98)* is spasms which contort the face in to the so-called 'sardonic grin'. There is nothing funny about this, or the other potentially fatal symptoms, which is why immunization — and keeping your protection up to date — is essential. Gardeners are particularly at risk from skin wounds being contaminated by soil containing the tetanus organism.

You should have tetanus immunization every ten years. A way of remembering is to renew the jab on every tenth birthday: for example at 10, 20, 30 and 40.

EXPRESSIONLESS FACE

Parkinson's disease is the classic reason for an expressionless, immobile face. However, a number of conditions can give rise to a similar appearance as a result of damage to the part of the brain that controls facial, and other, movement.

PROBABLE
PARKINSON'S DISEASE
DEPRESSION

The Face

POSSIBLE
DRUGS
SCLERODERMA

RARE
HEPATOLENTICULAR DEGENERATION

PROBABLE

■ PARKINSON'S DISEASE
A slowly progressive disease of the middle-aged and elderly.
* Tremor.
* Rigidity and some muscle pain.
* Slow movement.
* Immobile, mask-like face.
* Difficulty in writing.
* Occasional swallowing disorders.

Can be controlled with medication.

■ DEPRESSION
A depressed person may progressively lose the expression from his or her face. A dull, saddened, flat face is characteristic of depression. *See also page 389.*

POSSIBLE

■ DRUGS
Drugs that may cause some (but not necessarily all) of the symptoms of Parkinson's disease include phenothiazines and butyrophenones. Both these groups of drugs are commonly used as tranquillizers.

■ SCLERODERMA
A multi-system disease, usually afflicting women, which is likely to have already been diagnosed; *see page 123.*
* Stiffness of hands leading to rigidity.
* Smooth, hard, shiny skin.
* Difficulty in opening mouth.
* Immobile face with loss of expression.
* Alimentary tract, heart and kidneys may become involved.

RARE

■ HEPATOLENTICULAR DEGENERATION
Wilson's disease. An inherited disorder, usually showing itself during the teens.
* Parkinson's disease symptoms, plus:
* Liver damage leading to jaundice in some cases.
* Yellow-brown rings on the eyes.

PART OF THE FACE PARALYSED

Excluded here is immobility of the entire face, covered under *EXPRESSIONLESS FACE, page 105.*

PROBABLE
BELL'S PALSY
STROKE

POSSIBLE

INJURY
POLIOMYELITIS

RARE

TUMOURS
HERPES
GUILLAIN BARRE SYNDROME
MOTOR NEURONE DISEASE

PROBABLE

■ BELL'S PALSY
The cause is unknown, but the facial nerve is damaged on one side. The affected individual may note the symptoms on waking up one morning, or after having been out in cold weather, or in a draught:
* May be a dull ache on the affected side.
* Cannot close eye.
* Mouth drawn to the side, away from the damaged nerve
* Saliva may dribble from the affected side.
* Cannot smile properly or bare the teeth.
* Occasionally, taste sensation to one side of the tongue is affected.
* With luck, recovery commences within seven to ten days, but may take several weeks.

If you suspect Bell's palsy, see a doctor as soon as possible.
Some doctors believe that high doses of steroids, given early enough, may improve the chances of recovery.

■ STROKE
Any stroke may damage part of the brain that controls the nerve that makes the facial muscles work. Different types of stroke may affect the face in slightly different ways so that a number of symptoms can be present to a greater or lesser degree. These include:
* Difficulty or inability to wrinkle the forehead.
* Difficulty or inability to blink or close the eye.
* Difficulty or inability to smile symmetrically.
* Difficulty or inability to bare the teeth.
* Difficulty or inability to whistle.
* Saliva may leak out of the affected side of the mouth.
* The body will be affected on the same side as the face: for example, weakened left hand and face paralysed on left-hand side.

Paralysis of the face is unlikely to occur in the absence of other symptoms — which may help to determine the diagnosis.

POSSIBLE

■ INJURY
All or part of the facial nerve, which controls movement of the facial muscles, may be damaged — sometimes permanently. The symptoms are the same as for Bell's palsy (*see above*). Knife wounds to the face may be a cause.

■ POLIOMYELITIS
'Polio' can also affect the facial nerve, with similar results to *BELL'S PALSY, this page.*

The Face

RARE

■ TUMOURS
Primary or secondary cancerous tumours developing in the part of the brain that controls facial movement or that involve or press on the facial nerve, may cause a mixture of symptoms similar to those of *STROKE* or *BELL's PALSY*, *page 107.*

■ HERPES
A herpes infection of the mouth, palate or ear can damage the nerve supply to the face causing symptoms similar to BELL'S PALSY, *page 107.* This is known as Ramsey-Hunt syndrome.

■ GUILLAIN-BARRE SYNDROME
A disease of the neurological system with many different symptoms, ranging from mild to severe. Most cases recover, but this may take many months.
* Altered sensation in the arms and legs.
* Shoulder and back pain.
* Facial palsies.
* Muscles of respiration may be so weakened that artificial ventilation is required.
* Swallowing may be affected and tube-feeding may be needed while recovery progresses.

■ MOTOR NEURONE DISEASE
See page 123.

FACIAL PAIN

Covered here are causes of pain that have no *visible* symptoms, so, for example, shingles is excluded.

PROBABLE
DENTAL DISEASE
REFERRED PAIN

POSSIBLE
MIGRAINE
POST HERPETIC NEURALGIA
TRIGEMINAL NEURALGIA

RARE
CANCER
PAGET'S DISEASE
PSYCHOGENIC FACIAL PAIN

PROBABLE

■ DENTAL DISEASE
Check teeth and gums first if local face pain develops with no obvious cause. Is it an abscess? If in doubt, always check with your dentist.

■ REFERRED PAIN
Because the body's 'wiring'— its nervous system — is interconnected, pain arising in one place can travel onwards or 'be referred' to another. If the teeth and gums appear normal, then pain in the face may arise from elsewhere in

the head, for instance the facial sinuses.

POSSIBLE

■ MIGRAINE
See page 112, for full details. Facial pain can be felt as part of a migraine attack.
* The pain will usually be severe and piercing.
* Only one side of the face will be affected.

■ POST-HERPETIC NEURALGIA
Persistent burning pain at the site of a previous attack of shingles; *see page 240.*
* Normally in elderly patients.
* Pain is so severe that suicide may be considered.
* Even touching the site may start an attack of pain.

■ TRIGEMINAL NEURALGIA
Also called tic douloureux. Pain in the face in an area supplied by the trigeminal nerve [diagram].
* Stabbing, intermittent facial pain.
* Can be triggered by touch, or for no reason.
* Attacks come in bouts.

Many different treatments have been tried, some with more success than others. A specialist opinion is needed if the diagnosis is made, as the symptoms can be incapacitating.

RARE

■ MALIGNANT DISEASE
A doctor will consider the possibility of a cancerous tumour of the nose, mouth, sinuses or pharynx, particularly if the individual is an elderly smoker.

Trigeminal neuralgia

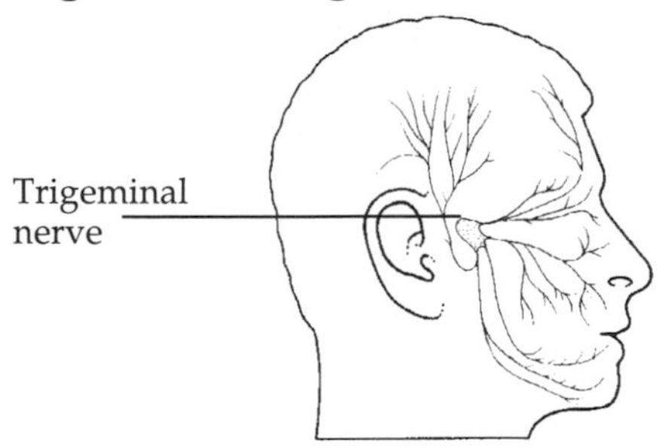

■ PAGET'S DISEASE
This disease *(see also page 437)* can cause local pain in the bones affected, including those of the face.

■ PSYCHOLOGICAL OR ATYPICAL
In a few individuals no cause of pain is ever found, despite full investigation and assessment. This pain is described as 'atypical'. Recent research by dental experts and pain specialists has found that tricyclics, a group of drugs generally used to treat depression, can be helpful to patients with 'atypical facial pain'.

It is certainly worth trying these drugs before accepting that "only psychotherapy will help".

THE HEAD

OVER-SIZED HEAD

There are two possibilities: hydrocephalus and Paget's disease. For details of the latter, *see page 437.*

In hydrocephalus, a problem of new-born and very young babies, there is a drainage failure of the cavities within the brain. The result is increased pressure in the skull, with:

* Progressive enlargement of the head.
* Bulging fontanelles.

The increased pressure damages the brain and can cause:

* Intellectual impairment.
* Epilepsy.
* Physical impairment.
* Vulnerability to infection.

Hydrocephalus needs specialist treatment: the fluid can be drained away to the stomach (abdomen) by a tube set permanently below the skin on the scalp.

BULGING OR SUNKEN PLACES ON HEAD

Several causes of bulges in the head are worth considering in their own right, separately from lumps, bumps and swellings that can occur anywhere on the body, and which are covered in detail in other major sections of this book.

One somewhat specialized area should also be mentioned in this context: the fontanelles. These are the soft 'gaps' that can be felt in babies' heads at the points where the skull bones have not yet fused into a consistent bony covering. The smaller, posterior fontanelle closes soon after birth, while the larger one, the anterior fontanelle, usually closes by one and a half years of age.

The size of the fontanelles varies enormously from child to child. Your doctor will often feel the fontanelle if your child is unwell. A bulging fontanelle can indicate raised pressure in the head — as in meningitis. It can also mean only that your baby is screaming the house down. It is best to check any changes or concerns regarding the fontanelle with your doctor.

PROBABLE
DEHYDRATION

POSSIBLE
PAGET'S DISEASE

RARE
HYDROCEPHALUS
RAISED INTRACRANIAL PRESSURE

PROBABLE

■ DEHYDRATION

A baby who is short of fluid, typically after a bout of diarrhoea, will show:

* Sunken eyes.
* Sunken fontanelle.
* Loss of skin elasticity.
* Listless, apathetic behaviour.

* Dry lips and mouth.
Dehydration is a serious condition in any baby or child; if you suspect it, see a doctor urgently. It can be effectively treated, but time is of the essence.

POSSIBLE

■ PAGET'S DISEASE
See page 437.

RARE

■ HYDROCEPHALUS
See under OVER-SIZED HEAD, page 110.

■ RAISED INTRACRANIAL PRESSURE
A tumour or infection raises the pressure inside the skull. It is normal for the fontanelles to bulge outwards when a baby cries or strains, say when coughing. But if intracranial pressure is raised, the fontanelle bulges permanently. There may well be other symptoms such as vomiting and headache. See a doctor.
When the fontanelle is closed, after around 18 months, it cannot bulge. After this time the main features of raised intracranial pressure will be vomiting and headache.

BLOOD VESSELS STAND OUT IN HEAD

An obvious feature of temporal arteritis; *see page 113.*

HEAD TWISTING TO ONE SIDE

Stiff neck? *See STIFFNESS OR PAIN IN NECK, page 135.* A common cause is torticollis, also considered in detail on *page 135.*

HEADACHE AND FITS OR CONVULSIONS

See CONVULSIONS, page 383.

HEADACHE

It is so rare for headache to be the symptom of grave underlying disease, such as a brain tumour, that worrying about it — though understandable — is usually a waste of time: better to worry about other aspects of your health which really might be significant, such as smoking or excess alcohol or cholesterol intake. As a rough rule of thumb, even the most vicious, throbbing headache is in all likelihood `innocent': the headache that signifies a brain tumour is something else entirely, and will almost always be accompanied by other symptoms. Ninety-eight per cent of all headaches that doctors treat are caused by tension or sinus trouble.

THE HEAD

PROBABLE
TENSION HEADACHE
SINUSITIS
MENSTRUATION- OR MENOPAUSE-RELATED
INFECTION

POSSIBLE
MIGRAINE
CLUSTER HEADACHE
TEMPORAL ARTERITIS
EYE, EAR, NOSE, THROAT, OR DENTAL DISEASE
DRUGS
TOXIC FUMES

RARE
MENINGITIS
SUBARACHNOID HAEMORRHAGE
BRAIN TUMOUR
SUBDURAL HAEMORRHAGE
BRAIN ABSCESS

PROBABLE

■ TENSION HEADACHE
Often develops in people with work or family problems. May also arise if an individual finds him- or herself under pressure, whatever the circumstances. The source of tension is not always obvious.
* May be intermittent for weeks and months in a previously fit individual.
* Normal periods in between.
* Band-like, crushing pain around head.
* No other physical abnormalities present.
* Disappears after a variable length of time.

■ SINUSITIS
See page 58. Any inflammation of the sinuses (air-spaces in the facial bones) can cause headache. This can be due to infection, catarrh and even hay fever.

Tends to be a remorseless, low-grade, throbbing pain.

■ MENSTRUATION- OR MENOPAUSE-RELATED
Alterations of body hormone production, either naturally, during, before or after a period, can cause variable headaches. Your doctor may be able to advise you on treatments or check-ups from which you might benefit.

■ INFECTION
Viral infections of any kind are notorious for producing multiple symptoms of which headache, often dull and persistent is but one. Other features are:
* Fever.
* Muscle and joint pain.
* Malaise.

These are in addition to other, more specific, symptoms, typically sore throat.

POSSIBLE

■ MIGRAINE
Recurrent, severe headaches, often but not always accompanied by

visual disturbance. Often starts in adolescence. Many different symptoms are described, including:
* Vision affected before the headache starts.
* Occasionally numbness or weakness of one limb before the headache starts.
* Pain starts on one side of the head, but may spread.
* The pain throbs.
* A wish to avoid light.
* Vomiting may occur.
* May last for a couple of days, but normally four to 12 hours.

The cause is not not fully understood but probably related to abnormal blood flow in the fine vessels of the scalp. Some relief is available from modern medications — see your doctor.

■ <u>CLUSTER HEADACHE</u>
* Commonest in men.
* Tends to be one-sided.
* Often severe.
* May occur at night.
* Occurs several times within a period of a few weeks, then disappears, returning some months later.
* Is harmless.

■ <u>TEMPORAL ARTERITIS</u>
Inflammation of the temporal arterywhich runs along the side of the face. Commonest in elderly males.
* Severe pain on the side of the face.
* Skin over the artery is inflamed.
* Artery is thickened and painful to touch.
* There may be fever and malaise.

If suspected, urgent medical treatment is needed, as the eye may become involved.

Temporal arteritis

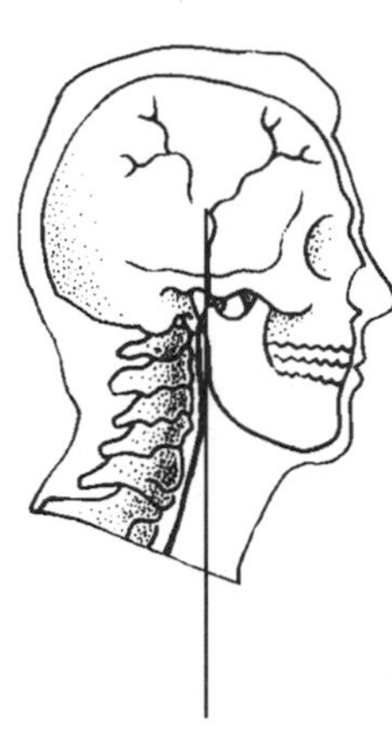

■ <u>EYE, EAR, NOSE, THROAT, OR DENTAL DISEASE</u>
See those sections for full detail. All these organs can produce pain that is referred to the head. The pain may be dull and persistent. These possibilities should therefore be excluded if a headache persists for longer than expected.

■ <u>DRUGS</u>
Including cigarettes and alcohol. The system is poisoned by the body's inability to eliminate the broken-down by-products.

Some prescription drugs can cause headache, too. You must reasonably suspect this if the headache is noted after taking the drug. One such drug is the anti-angina medication, glyceryl trinitrate, which gives some people a throbbing headache.

The Head

If headaches coincide with taking a prescribed drug, always report it to your doctor — there may well be an alternative to try instead.

■ TOXIC FUMES
Dry-cleaning agents, tar and diesel fumes are among regular culprits. Some people suddenly develop a sensitivity to fumes, even having worked with them for years.

Low-grade poisoning with carbon monoxide from a faulty central heating boiler can cause headaches.

RARE

■ MENINGITIS
An infection of the membranes that enclose the brain and spinal cord. If you suspect it, see a doctor immediately.
* Severe headache.
* Stiff neck; bending the neck worsens the pain.
* Reduced level of consciousness.
* Photophobia — fear of light.
* Vomiting.
* Fever.
* Very ill.
* A rash may appear.

■ SUBARACHNOID HAEMORRHAGE
A leakage of blood from a vessel into the liquid that bathes the spinal cord and brain. The following may occur:
* Sudden onset of severe headache after a period of exertion — often described as being like a blow on the back of the head. However:
* The headache may have a slower, more insidious, onset.
* Vomiting.
* Stiff neck.
* Mental confusion.
* Speech difficulties.
* Limb weakness.
* Visual disturbances.
* Convulsions.

If suspected, see a doctor urgently.

■ BRAIN TUMOUR
Because the adult skull is rigid, a growth within it can increase the internal pressure, giving rise to headache. However, not every brain tumour has this effect.
Brain tumours can be primary — a pituitary tumour is an example — or secondary, that is, having spread from elsewhere in the body, for example from a primary breast cancer. There will almost always be a range of symptoms:
* Gradually increasing, dull headache.
* Vomiting.
* Impaired consciousness.
* Pulse becomes slower.
* Respiration rate becomes slower.
* Convulsions may occur.
* Vision may be affected.
* Headache often present when you wake in the morning.

If the first three symptoms develop in an individual, along with other signs of neurological damage, say weakness or numbness of a limb, urgent medical assessment is needed. The symptoms can be relieved, even if the tumour itself cannot be removed.

■ SUBDURAL HAEMORRHAGE
Blood collects between the layers of tissue covering the brain,

causing raised pressure. May happen in the elderly after an (apparently)
insignificant fall. Symptoms may develop some weeks later and include:

* Headache, often minor.
* Periods of sleepiness and unconsciousness.
* Increased confusion.
* Possibly speech difficulties.
* Possibly convulsions.

May often be mistaken for 'getting old' — so not to be discounted if someone has recently received a blow to the head.

■ BRAIN ABSCESS
Infection enters the brain in one of several ways: a broken skull-bone with overlying skin damage; from ear, throat, sinus and lung infection; or occasionally from facial infection.

* Symptoms of the initial infection, for example, earache.
* Progressive headache.
* Progressive drowsiness.
* Fever.
* Vomiting.
* Malaise.
* Anorexia.
* Convulsions.

HEADACHE WITH HIGH FEVER

The commonest illnesses which give fever combined with headache are common viral infections such as influenza and glandular fever. There are, however, several rare but dangerous infections which may also be responsible for similar symptoms. Don't read this summary without also reading the sections on fever, *pages 440-51.*

PROBABLE
COMMON INFECTIONS, *see FEVER, pages 440-51*

POSSIBLE
TEMPORAL ARTERITIS, *page 113*
SINUSITIS, *page 58*
DISEASES OF EYE, EAR, NOSE, THROAT, TEETH, *see pages 13-29, 116-31 and 93-5*
MALARIA, *page 453*

RARE
MENINGITIS, *page 440*
BRAIN ABSCESS, *this page*
BRUCELLOSIS, *page 448*
TYPHUS FEVER, *page 454.*
WEIL'S DISEASE, *page 453*

HEADACHE PLUS CHILLS AND FEVER

See FEVER, pages 440-51

HEADACHE: BABIES AND CHILDREN

Babies and children can get headaches for the same reasons as adults. But in seeking the cause, you should consider two other factors:

First, babies and young children, say up to the age of five or even six, are notoriously inexact about where pain is coming from. 'Head pain' often turns out to be earache or sore throat. So, explore every possibility before settling for headache.

Second, complaining of recurrent headaches can be characteristic of a child who is unhappy or under stress: typically he or she is going through a bad patch at schoool. You can detect no other symptoms; and if illness or disease can really be ruled out, then you should find out what is causing the problems. Removing the cause can make the headaches vanish overnight.

RECURRING HEADACHE

See HEADACHE WITH HIGH FEVER, page 115.

SLURRED OR UNCLEAR SPEECH

Hoarseness is covered separately on *page 117.* Listed here are the main causes of impaired speech; but bear in mind that impaired speech is not always a feature of these conditions, and that their other symptoms usually predominate. Look up specific entries elsewhere in the book for further details.

PROBABLE

ALCOHOL AND DRUGS
SEPTAL DEVIATION
INJURY
COMMON COLD
ADENOIDS
STUTTERING
LISPING AND ROLLING Rs

POSSIBLE

CLEFT PALATE
NEUROLOGICAL DISEASE
CHRONIC SINUSITIS
BENIGN TUMOURS

RARE

MALIGNANT TUMOURS OF THE NOSE

PROBABLE

■ ALCOHOL AND DRUGS
Temporary slowness and slurring.

■ SEPTAL DEVIATION
Muffled or nasal quality to speech. *See page 61.*

■ INJURY
Muffled or nasal quality to speech. *See page 54.*

■ COMMON COLD
Muffled or nasal quality to speech. *See page 454.*

■ ADENOIDS
Muffled or nasal quality to speech. *See page 60.*

■ STUTTERING
Tends to begin as a child begins to learn to talk, from two years onwards.

■ LISPING AND ROLLING Rs
Not necessarily a speech impairment, but a variation of normal. Common when children first learn to speak, and tends to disappear by the age of six. If marked or persistent, speech therapy may be appropriate. Indeed, early attention from a speech therapist can prevent speech disorders becoming permanent.

POSSIBLE

■ CLEFT PALATE
See page 87.

■ NEUROLOGICAL DISEASE
Any disease that can affect control of the tongue, soft palate and related structures will give slurred and unclear speech. Motor neurone disease, multiple sclerosis and Parkinson's disease are examples.

■ CHRONIC SINUSITIS
May give a muffled or nasal quality to speech. *See page 129.*

■ BENIGN TUMOURS
Including nasal polyps, may give a muffled or nasal quality to speech.*See page 58.*

RARE

■ MALIGNANT TUMOURS OF THE NOSE
See CANCER OF THE NOSE, page 59.

HOARSE VOICE - OR NO VOICE

Severe cases of hoarseness may suffer complete loss of voice; mild cases merely a temporary thickening or roughening. The causes can be divided into three main categories: those affecting the vocal cords themselves; those affecting the nerves supplying them; and those caused by other disease of the larynx. All cases of hoarseness lasting more than 10 days must be reported to a doctor. *See also PROBLEMS WITH SWALLOWING PLUS HOARSE VOICE, page 121.*

THE THROAT

Throat, larynx and speech

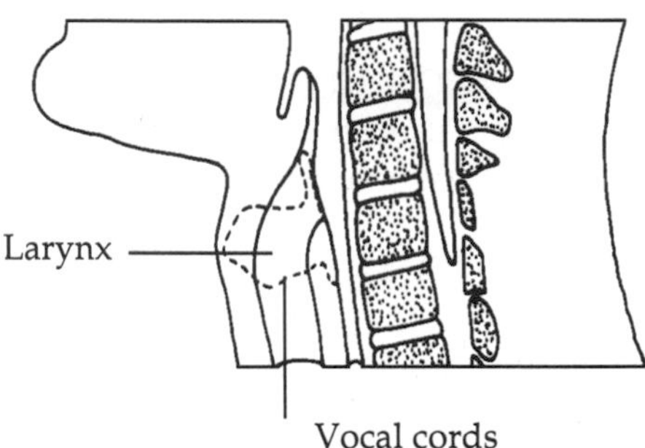

PROBABLE
SMOKING, DRINKING, EXCESSIVE TALKING/SHOUTING
LARYNGITIS
COMMON COLD

POSSIBLE
VOCAL NODULES
SURGERY
MYXOEDEMA
EPIGLOTTITIS
CANCER OF THE LARYNX
INHALATION

RARE
FOREIGN BODIES
THORACIC AORTIC ANEURYSM
CANCER
AFTER RADIOTHERAPY
SARCOIDOSIS
MYASTHENIA GRAVIS

PROBABLE

■ SMOKING, DRINKING, EXCESSIVE TALKING OR SHOUTING

Obvious and familiar when combined, but also capable of inflaming the vocal cords in isolation.
* Hoarseness.
* Sore throat.
* Settles in three to four days.

If you keep up these insults to your vocal cords, recovery may be slow, indeed you may suffer total loss of voice. Rest (not talking) is the only answer.

■ LARYNGITIS
See page 125.

■ COMMON COLD
May occasionally involve the larynx, resulting in hoarseness.
See also page 454.

POSSIBLE

■ VOCAL NODULES
Also called Singer's nodes. Typically in singers pitching their voice higher than their natural range.
* Progressive hoarseness.

The nodules often need to be removed by surgery.

■ SURGERY
Surgery to the neck, particularly to the thyroid gland, may damage the recurrent laryngeal nerve. Recovery takes a few weeks but the hoarseness can be permanent. If so, there are methods of improving the speech.

After any operation where a breathing tube as been passed down the throat, slight hoarseness and a sore throat is usual.

■ MYXOEDEMA
Swelling around eyes and feet as a result of an underactive thyroid gland, plus highly distinctive, deep, gruff voice.

■ EPIGLOTTITIS
See page 139.

■ CANCER OF THE LARYNX
See page 125.

■ INHALATION
Of smoke or chemicals can cause temporary hoarseness.

RARE

■ FOREIGN BODIES
See page 122.

■ THORACIC AORTIC ANEURYSM
The aorta is the main artery in the chest. An aneurysm is a swelling due to weakness of the wall. This can cause hoarseness by local pressure on the recurrent laryngeal nerve.

■ CANCER
Any malignant tumour in the chest, but especially on the oesophagus or lung, may press on or invade the recurrent laryngeal nerve causing hoarseness.

However, this symptom is usually one of the last to occur.
See NOTICEABLE BLOOD VESSELS IN THE NECK, SWOLLEN LYMPH NODES IN NECK, PROBLEMS IN SWALLOWING, pages 131, 137 and this page.

■ AFTER RADIOTHERAPY
Radiotherapy is sometimes used to treat cancer of the larynx, leaving the patient hoarse.

■ SARCOIDOSIS
A disease (cause unknown) giving enlarged lymph nodes and deposits in various tissues, including larynx, hence hoarseness.

■ MYASTHENIA GRAVIS
See page 122.

CLEARING THE THROAT

See PHLEGM IN THE THROAT, page 128.

PROBLEMS WITH SWALLOWING

PROBABLE
TONSILLITIS
PHARYNGITIS

POSSIBLE
GLOBUS HYSTERICUS
OESOPHAGITIS
ACHALASIA

RARE
CONGENITAL ATRESIA OF THE OESOPHAGUS
CANCER OF THE OESOPHAGUS
CANCER OF THE STOMACH

THE THROAT

PROBABLE

■ TONSILLITIS AND PHARYNGITIS,
see pages 138 and 124.

POSSIBLE

■ GLOBUS HYSTERICUS
Often seen in young women with a history of anxiety-related illness: a certain belief that there is something stuck in the throat; sensation of choking. Requires full medical examination and, if all is normal, strong reassurance.

■ OESOPHAGITIS
See this page .

■ ACHALASIA
A narrowing of the gullet at the lower end. Appears in young adults.
* Difficulty in swallowing.
* Regurgitation of undigested food into the mouth .
* Vomiting.
* Loss of weight.
* Occasionally, chest infections with fever.

RARE

■ CONGENITAL ATRESIA OF THE OESOPHAGUS
At birth:
* All feeds regurgitated.
* Frothy saliva from mouth.
* Difficulty breathing while being fed.
*Episodes of cyanosis (blueness).
* Pneumonia.

■ CANCER OF THE OESOPHAGUS AND CANCER OF THE STOMACH
See page 121.

PROBLEMS WITH SWALLOWING PLUS REGURGITATION OR VOMITING

PROBABLE
OESOPHAGITIS

POSSIBLE
PEPTIC STRICTURE
PHARYNGEAL POUCH

RARE
CANCER OF THE OESOPHAGUS
STOMACH CANCER
OTHER CANCERS
THORACIC AORTIC ANEURYSM

PROBABLE

■ OESOPHAGITIS
Caused by stomach acid flowing back up into the gullet.
* Burning pain on swallowing.
* Food and fluid regurgitated.
* Bitter taste in mouth.
* Heartburn.
* Pain in middle of chest, at front or at back, or down arms.
* Food 'sticks' behind breast bone.
* Aggravated by hot or spicy foods and alcohol.
Relieved by antacids.

POSSIBLE

■ PEPTIC STRICTURE
A narrowing of the gullet caused by long-standing reflux oesophagitis.
* Food regurgitated with fluid.
* Heartburn.
* Associated with weight loss after prolonged period.
* Chest infections associated with regurgitation.
* May be associated with hiatus hernia; *see page 143*.
* May be a long-standing history of reflux oesophagitis.

■ PHARYNGEAL POUCH
See page 134.

RARE

■ CANCER OF THE OESOPHAGUS
Commonest in 50-plus age group.
* Difficulty in swallowing.
* Liquids swallowed more easily than solids.
* Some regurgitation of food.
* Rarely pain.
* Weight loss.
* Poor appetite.
* Fatigue.
* Anaemia (particularly in women).
* Hoarse voice.
* Occasional chest infection with fever — due to regurgitation.

■ STOMACH CANCER
Similar symptoms to oesophageal cancer, but there may also be:
* Abdominal pain.
* Poor appetite, developing earlier.
* A feeling of fullness soon after eating very little.
* Symptoms of indigestion which persist, do not respond to usual treatment, or become more severe.
* Feeling bloated.
* A previous ulcer.
* Anaemia.
* In later stages, occasional difficulty in swallowing.

■ OTHER CANCERS
Secondary tumours or large primary tumours outside the oesophagus, but within the chest, can compress the oesophagus giving rise to:
* Difficulty in swallowing.
* Weight loss.
* Poor appetite.
* Weakness.

All in addition to the symptoms of the primary tumour.

■ THORACIC AORTIC ANEURYSM
See page 119.

PROBLEMS WITH SWALLOWING PLUS HOARSE VOICE

Hoarseness which persists in the absence of other symptoms can be a sign either of laryngeal polyps or of cancer. Early treatment will significantly affect the outcome for the better. Seek your doctor's advice as early as possible.

PROBABLE
LARYNGITIS

POSSIBLE
FOREIGN BODY IN GULLET

RARE
MYASTHENIA GRAVIS
CANCER OF THE OESOPHAGUS

PROBABLE

■ LARYNGITIS
See page 125.

POSSIBLE

■ FOREIGN BODY (FOR EXAMPLE A FISH BONE) IN GULLET
* Pain and discomfort on swallowing.
* Hoarseness.
* Feeling of 'something in the throat'.

RARE

■ MYASTHENIA GRAVIS
A disorder causing weakness and tiring of the muscles.
* Muscular weakness.
* Drooping eyelids.
* Double vision.
* Hoarse, weak voice.
* Difficulty in swallowing.
* Possibly weight loss.

■ CANCER OF THE OESOPHAGUS
See page 121.

PROBLEMS WITH SWALLOWING PLUS WEIGHT LOSS

This combination of symptoms is likely to be an indication of serious illness. Seek help soon, since early intervention will significantly improve your chances of recovery. Smoking and drinking to excess will increase the risk of oesophageal problems and cancer of the stomach.

PROBABLE
OESOPHAGEAL STRICTURE
CANCER OF THE OESOPHAGUS

POSSIBLE
OESOPHAGEAL BENIGN TUMOUR
MULTIPLE SCLEROSIS
MOTOR NEURONE DISEASE
PARKINSON'S DISEASE
PSEUDOBULBAR AND
BULBAR PALSY

RARE
CHAGAS' DISEASE
MYASTHENIA GRAVIS
SCLERODERMA
SYSTEMIC LUPUS
ERYTHEMATOSIS
CANCER OF THE STOMACH

PROBABLE

■ OESOPHAGEAL STRICTURE
See PEPTIC STRICTURE, page 121.
The symptoms are the same, but can be caused by, for instance, accidental or deliberate swallowing of toxic chemicals.

■ CANCER OF THE OESOPHAGUS
See page 121.

POSSIBLE

■ BENIGN TUMOUR OF THE OESOPHAGUS
Such as a fibroma, leiomyoma or haemangioma.
* Intermittent difficulty in swallowing.
* Sensation of 'something' in the gullet.
* Health otherwise good.
* Minimal weight loss, unless tumour is large.

■ MULTIPLE SCLEROSIS
In addition to motor and sensory changes *(see page 406)*:
* Difficulty in swallowing.
* Some risk of regurgitation of food into chest.
* Gradual weight loss.

■ MOTOR NEURONE DISEASE
Progressive muscular weakness with:
* Difficulty in starting to swallow because of poor tongue muscle control.
* Risk of inhaling food or fluids.
* Gradual weight loss.
See also page 406.

■ PARKINSONS'S DISEASE
In addition to the tremor, mask face and slowness of movement:
* Difficulty in starting to swallow.
* Occasional choking.
* Weight loss.

■ PSEUDOBULBAR AND BULBAR PALSY
These conditions are usually set off by a stroke (pseudobulbar palsy) or motor neurone disease (bulbar palsy). They cause:
* Difficulty in speech.
* Difficulty in swallowing.
* Regurgitation of food into nose.
* If prolonged, weight loss.

RARE

■ CHAGAS' DISEASE
Common in South America. Caused by infection with *trypanosoma cruzi*. Symptoms are similar to those of ACHALASIA; *see page 120.*

■ MYASTHENIA GRAVIS
See page 122.

■ SCLERODERMA
A disease which can affect many organs and which will usually have been diagnosed already. Commonest in women in their 30s and 40s.
* Associated with pain because of oesophagitis; *see page 120.*
* Slow weight loss.

■ SYSTEMIC LUPUS ERYTHEMATOSIS *See page 448.*

■ CANCER OF THE STOMACH
See page 121.

PROBLEMS WITH SWALLOWING PLUS PAIN

PROBABLE
TONSILLITIS
PHARYNGITIS
LARYNGITIS

POSSIBLE
CANDIDIASIS
OESOPHAGITIS
OESOPHAGEAL SPASM
ULCERS OF TONGUE AND MOUTH
GLOSSITIS
HERPES SIMPLEX

RARE
CANCER OF THE OESOPHAGUS
CANCER OF THE LARYNX

PROBABLE

■ TONSILLITIS
See page 138.

■ PHARYNGITIS
The pharynx lies behind the tonsils at the back of the mouth, above the voice box and gullet.
* Pain on swallowing.
* Back of throat is noticeably red.
* Possibly enlarged lymph nodes — similar to tonsillitis, but tonsils not inflamed.

If you have had tonsils removed, pharyngitis may develop in response to an infection which would otherwise have caused tonsillitis.

■ LARYNGITIS
See page 125.

POSSIBLE

■ CANDIDIASIS
* Discomfort making swallowing difficult.
* White patches seen at the back of the throat and sides of mouth.
* Commonest in the immuno-suppressed and the elderly.

■ OESOPHAGITIS
Similar to reflux oesophagitis, but the main symptom is:
* Burning pain behind the breast bone within a few seconds of swallowing plus:
* Spread of pain to the arms.
* Heartburn.
* Aggravated by spicy foods or alcohol.

■ OESOPHAGEAL SPASM
Spasm of the muscles of the gullet.
* Chest pain initiated by eating or emotional stress.
* The condition can be mild or severe.
* Pain varies in intensity during an attack.
* Can be painless.
* Intermittent difficulty in swallowing, often at the same time as the pain.

■ ULCERS OF TONGUE AND MOUTH
See pages 96 and 97.

■ GLOSSITIS
Swollen, painful tongue, occasional fever, sometimes associated with riboflavine deficiency, *page 84*.

■ HERPES SIMPLEX
A viral infection causing pain and formation of fluid-filled spots or ulcers. May be present in mouth, throat or oesophagus.
* Severe pain associated with the herpes sore.
* Vesicles and intensely painful ulcers seen in mouth.
* Feeling very unwell.
* Fever.

RARE

■ CANCER OF THE OESOPHAGUS
See page 121.

■ CANCER OF THE LARYNX
* Persistent hoarseness.
* Occasionally pain on swallowing because of spread or ulceration.

PROBLEMS WITH SWALLOWING PLUS FEVER

PROBLABLE
TONSILLITIS
LARYNGITIS

RARE
LUDWIG'S ANGINA
CANCER OF THE OESOPHAGUS

PROBABLE

■ TONSILLITIS
Tonsils at the back of the mouth, either side of the throat, become inflamed.
* Enlarged tonsils.
* Occasional white spots on tonsils.
* Reddening in the throat.
* Pain on swallowing.
* Occasionally, associated cough.
* Fever.
* Enlarged lymph glands in neck may be tender.

■ LARYNGITIS
Infection involving the larynx — the 'voice box' in the neck.
* Hoarse voice, or difficulty in speaking at all.
* Fever.
* Pain on swallowing, but less severe than with tonsillitis.

RARE

■ LUDWIG'S ANGINA
Severe infection of the floor of the mouth.
* Severe pain.
* Can cause breathing difficulty — because of swollen upper airways.
* Pain on swallowing.

The condition is usually associated with poor oral hygiene, and problems with infected teeth or gums.

■ CANCER OF THE OESOPHAGUS
See page 121.

THE THROAT

SWOLLEN THROAT

See SWOLLEN LYMPH NODES IN NECK, page 137.

LUMP IN THROAT

See PROBLEMS WITH SWALLOWING, pages 119-25.

SORE THROAT

Common reasons for a sore throat are covered under *PROBLEMS WITH SWALLOWING PLUS PAIN, page 124.*

If you think you have this symptom in isolation, *see SWOLLEN LYMPH NODES IN THE NECK, page 137; ISOLATED LUMPS AND SWELLINGS IN OR ON THE NECK, page 132; STIFFNESS OR PAIN IN THE NECK, page 135; PROBLEMS WITH SWALLOWING PLUS PAIN, page 124 and ULCERS IN MOUTH, page 127.*

It is however most likely to occur along with fever. *See below.*

SORE THROAT WITH FEVER

PROBABLE
COMMON COLD — UPPER RESPIRATORY TRACT INFECTION
TONSILLITIS
LARYNGITIS
PHARYNGITIS

POSSIBLE
INFECTIOUS MONONUCLEOSIS
DENTAL INFECTION

RARE
GLOSSITIS
LUDWIG'S ANGINA
ADVERSE DRUG REACTION

Smoking
Smokers are likely to suffer from exaggerated symptoms if they have any of the conditions listed below. They are also likely to take longer to recover than non-smokers; and are at greater risk of developing complications, such as secondary infections of the ears or chest.

PROBABLE

■ COMMON COLD
See page 454.

■ TONSILLITIS
See page 138.

■ LARYNGITIS
See page 125.

■ PHARYNGITIS
See page 124.

POSSIBLE

■ INFECTIOUS MONONUCLEOSIS
See page 138.

■ DENTAL INFECTIONS
See page 138.

RARE

■ GLOSSITIS
See page 125.

■ LUDWIG'S ANGINA
See page 125.

■ ADVERSE DRUG REACTION
Sore throat, inflammation of the mucous membranes of the mouth and fever are the commonest symptoms of adverse drug reactions.

ULCERS IN MOUTH

PROBABLE
APHTHOUS ULCER
HERPES SIMPLEX

POSSIBLE
ERYTHEMA MULTIFORME

RARE
CANCER OF THE MOUTH OR THROAT
SYPHILIS
PEMPHIGUS
CROHN'S DISEASE
BEHCET'S SYNDROME
LEUKAEMIAS/MYELOMAS
TUBERCULOSIS

PROBABLE

■ APHTHOUS ULCER
* Small and multiple (or larger and solitary).
* Anywhere in mouth or on tongue, typically behind lower lip at the front.
* Extremely painful; aggravated by acid fruits.
* May be aggravated by sharp dentures or other dental problems.
* Often appears at times of stress.

Most heal after a few days, but larger ones take longer, though rarely more than eight to ten days. Treatments for apthous ulcers are often unsatisfactory. Pain relieving gel or tablets may be bought from a chemist.

■ HERPES SIMPLEX
See page 125.

POSSIBLE

■ ERYTHEMA MULTIFORME
Irregular red marks. May be associated with a reaction to drugs or an infection. Commonest in children and young women.
* Itchy rash anywhere on body; not unlike measles rash.
* Pale-centred wheals, sometimes called 'target lesions'.
* Sore throat.
* Headache.
* Fever.
* Ulceration in the mouth and throat.

There is a severe form of the condition, called Stevens-Johnson syndrome.

The Throat

RARE

■ CANCER OF THE MOUTH OR THROAT
May occur anywhere in mouth or throat. Tobacco users at risk, especially pipe-smokers, tobacco-chewers. Suspicion is aroused by:
* Long-standing, large ulcers (more than two weeks).
* Ulcer with irregular shape.
* Ulcers on surfaces of polyps.
* Ulcers with raised edges.
* Feeling unwell.
* Bad breath.
* Enlarged lymph nodes in neck .

■ SYPHILIS
Ulcers in the throat can mean primary, secondary or tertiary syphilis. Ulcers are likley to be:
* Single.
* Shallow.
* Hard at the base.
* Painless.
* Non-bleeding.
And they have:
* A raised, reddened margin.
* Enlarged lymph nodes may be present.

■ PEMPHIGUS
A skin disease in which fluid-filled sacs appear on the skin at sites of pressure and trauma.
* Fluid-filled sacs in the mouth.
These burst, forming:
* Ulcers which may remain for weeks.

■ CROHN'S DISEASE
The following symptoms always accompany other signs of gut disease.
* Aphthous-type ulcers. *See page 127.*

Recurrent diarrhoea, with or without weight loss, in an otherwise fit person who has aphthous ulcers suggests the possibility of Crohn's disease.

■ BEHCET'S SYNDROME
Most common, though still rare, in some Middle Eastern countries.
* Recurrent major ulceration in mouth and throat.
Followed by:
* Ulcers on the genitals.
* Eye inflammation.

■ LEUKAEMIAS/MYELOMAS
* Ulceration in the mouth.
* Persistent sore throats.
* Infections.
* Feeling unwell.
* Bruise easily.
See also page 424.

■ TUBERCULOSIS
* Small ulcers.
* Sore throat.
* Difficulty in swallowing.
* Excessive salivation.
See also page 447.

PHLEGM IN THE THROAT

Which, typically, you are always trying to clear.

PROBABLE
VASOMOTOR RHINITIS
ALLERGIC RHINITIS
CHEST INFECTION

POSSIBLE
SINUSITIS
NASAL POLYPS

RARE
CANCER OF THE NASAL FOSSA OR NASOPHARYNX

PROBABLE

■ VASOMOTOR RHINITIS
More or less constant production of mucous in the nasal passages.
* Clear discharge from front of nose. The mucous also dribbles into the throat from the back of the nose (the two are connected). This last is known as post-nasal drip.
* Brought on by by change of environment or atmosphere.
* Difficulty in breathing through nostrils.
* Not associated with other symptoms of *ALLERGIC RHINITIS* ; *see below.*

■ ALLERGIC RHINITIS
You are likely to have a known allergy, typically to pollen, dust or animals.
* Clear discharge from front of nose and into throat.
* Difficulty in breathing through the nostrils.
* Watery eyes.
* Sneezing.
* Wheezing.

A family history of asthma, eczema or hay fever is often found in those with this condition.

There is some evidence that modern living, with its double glazing, central heating and indoor life, has increased the volume of house dust generally, and that rhinitis is, as a consequence, much more common.

■ CHEST INFECTION
Particularly in patients with chronic chest conditions, for example, bronchitis, cystic fibrosis, bronchiectasis. Smokers are also a high-risk group.
* Persistent coughing up of green or yellow phlegm.
* Fever
* Feeling unwell.
* Sometimes, difficulty in breathing.

Normally requires antibiotics.

POSSIBLE

■ SINUSITIS
Any of the nasal sinuses may become infected causing local pain/discomfort.
* Persistent nasal discharge (green or yellow).
* Headache.
* Pain over affected sinus.
* Fever.
* Bad breath.

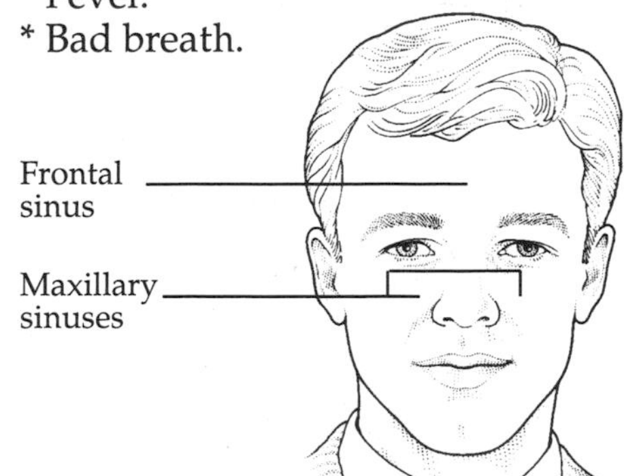

THE THROAT

■ NASAL POLYPS
Polyps are fleshy growths or tumours, almost never malignant. Often multiple.
* Can sometimes be seen by looking into nose.
* Obstruction in nose.
* Clear discharge occasionally.
* Loss of sense of smell.
Often associated with allergies.

RARE

■ CANCER OF THE NASAL FOSSA OR NASOPHARYNX
Most common in the elderly.
* Foul smelling and tasting nasal discharge.
* Persistent pain.
* Bad breath.
* A lump may be seen in the mouth or nose; or a facial swelling may develop.
* Toothache may develop.
* Bloodstained nasal discharge or sputum.

WHITE SPOTS VISIBLE IN MOUTH AND THROAT

PROBABLE
CANDIDIASIS
TONSILLITIS

POSSIBLE
KOPLIK'S SPOTS
LICHEN PLANUS
LEUKOPLAKIA

RARE
KERATOSIS PHARYNGIS

PROBABLE

■ CANDIDIASIS
Otherwise known as thrush or monilia. Most commonly seen in new-born babies or infants. (It has been known for parents to mistake thrush for milk on the inside of a baby's cheek; but the white patches are hard to remove and doing so will cause the baby some discomfort.)
* White patches in mouth.
* Associated reddening.
* Lips, tongue and cheek may be painful.
* Patches may be dislodged, but not always easily.
Often associated with antibiotic therapy, general ill-health and immuno-suppression.

■ TONSILLITIS
See page 138

POSSIBLE

■ KOPLIK'S SPOTS
A sure sign of measles *(see page 444).*
* White spots inside the mouth opposite the molar teeth.
* Spots are about the size of a grain of salt with surrounding reddening.
Other symptoms of measles are:
* A red rash starting by the ears spreading over seven days to

the body and limbs.
* Runny nose.
* Reddened eyes.
* Cough.

■ LICHEN PLANUS
Irregular, small, shiny patchy changes in the skin, occurring all over the body, including the genital area. Commonest in the middle-aged.
* Multiple fine white lines on lips, tongue and cheek.
* White spots in the same region.
* Sometimes ulcers between the spots and lines.

■ LEUKOPLAKIA
* White patches on the tongue or lining of the mouth.
* Cannot be scraped off.
* Occasionally disappear leaving a red base.
* Possibly localized hardening under the patch.

Associated with smoking (particularly pipe-smoking), and rubbing dentures. Also, it is increasingly found in people with AIDS.

RARE

■ KERATOSIS PHARYNGIS
* Small white or creamy lumps seen on tonsil surface.
* Frequently no other symptoms.

Persistent, white patches in the mouth that persist can be a sign of serious illness, and should not be ignored.

Consult your doctor if:
* Patches persist.
* They cannot be removed easily.

Seeking professional help early is always worthwhile.

NOTICEABLE BLOOD VESSELS ON THE NECK

Newly developed, visible blood vessels are a sign of underlying disease that need careful investigation, and probably tests, before treatment can be started.

PROBABLE
HEART FAILURE

POSSIBLE
MALIGNANT TUMOUR WITHIN THE CHEST
PERICARDIAL EFFUSION

RARE
BENIGN TUMOUR WITHIN THE CHEST
CONSTRICTIVE PERICARDITIS

PROBABLE

■ HEART FAILURE
The pump fails to pump blood adequately, typically after a heart attack. May be associated with one or more of the following:
* Prominent symmetrical veins on each side of the neck, that distend more as the patient lies flat.

The Neck

* The prominence varies with respiration and heart beat.
* Shortness of breath worse on lying flat.
* Shortness of breath on walking.
* Bluish discolouration of face.
* Swelling of ankles and legs.

POSSIBLE

■ MALIGNANT TUMOUR WITHIN THE CHEST
Malignant tumours (primary or secondary) within the chest can compress the great veins inside the chest giving rise to:
* Symmetrical prominent veins on head neck and upper chest unaffected by bodily position.
* Face may appear congested and reddened.
* The face, neck and upper chest may be swollen.
* Breathing may be normal.

In addition, there may well be the following general symptoms of:
* Weight loss.
* Poor appetite.
* Weakness.
* Feeling unwell.

■ PERICARDIAL EFFUSION
Fluid distends the sac around the heart. May be caused by infection, auto-immune disease, tumour or after a heart attack and can cause:
* Shortness of breath when lying flat.
* Prominent neck veins (symmetrical).
* Tightness in the chest, varying with movement.
* Fever (with infection).
* Feeling unwell.

RARE

■ BENIGN TUMOUR WITHIN THE CHEST
Large benign tumours within the chest can compress the great veins inside the chest giving rise to the same symptoms as malignant tumour(s) — *see above.*

■ CONSTRICTIVE PERICARDITIS
Increasing rigidity of the sac round the heart. Caused by tuberculosis, or other infection or injury, often many years previously.
* Rapid pulse (sometimes irregular).
* Low blood pressure.
* Tiredness.
* Prominent neck veins — more prominent on breathing in.
* Fluid in the abdomen.
* Liver enlargement.

ISOLATED LUMPS OR SWELLINGS IN OR ON NECK

Isolated lumps may be associated with a number of structures in the neck in addition to the lymph nodes (*see page 137: read with this*). These include the skin, and the salivary or thyroid glands. A few are present from birth.

PROBABLE
BOIL
SEBACEOUS CYST
LIPOMA

POSSIBLE
DIFFUSE THYROID ENLARGEMENT
ISOLATED THYROID NODULE (BENIGN)
SUBMANDIBULAR DUCT STONE

RARE
CERVICAL RIB
DIFFUSE THYROID ENLARGEMENT (MALIGNANT TUMOUR)
ISOLATED THYROID NODULE (MALIGNANT)
THYROGLOSSAL CYST
PHARYNGEAL POUCH
STERNOMASTOID TUMOUR
SUBMANDIBULAR TUMOUR

PROBABLE

■ BOIL
A skin infection commonly originating in a hair follicle or follicles.
* Painful.
* Localized reddening.
* Skin warm to the touch.
* Localized swelling.
* A yellow centre that may discharge pus.

■ SEBACEOUS CYST
* Superficial.
* Painless (unless infected).
* Present for many years.
* Slowly increases in size.
* Has a central 'punctum' — the opening to the blocked sweat gland that causes the cyst.

■ LIPOMA
A benign fatty tumour which can be superficial or extend under the skin. Same characteristics as a sebaceous cyst except:
* No punctum.

POSSIBLE

■ DIFFUSE THYROID GLAND ENLARGEMENT
The thyroid gland lies on both sides of the neck below the Adam's apple.

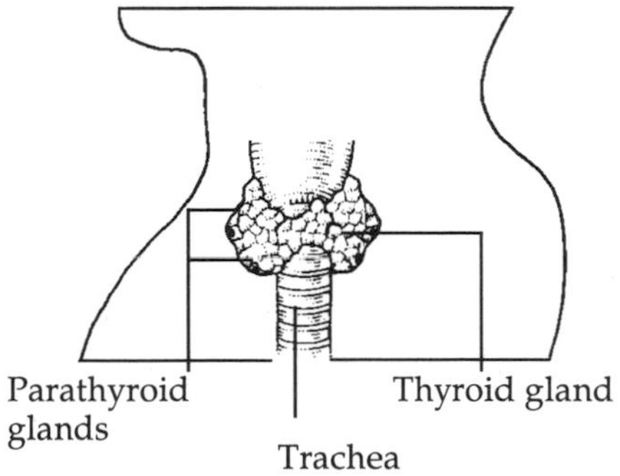

* Movement of swelling up and down on swallowing.
* Diffuse swelling — no separate lumps.
* No other symptoms.

Other causes of diffuse thyroid swelling can be divided into those causing excess thyroid hormone secretion, and those causing an underactive thyroid. Both require professional attention. Further details, *pages 479 and 461*.

■ ISOLATED THYROID NODULE — BENIGN
A localized lump within the thyroid, which can be benign or

THE NECK

malignant - *see below*.
* Can be felt either side of the neck below the Adam's apple.
* Moves up and down on swallowing.

May be associated with signs of overactive or underactive thyroid; *see above*.

■ SUBMANDIBULAR DUCT STONE

Beneath the jaw, each side of the tongue, are two salivary glands, the submandibular glands. Stones may form in the ducts of the glands, or the body of the gland, causing:
* Painless swelling (normally on one side).
* The swelling increases when eating and
* Reduces between meals.
* Swelling can sometimes be felt in the mouth, under the tongue.

RARE

■ CERVICAL RIB

See page 136.

■ DIFFUSE THYROID GLAND ENLARGEMENT (MALIGNANT TUMOUR)

Features of thyroid enlargement plus:
* Irregular symmetric enlargement.
* Movement of swelling up and down on swallowing may be lost.
* Trachea (wind pipe) may be compressed, causing difficulty in breathing.

■ ISOLATED THYROID NODULE — MALIGNANT

A localized lump within the thyroid gland.
* Moves up and down on swallowing.

May have no other symptoms, but can cause:
* Hoarseness.
* Pain.
* Drooping of one eyelid (Horner's syndrome).

■ THYROGLOSSAL CYST
* Lies in the middle of the neck at the front.
* Near the surface.
* Moves up if the tongue is stuck out.
* Painless.

■ PHARYNGEAL POUCH

A swelling on one side of the neck caused by a defect in the upper gullet.
* Varies in size.
* Causes variable difficulty in swallowing.
* Enlarges while eating or drinking.
* May 'gurgle' as fluid empties from it.
* Old food may regurgitated.
* Can be emptied by direct pressure on it.
* Not painful, but can be uncomfortable as it increases in size.

■ STERNOMASTOID TUMOUR

Present from birth — not a true tumour:
* Lump sited in the middle of the muscle at the side of the neck.
* The face is turned away from the side of the lesion.

■ SUBMANDIBULAR TUMOUR

May be benign or malignant.

* One-sided enlargement of gland.
* Progressive.
* May become painful.
* Lymph nodes may be involved

STIFFNESS OR PAIN IN NECK

PROBABLE
ACUTE STIFF NECK
ACUTE NECK SPRAIN
WHIPLASH INJURY
WRY NECK (TORTICOLLIS)

POSSIBLE
CERVICAL SPONDYLOSIS
CERVICAL RIB
RHEUMATOID ARTHRITIS

RARE
CERVICAL SPINE INFECTION
MENINGITIS
PROLAPSED CERVICAL DISC
SPINAL CORD TUMOURS

PROBABLE

■ ACUTE STIFF NECK
* Associated with sleeping in awkward position; also with exposure to cold.
* Pain on movement localized to neck.
* Neck movements limited by pain and muscle spasm.

■ ACUTE NECK SPRAIN
* Associated with sudden twisting/turning or bending.
* Extreme pain on any movement.
* Pain in upper back and head.
* Marked muscle spasm limiting neck movement.

■ WHIPLASH INJURY
Typically present after a car crash (hit from behind or from the front).
* Pain in neck and upper back.
* Neck held stiffly.
* Pain may have taken a few hours to develop after injury.
* Pain and stiffness may persist for weeks.
* May have pain and weakness in arms.
* Reduced range of neck movement.

■ WRY NECK (TORTICOLLIS)
* Head pulled down on affected side.
* Chin points towards the opposite shoulder.
* The affected muscle is a solid band.
* Neck movements are considerably restricted.

Typically, the condition occurs on waking: suddenly, you cannot move your neck freely. Wears off in a day or two.

POSSIBLE

■ CERVICAL SPONDYLOSIS
Caused by degeneration of the lower cervical intervertebral discs.

THE NECK

Sufferer is typically middle-aged.
* Pain in neck and back.
* Painful over neck.
* Worse on waking.
* Slight limitation of movement.

Occasionally:
* Pain in arms.
* Numbness in arms.
* Weakness in arms.

Prolapsed lower cervical intervertebral disc

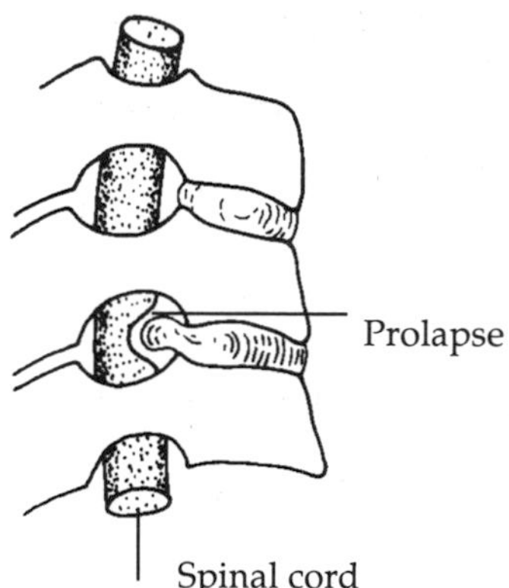

■ CERVICAL RIB

Some people are born with an extra rib, or with fibrous material which constricts nerves and arteries in the neck. Symptoms may appear in the late twenties.
* May be a palpable lump in the neck.
* Neck is rarely painful.
* Pain behind collar bone.
* Pain on the inner side of the arm after or when carrying shopping.
* Intermittent coldness and blueness of fingers.

■ RHEUMATOID ARTHRITIS

Patients with known rheumatoid arthritis may get degenerative changes in the neck.
* Pain is common.
* Range of movement is reduced.
* Weakness and sensory changes may be present in upper and occasionally lower limbs.

RARE

■ CERVICAL SPINE INFECTION

Tuberculous infection still occasionally occurs.
* Mild neck pain.
* Pain on any movement.
* Head may be held in hands.
* Stiffness, with reduced movement.

Occasionally there may be sudden paralysis as the spinal cord gets involved.

■ MENINGITIS

Infection of the lining of the brain and spinal cord. Usually other marked symptoms, such as fever, will be present.
* Neck stiffness — inability to bend the neck forward because of pain and muscle spasm.
* Headache.
* Feeling unwell.
* Fever
* Fine purple rash.

If meningitis is suspected, call a doctor immediately.

■ PROLAPSED CERVICAL DISC

May be caused by sudden movements, and degeneration of the intervertebral discs. There is a sudden onset of symptoms which may include:
* Neck pain and stiffness.
* Pain and altered sensation in the arms.

* Muscular spasm of the neck and upper back.
* Symptoms may resolve and then return.

■ SPINAL CORD TUMOURS
Progressive onset of symptoms may include:
* Altered sensation in arms and legs.
* Areas of numbness.
* Weakness in arms and legs.
* Wasting of muscles.
* Ability to pass urine may be affected.

SWOLLEN LYMPH NODES IN NECK

Most people have temporarily enlarged lymph nodes (also known simply as glands) in the neck at some time. This is generally associated with infection or inflammation, either locally, or of the whole body. Sometimes just one is enlarged, giving a single swelling. Occasionally, recurring or persistent enlargement may indicate more serious underlying disorders.

Enlarged lymph nodes need to be distinguished from other lumps in the neck, such as enlarged salivary glands — *see ISOLATED NECK LUMPS OR SWELLINGS IN OR ON NECK, page 132.*

Lymph nodes of the neck

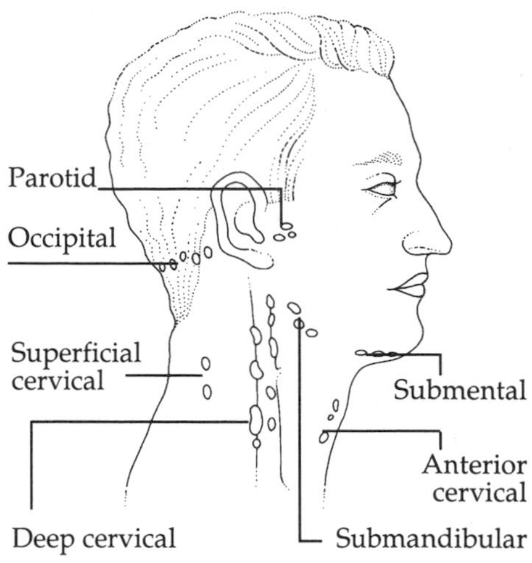

PROBABLE
COMMON COLD
LOCAL INFECTION OR INFLAMMATION (eg acne, impetigo, sebaceous cyst)
TONSILLITIS
DENTAL INFECTION

POSSIBLE
GLANDULAR FEVER
GERMAN MEASLES
TOXOPLASMOSIS
PERITONSILLAR ABSCESS
EPIGLOTTITIS

RARE
TUBERCULOSIS
CANCER (of mouth and upper respiratory passages)
LEUKAEMIAS/LYMPHOMAS
HIV/ARC/AIDS

THE NECK

PROBABLE

■ COMMON COLD
Or upper respiratory tract infection (URTI). These can occur alone or in combination:
* Tender lymph nodes enlarged symmetrically below ears and under jaw.
* Fever.
* Malaise.
* Sore throat
* Cough.
* Runny nose.
* Earache.
Usually cures itself.

■ TONSILLITIS
* Tonsils enlarged
* Throat looks red.
* Tender lymph nodes enlarged below and behind jaw.
* Often enlarged more on one side than the other.
* White spots often apparent on tonsil surface (pus emerging from tonsil).
* Fever.
* Feeling unwell.
Could require antibiotics. Your doctor may take swabs from the tonsils, particularly if the surface is purulent. Frequent attacks may necessitate referral to a specialist throat surgeon.

■ LOCAL INFECTION OR INFLAMMATION (EG ACNE, IMPETIGO, SEBACEOUS CYST)
* Nearest lymph nodes will be enlarged and may be painful.
* Pain and tenderness in scalp (look in hair).
* If a lump is present it may be an infected sebaceous cyst.
* If an area is scaly/reddened/weeping/itchy, consider impetigo, dermatitis, eczema/psoriasis — see your doctor to distinguish which.

■ DENTAL INFECTION
Diseases of the gums or teeth may be associated with lymph node enlargement.
* Enlarged tender nodes which tend to be those nearest the affected tooth.
* Toothache.
* Bleeding gums (gingivitis).
* Teeth with loose fillings.
* Dental abscess (painful tooth/gums and local swelling).

POSSIBLE

■ GLANDULAR FEVER — INFECTIOUS MONONUCLEOSIS
Caused by infection with the Epstein-Barr virus and sometimes known as 'kissing disease'. A disease of children and young adults.
* Generalized lymph node enlargement and tenderness, but neck nodes, including those at the back of the head, may be worst affected.
* Fever.
* Sore throat.
* Feeling unwell.
* Symptoms may last for a few days to a few weeks.
* Characteristic changes in the blood: your doctor may confirm the diagnosis with a blood test.
* Spleen may become enlarged in up to 50 per cent of cases.

■ GERMAN MEASLES
Rubella. Commonest in children.

* Runny nose.
* Red rash, mainly on body.
* Enlarged, tender neck lymph nodes, particularly over the back of the scalp, just above the neck.
* In teenage and adult females there may be pains in the joints of the hands.

■ TOXOPLASMOSIS
A parasite which infects 50 per cent of us. Mostly cures itself in one to three weeks. Acquired by eating infected, raw or lightly cooked meat (or through contact with cat faeces). Only about 20 per cent of people affected actually have symptoms.
* Fever.
* Enlarged lymph nodes — neck nodes predominant — which may also be tender.
* Feeling unwell.

Diagnosis is confirmed by blood test or by removing a lymph node and examining it under a microscope.

If a pregnant mother develops toxoplasmosis there is a risk of the baby being damaged. Brain and eyes are primarily affected. In many countries there is routine screening for toxoplasmosis, but not in the U.K.

Avoiding toxoplasmosis in pregnancy:
– Never eat raw or uncooked meat.
– Wash all fruit, vegetables and salads well.
– Do not empty cat litter trays. (If you must do so, wear protective gloves.)
– Wear gloves for gardening.

■ PERITONSILLAR ABSCESS
Similar signs to tonsillitis, but:
* Pain on opening mouth also present because abscess or 'quinsy' has developed. Requires surgical drainage.

■ EPIGLOTTITIS
* Very painful throat.
* Pain on swallowing.
* Lymph nodes may be enlarged.
* Fever.

A doctor should see any child suspected of having epiglottitis immediately.

RARE

■ TUBERCULOSIS
* Isolated non-tender lymph node enlargement, commonest in immigrants.
* Redness.
* Skin overlying node(s) breaks down.
* Intermittent fever.

Skin tests and blood tests, or biopsy of the node, confirms the diagnosis. Drug treatment required.

■ CANCER OF THE MOUTH OR UPPER RESPIRATORY PASSAGES (INCLUDING LARYNX)
All these cancers can cause enlarged lymph nodes, often as a result of the cancer spreading. These are diseases especially of smokers in the 50-plus age range.
* Persistently enlarged but painless lymph nodes.
* Other lump developing in mouth/tongue or palate.
* Change in voice.
* Weight loss.

THE NECK

* Feeling unwell.
* Persistent pain in mouth or neck.
* Dentures not fitting.
* Anaemia.

■ CANCER ELSEWHERE IN THE BODY
* Enlarged painless lymph nodes above the collar bone may suggest spread of a tumour from within the chest or abdomen, but would normally be accompanied by other symptoms from those areas.

■ LEUKAEMIAS
Some or all of the following in combination:
* Enlarged painless lymph nodes in the neck or elsewhere.
* Persistently feeling unwell.
* Palour, due to anaemia.
* Shortness of breath.
* Fatigue.
* Bruising.

■ LYMPHOMAS
May have no symptoms apart from:
* Painless, generalized enlargement of lymph nodes.

Later stages include:
* Fever.
* Weight loss.
* Anaemia.

■ HIV/ARC/AIDS
HIV stands for the human immunodeficiency virus, which tends to infect people for years without making them ill. Eventually, however, it causes ARC — an AIDS-Related Complex and finally full-blown AIDS. The symptoms listed below cover the whole range from ARC to AIDs.
* Enlarged lymph nodes.
* Fever.
* Feeling unwell.

Anyone in a high-risk group for HIV infection should report persistently enlarged lymph nodes to their doctor. Effectiveness of treatment depends on early diagnosis.

Persistent symptoms
If enlarged lymph nodes persist in the neck for more than two weeks, and particularly if other symptoms are present, you must see your doctor.

THE ABDOMEN – DIGESTIVE AND URINARY SYSTEMS

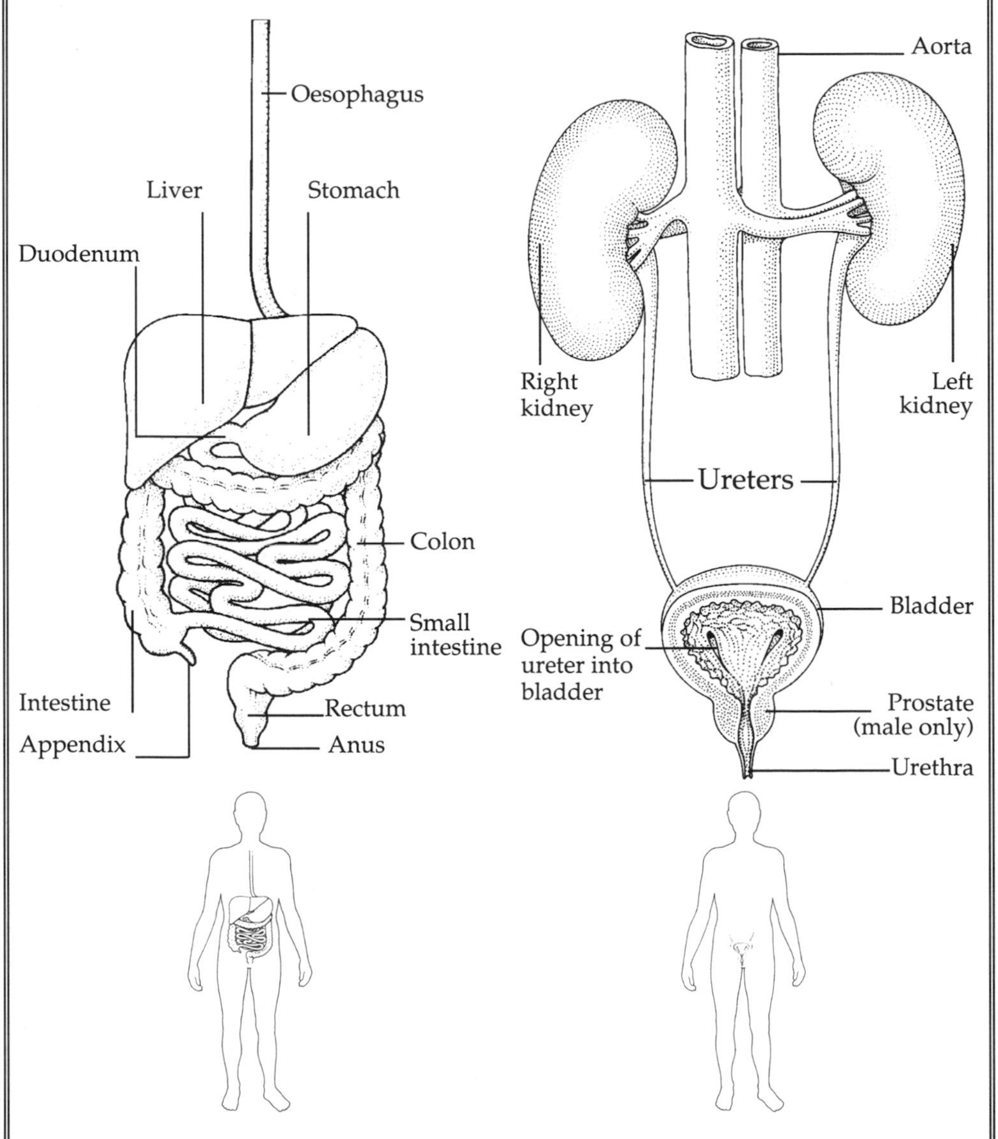

ABDOMEN: DIGESTIVE SYSTEM

THE ABDOMINAL CAVITY INTRODUCTION

It lies below the rib cage and above the pelvic bones. The terms tummy, stomach and gut are often used, the latter two incorrectly since they are organs that lie within the abdominal cavity.

The abdomen contains the organs of digestion and absorption; part of the oesophagus; the stomach, then the duodenum and the rest of the small bowel (jejunum and ileum, including appendix); the large bowel (colon and rectum). It also contains organs connected to the gut which supply the chemicals necessary for digestion: liver, pancreas, gall bladder and biliary tract.

The abdomen also contains organs covered in other sections of this book, including the kidneys, ureters and bladder, which are concerned with excreting urine; and the adrenal glands, which are responsible for secreting hormones that control many of the body's functions.

In men, there are also the prostate gland and the seminal vesicles, part of the reproductive system; and likewise in women, the uterus or womb, the Fallopian tubes and the ovaries.

VOMITING

Vomiting can be forceful or it can be passive, as when one regurgitates food into the mouth.

Sometimes bitter gastric or duodenal juices are vomited, sometimes undigested food, and sometimes blood (either fresh or old — sometimes called 'coffee grounds' because of its appearance). In order to diagnose the underlying cause, you have to take precise note, however disagreeable, of the nature of the vomit. Excluded from this section are the all-too-familiar and obvious causes of vomiting: too much to drink, too much rich food to eat; and travel sickness.

PROBABLE

GASTROENTERITIS/ FOOD POISONING
ACUTE GASTRITIS
PREGNANCY
MIGRAINE

POSSIBLE

PEPTIC ULCER
HIATUS HERNIA AND OESOPHAGITIS
OESOPHAGEAL VARICES
CANCER OF THE STOMACH
INTESTINAL OBSTRUCTION
POST-GASTRECTOMY SYNDROME
PYLORIC STENOSIS

ABDOMEN: DIGESTIVE SYSTEM

RARE
CHRONIC PANCREATITIS
BRAIN TUMOURS
RENAL FAILURE
BULIMIA
BOTULISM
CHOLERA

Terminology
'Gastric contents' means typical vomit: partially digested and undigested food, pinkish-yellow, frothy, foul-smelling.

'Duodenal contents' means bile-stained (green), thin fluid, mixed with slime and clear secretions.

PROBABLE

■ GASTROENTERITIS/ FOOD POISONING
Gastric or duodenal contents. Likely to be viral or can occur as part of food poisoning. Abdominal pain may be a feature.

Vomit is likely to contain partially-digested and undigested food, and will look like 'typical vomit' at first. After several vomits, clear, greeny-yellow liquid and slime.

See page 168.

■ ACUTE GASTRITIS
Gastric and duodenal contents with old blood, which appears as streaks of brown staining or looking like coffee granules. This is likely after a very heavy drinking bout. Abdominal pain might be a feature. *See page 172.*

■ PREGNANCY
Gastric and duodenal contents. Other symptoms of pregnancy will be pronounced:
* Nausea on waking.
* Tendency to acid stomach and heartburn.

See also page 148.

■ MIGRAINE
Gastric and duodenal contents. *See page 112.* Other migraine symptoms will be present.

POSSIBLE

■ PEPTIC ULCER
Gastric and duodenal contents. *See page 170.*

■ HIATUS HERNIA and OESOPHAGITIS
* A feeling akin to regurgitation.
* A feeling of acid in the lower throat; bilious taste.
* Symptoms of heartburn.
* If severe, vomiting undigested food; also,
* Vomiting old blood, sometimes fresh.

■ OESOPHAGEAL VARICES
Fresh or old blood. *See page 159.*

■ CANCER OF THE STOMACH
Vomiting can be a late feature of stomach cancer and may be present with other signs of cancer, such as malaise, marked weight loss and anaemia..

Gastric and bowel contents.
* Likely to follow a progressive

feeling of fullness after eating small quantities.

See also STOMACH DISEASE, page 164.

■ INTESTINAL OBSTRUCTION
* Pain in abdomen that comes and goes.
* No wind or faeces passed rectally.
* Abdomen becomes distended.
* You feel bloated.

Gastric and bowel contents, occasionally like diarrhoea.

See also page 151.

■ POST-GASTRECTOMY SYNDROME

See page 169.

Duodenal contents.

■ PYLORIC STENOSIS

This is a narrowing of the outlet from the stomach. Usually the only ones to be affected by this condition are young children (at about six years of age) or older inviduals with long-standing ulcers. In children, the term hypertrophic pyloric stenosis is used to describe the thickening of the muscle in the wall of the pylorus.

Gastric contents.

RARE

■ CHRONIC PANCREATITIS

See PAIN IN THE ABDOMEN AND DIARRHOEA, page 168.

Gastric contents.

■ BRAIN TUMOURS

See BRAIN SECTION, page 114.

Gastric contents.

■ RENAL FAILURE

Acute or chronic.
* Mental confusion.
* Headache.
* Breath smelling of urine.
* Vomiting gastric contents.
* Coma.

■ BULIMIA

See ANOREXIA NERVOSA, page 424.

■ BOTULISM

A dangerous but extremely rare form of food poisoning.
* Malaise.
* Nausea.
* Dizziness.
* Vomiting gastric and duodenal contents.
* Abdominal cramp and diarrhoea.
* Breathing problems.
* Pupils wide open.
* Collapse leading to coma.

■ CHOLERA

See page 168.

VOMITING BLOOD

See ABDOMINAL PAIN PLUS VOMITING BLOOD, page 171.

VOMITING AND HEADACHE

See especially MIGRAINE, page 112; also other causes of headache and headache with fever, pages 111-16.

REGURGITATION

See VOMITING, page 142.

PROMINENT BLOOD VESSELS ON THE ABDOMEN

Unusually large surface veins sometimes develop on the skin of the abdomen. They are may be a sign of an abnormality of underlying blood vessels, and can be caused by blockage of vessels; pressure from some types of abdominal distension; or local pressure on veins, from growths.

Other symptoms that may be present if any of these causes apply are:

* Leg swelling, sometimes one-sided.
* Lower abdominal wall veins most prominent.
* Caput medusae — distended veins radiating out from the umbilicus.

Some conditions (all rare) that can cause these symptoms are:

Acute pancreatitis – page 150.
Cirrhosis of the liver – see page 150.
Malignant ascites – see page 150.
Ovarian cyst – see page 171.
Cancer of the kidney – see HAEMATURIA, page 185. A tumour grows into the renal vein and blocks the main vein in the abdomen.

GENERALIZED SWELLING OF THE ABDOMEN IN BABIES AND CHILDREN

PROBABLE
NORMAL VARIANT
CONSTIPATION

POSSIBLE
CYSTIC FIBROSIS
COELIAC DISEASE
PREMATURITY

RARE
HIRSCHSPRUNG'S DISEASE
KWASHIORKOR

PROBABLE

■ NORMAL VARIANT
The pot-bellied child is simply made that way and because the tummy bulges in childhood, it will not necessarily do so in adulthood.

■ CONSTIPATION
In some toddlers and children there is a strong psychological element to constipation. It may well develop at potty-training, when the child resists parental exhortation to pass stools; and it can develop into a life-long habit.

Clothes may get soiled with faeces — 'apparent diarrhoea' — as a result of hardened stools

Abdomen: Digestive System

building up in the rectum: watery material leaks past the solid mass.

See also CONSTIPATION, page 161.

Whatever you do, don't allow potty training to become a battleground between you and your child. A relaxed approach is usually best. All children will learn in time to control their bowels and bladder. Most problems are caused by over-zealous carers pushing a child to be 'clean' before he or she is ready. If you are in any doubt, take advice from your GP or health visitor.

POSSIBLE

■ CYSTIC FIBROSIS
Most symptoms of this hereditary disease are caused by abnormal body secretions.
* Failure to thrive, but healthy appetite.
* Thin, with distended abdomen.
* Recurrent chest infections.
* Large amounts of smelly faeces.
* Finger clubbing.
* Occasionally the rectum may slip out through the anus (rectal prolapse).

■ COELIAC DISEASE
Caused by an allergy to gluten, a component of cereals. Normally, the child will be underweight and will not grow as expected.
* Often, the child has a fair complexion.
* Child is unhappy.
* Appetite is poor.
* Muscles are wasted.
* Abdomen is distended.
* Occasional diarrhoea and vomiting.

Treatment is a gluten-free diet for life, and a complete recovery can be expected.

■ PREMATURITY
Premature babies may become constipated with bowel distension due to the presence of meconium, the greenish bowel contents present at birth. This stage usually passes quickly.

RARE

■ HIRSCHSPRUNG'S DISEASE
Part of the bowel fails to develop proper nervous tissue and fails to work correctly, resulting in the progressive distension of the large bowel by faeces. Large quantities may be retained. The tummy may be not so much swollen as massive. Symptoms of constipation appear soon after birth, but the diagnosis may not be made for years.

■ KWASHIORKOR
Malnutrition caused by insufficient protein. All too common in underdeveloped countries, especially in poor, rural areas in the tropics.
* Unhappy child.
* Distended abdomen.
* Swelling of face and limbs.
* Dry, thin hair.
* Pigmented areas of skin.
* Occasional diarrhoea.

GENERALIZED SWELLING OF THE ABDOMEN

Described by doctors as distension. The common causes are fat, wind, faeces, fluid or, in a woman, a baby. Doctors often find it difficult to decide whether there really is distension.

This section does not deal with isolated lumps or bumps felt in the abdomen and it excludes pregnancy.

These aside, there are *many* causes of abdominal swelling: some, as one would expect, are harmless, and some suggest serious underlying disease.

It is important to consider whether symptoms associated with abdominal swelling are new and uncomfortable (such as pain and indigestion) or have built up slowly, possibly during a period when your personal circumstances altered (for example, reduced exercise, 'comfort eating', family crisis or bereavement). Usually it will be clear to you whether your symptoms are part of a long, even lifelong, history of abdominal discomfort, or are new and therefore more likely to suggest an illness.

PROBABLE

OBESITY
WIND
POOR MUSCLE TONE
CONSTIPATION

POSSIBLE

PREGNANCY
IRRITABLE BOWEL SYNDROME
DIVERTICULAR DISEASE
HEART FAILURE
PERFORATED VISCUS
BOWEL CANCER

RARE

ACUTE PANCREATITIS
CIRRHOSIS OF THE LIVER
MALIGNANT ASCITES
OVARIAN CYST
INTESTINAL OBSTRUCTION
ULCERATIVE COLITIS

PROBABLE

■ OBESITY
An obvious, and extremely common diagnosis, but worth considering in its own right. Fat does not just accumulate below the skin, it accumulates in the body cavities.Work out your correct weight for height and age, or ask your doctor what it should be. Then compare every stone you are overweight with the bulk created by 28 half-pounds of butter. It all has to be stored somewhere.

ABDOMEN: DIGESTIVE SYSTEM

■ WIND

Doctors call it flatus. Produced by the fermentation of food in the gut. Most of us are aware of those foods that cause most wind.

■ POOR MUSCLE TONE

Many women develop protruding abdomens after childbirth. Often, intensive exercise is needed to get the abdominal wall muscles to revert to their original tone, and sometimes they never do.
Men can also find that they acquire a 'pot belly', either when they stop exercising or when they indulge in the steady consumption of beer.

■ CONSTIPATION

Most people have one bowel movement a day for most of their lives. Constipation is a term individuals may use if they believe they are not passing stools either easily or frequently enough. In fact, constipation should be divided into three types.

First, that in which hard, pellet-like or rock-like stools are passed, a common condition caused by change in diet and/or lifestyle, often in younger people and in children.

Second, there are people who have bowel movements at long intervals — say every week or fortnight. This has been their pattern for a long time, but they describe themselves as constipated. In fact, there is nothing essentially wrong: they are a variant of normal.

The third type is constipation of sudden onset, often in the elderly. Sometimes it is impossible even to pass wind. This may suggest an underlying disorder: report it to a doctor — it must be investigated.

Most people have regular bowel movements (even though they may be preoccupied, perhaps even obsessed, by variations). Often, bowel movements occur at about the same time every day. However, it is not necessarily abnormal not to have such a regular habit. What is always important is a *change from your usual pattern.* It is this that should be reported to your doctor.

POSSIBLE

■ PREGNANCY

Again, an apparently obvious diagnosis, but some women are taken unawares by pregnancy. Enough to say that an enlarging abdomen, missed periods, dyspeptic symptoms, fullness and discomfort of the breasts, with or without morning sickness in a sexually active woman in the reproductive years are sound reasons for doing a home pregnancy test.

■ IRRITABLE BOWEL SYNDROME

Many people have severe bowel symptoms which, after investigation, are nothing to do with any specific abnormalities of the bowel. Irritable bowel syndrome (IBS) could then be suspected: it is a well-defined syndrome or set of symptoms, probably caused by abnormal motility of the gut. It

tends to come and go, and to be related to anything that affects the gut's activity, for example, stress, change of diet, unusual food. The typical picture is:
* Intermittent abdominal pain.
* Bowel upsets (diarrhoea and constipation).
* Passage of mucus.
* Abdominal distension.
* Wind.

■ DIVERTICULAR DISEASE

A diverticulum is a small pouch on the wall of the bowel. Most people develop them as they get older, but only a few will get symptoms. These usually arise if one of the diverticula becomes inflamed.
* Change of bowel habit.
* Steady or colicky abdominal pain, often on the left side.
* Abdominal distension.
* Pellet-like stools.
* Occasional passage of dark to bright red blood from the rectum.

If the inflammation becomes severe, with:
* Fever.
* Intense pain.
* A tender lump in the abdomen.

This condition is then called diverticulitis. It usually settles down with antibiotic treatment.

Decreasing the amount of food you eat allows the gut to rest and will also help.

■ HEART FAILURE

Severe untreated heart failure can result in the accumulation of fluid in the abdominal cavity in addition to several other symptoms. *See page 208.*

■ PERFORATED VISCUS

The major symptom of this condition is pain, which will dominate any discomfort or swelling of the abdomen.

Any of the hollow organs within the abdominal cavity can become inflamed or damaged. If the inflammation or damage is severe enough, the wall of the organ — typically the stomach, small bowel, colon or appendix — bursts. Gut contents leak into the abdominal cavity. This material contains organisms that can cause peritonitis — inflammation of the abdominal cavity — if treatment is delayed. This can be fatal.

The symptoms are similar whichever organ perforates, although initially the site of pain may be different. An inflamed appendix, a peptic ulcer and a diverticulum may all burst.
* Sudden onset of severe pain.
* Fever.
* Very tender abdomen (muscles of the abdominal wall appear rigid).
* Pale, sweating face, sunken eyes.
* Eventually, distension of the abdomen caused by leakage of gas and contents from the gut.
* Shock may develop. *See page 408.*

■ BOWEL CANCER

Includes cancer of colon and rectum. This can block the intestine, either gradually or suddenly. Though a common symptom is a change in bowel habit (type or frequency of stool), swelling (distension) of the abdomen may be caused by a build-up of food, fluid, faeces or wind. Other possible symptoms may include:
* Colicky, abdominal pain.

ABDOMEN: DIGESTIVE SYSTEM

* Possibly intermittent symptoms.
* Slime or mucus in stool.
* Abnormal stools.
* Blood in stools.

RARE

■ ACUTE PANCREATITIS

Abdominal pain will be a major and primary symptom of this condition. It is inflammation of the pancreas, which lies at the back of the abdominal cavity and produces chemicals, known as enzymes, which help with digestion of food. If inflamed, the pancreas can actually start digesting your own innards. There are mild or very severe, and sometimes fatal forms. People who drink excessive amounts of alcohol, or who have a history of gall bladder disease are at increased risk. Features include:
* Continuous, central abdominal pain.
* Pain may radiate to the back.
* Vomiting.
* Malaise.
* Slight jaundice may appear a couple of days after the initial attack.
* Bruising/discoloration around the umbilicus or flanks after two to three days.

Some individuals who collapse for no apparent reason are later found to have pancreatitis.

■ CIRRHOSIS OF THE LIVER

An irreversible degeneration of the liver that has many causes. Perhaps the most well known is alcohol abuse. Features of advanced cirrhosis are:
* Malaise, weakness.
* Weight loss.
* Anorexia.
* Swelling of the ankles.
* Abdominal distension due to fluid in the abdominal cavity — ascites.
* Vomiting, sickness.
* Vomiting blood, blood in stools.
* Jaundice.
* Mental deterioration.
* Easy bruising.
* Red vascular marks on skin (spider naevi).
* Clubbing of the nails. *See page 296.*

In men:
* Enlargement of the breasts.
* Shrinkage of the testes.

Other causes of cirrhosis, of which there are several different types, include:

Active chronic hepatitis.
Haemochromatosis.
Wilson's disease.
Primary biliary cirrhosis.
Budd-Chiari syndrome.
Chronic cardiac failure.

In most cases the individual is aware of the primary diagnosis before cirrhosis develops.

■ MALIGNANT ASCITES

Cancer of any organ within the abdominal cavity may lead to the formation of fluid in the abdominal cavity, or ascites. In addition to the symptoms of the original cancer individuals may develop:
* Tense, distended abdomen.
* Swelling of the ankles.
* Shortness of breath (due to pressure on the diaphragm).

■ OVARIAN CYST

Very occasionally, an enormous cyst may develop on an ovary, causing abdominal distension. It requires surgery.

■ INTESTINAL OBSTRUCTION
The intestine is a term for the stomach, the small and the large bowel. Blockage can occur for many reasons. The features are similar:
* Colicky, often central abdominal pain (site dependent on cause).
* Abdominal distension: if low, ileum or colon/rectum obstruction is likely.
* Vomiting may be an early feature of stomach or jejunal obstruction, later involving the ileum. It tends to be a late feature of colon obstruction.
* Constipation — no stools and often no wind.
* Loops of bowel may be seen undulating under the skin surface as they try to overcome the obstruction.
* Perforation may ultimately occur *(see PERFORATED VISCUS, page 149).*

Urgent medical attention is needed. Causes include:

Strangulated hernia
* Hernia (rupture) in groin may become painful and not be able to be pushed back.

Cancer
* Other features of cancer may have been present before, for example, altered bowel habit (constipation/diarrhoea), weight loss, anorexia, anaemia.

Inflammation
For example Crohn's disease, diverticular disease.
* A fibrous internal band, sometimes referred to as adhesions, common after abdominal surgery.
* Bowel gets twisted internally around fibrous tissue present from, or after, birth.

Volvulus
* Bowel twists on itself, causing a blockage.

Gall-stone
* Occasionally a gall-stone passes into the bowel and gets jammed in the narrowest part (the end of the ileum).

■ ULCERATIVE COLITIS
Chronic disease of the colon. Main features:
* Diarrhoea.
* In acute attacks, blood, mucous and pus is passed.
* Abdominal pain and fever in acute cases.
* As a complication of some cases, abdominal swelling.

OVERALL SWELLING OF THE ABDOMEN PLUS DIARRHOEA

PROBABLE
OBESITY
WIND

POSSIBLE
CONSTIPATION
IRRITABLE BOWEL SYNDROME
DIVERTICULAR DISEASE
FACTITIOUS DIARRHOEA
CROHN'S DISEASE

RARE
BOWEL CANCER
ULCERATIVE COLITIS

ABDOMEN: DIGESTIVE SYSTEM

PROBABLE

■ OBESITY
■ WIND *See pages 147 and 148.*

POSSIBLE

■ CONSTIPATION
Occasionally someone, especially an elderly person, can become so constipated that other gut contents leak out of the rectum past the impacted mass of faeces. This gives the impression of diarrhoea.

■ IRRITABLE BOWEL SYNDROME
■ DIVERTICULAR DISEASE
See pages 148 and 149.

■ FACTITIOUS DIARRHOEA
Some people take laxative medicine as a matter of habit and yet complain of diarrhoea. They may be doing so in order to lose weight, but sometimes doctors are faced with people who cannot explain why they take laxatives so often, or they may deny it altogether. So, this is worth considering for any individual who complains of diarrhoea, yet is otherwise well. Some laxatives cause associated abdominal distension and discomfort.

■ CROHN'S DISEASE
Tends to occur in young adults.
* Intermittent, colicky pain with or without diarrhoea.
* With or without weight loss.
* Spontaneously resolves and relapses.
* Sometimes taken for a 'grumbling appendix'.
* Occasionally intestinal obstruction due to narrowing of bowel.

Drug treatment and/or surgery may be needed. *See also page 128.*

RARE

■ BOWEL CANCER
See page 149.

■ ULCERATIVE COLITIS
See page 151.

OVERALL SWELLING OF THE ABDOMEN PLUS CONSTIPATION

PROBABLE
WIND
CONSTIPATION

POSSIBLE
IRRITABLE BOWEL SYNDROME
DIVERTICULAR DISEASE

RARE
BOWEL CANCER

PROBABLE

■ WIND
■ CONSTIPATION
See pages 148 and 161.

POSSIBLE

■ IRRITABLE BOWEL SYNDROME
■ DIVERTICULAR DISEASE
See pages 148 and 149.

RARE

■ BOWEL CANCER
Most bowel cancer originates in the rectum, colon or caecum. It may present in many ways, or be found incidentally on routine examination. It is possible to divide symptoms into right colon + caecum and left colon + rectum. *See also INTESTINAL OBSTRUCTION, page 151.*

Right colon plus caecum:
* Vague lower abdominal pain.
* Pain may localize to right side.
* Mass in right side of abdomen.
* Change in bowel habit often diarrhoea occasionally constipation).
* Anaemia and associated symptoms (*see page 419*) due to slow blood loss.

Left colon plus rectum:
* Increasing constipation.
* Intermittent diarrhroa.
* Colicky abdominal pain and distension.
* Blood present when passing stools.
* Mass in left side of abdomen.

Any persistent change in bowel habit in someone over 50 must be assessed by a doctor.

QUICKLY FEELING FULL ON EATING

■ POST-GASTRIC SURGERY
If surgery to remove a diseased stomach leaves only a small part behind, relatively small meals make you feel replete.

■ STOMACH CANCER
See STOMACH DISEASE, page 164.

WORMS

There are four types of worm that most commonly affect humans. In developed countries, the only type of worm normally seen is the threadworm.

Threadworms are an extremely common infestation among schoolchildren. Most children will have them at some time. Typically, a child wakes with an itchy anus at night and may be very distressed. Small, white, thread-like worms can be seen on the skin of the anus, and, less easily, in the stools.

Treatment is simple, with medicine which should normally be taken by all family members. The commonest source of threadworm infestation is garden soil. Washing hands and scrubbing nails helps prevent infection or re-infection.

ABDOMEN: DIGESTIVE SYSTEM

PROBABLE

■ THREADWORM
* Anal irritation.
* May prevent sleep.
* Worms observed in stools.

POSSIBLE

■ ROUNDWORMS — ASCARIS LUMBRICOIDES
* May be no symptoms.
* Worm observed in stools.
* Occasionally abdominal pain.
* Occasionally the lungs become inflamed.
* Occasionally an urticarial skin reaction develops; *see page 258.*

■ HOOKWORMS
* May cause chronic bleeding from small intestine.
* Anaemia.
* Malaise.
* Diarrhoea.

■ TAPEWORMS
* Abdominal discomfort.
* Increased appetite.
* Segments of worms seen in stools.

All types of worm infestation should be assessed and treated by a doctor.

TAR-LIKE STOOLS

See BLOOD FROM THE BACK PASSAGE, page 157.

PALE-COLOURED FAECES

Faeces are normally coloured brown by a mixture of the body's bile pigments and bacteria. Certain conditions hinder this pigmentation; and sometimes bile is excreted instead via urine, which then appears dark brown or yellow. There may also be jaundice and sometimes itching.

Jaundice occurs when pigments which are normally excreted in bowel or urine waste products build up in the body to such an extent that they colour the eyes and skin with a yellow tinge.

PROBABLE
GALL STONES
HEPATITIS

POSSIBLE
CANCER OF THE PANCREAS
CHRONIC PANCREATITIS
CIRRHOSIS OF THE LIVER
LIVER TUMOURS

RARE
JAUNDICE OF PREGNANCY
BILIARY ATRESIA
SCLEROSING CHOLANGITIS
CANCER OF THE BILE DUCTS

ABDOMEN: DIGESTIVE SYSTEM

PROBABLE

■ GALL STONES
See CHOLECYSTITIS, page 173.

■ HEPATITIS
Several different types of virus cause hepatitis. Some are more significant than others and so suspected hepatitis needs professional attention. In some cases, the disease is so mild it is assumed to be a cold or flu.
* Lethargy.
* Loss of appetite.
* Loss of desire for cigarettes and alcohol.
* Nausea.
* Joint pains.
* Variable rash.
* Right-sided upper abdominal pain.
* Fever.
* Diarrhoea.

The pale stools, dark urine and jaundice appear (if, indeed, they are going to) after a few days. In mild cases, jaundice may not be a feature.

POSSIBLE

■ CANCER OF THE PANCREAS
See DISEASED PANCREAS, page 165.

■ CHRONIC PANCREATITIS
See page 168.

■ CIRRHOSIS OF THE LIVER
See page 150.

■ LIVER TUMOURS
See LIVER DISEASE, page 165.

RARE

■ JAUNDICE OF PREGNANCY
Occurs in a small proportion of women. Normally harmless and appears in the final three months.

■ BILIARY ATRESIA
Failure of the biliary tract to develop properly in a foetus.
* Jaundice a few days after birth.
* Itching.
* Retarded growth.
* Cirrhosis develops.
* Malabsorption.

Liver transplants offer hope.

■ SCLEROSING CHOLANGITIS (ADULT)
For some unknown reason the bile ducts grow fibrous and shrink.
* Progressive jaundice.* Itching.
* Liver failure after a few years.

■ CANCER OF THE BILE DUCTS
Very rare. Causes jaundice with pale faeces and dark urine associated with other signs of cancer, such as weight loss.

DIARRHOEA

Can be difficult to define: perhaps the most useful criterion is whether the passage of stools is loose enough or frequent enough to be inconvenient.

Diarrhoea may be watery; green-yellow; bloody (bright red, dark or tarry); a normal colour; or mixed with mucus and pus. Strictly speaking, blood passed via the anus is not diarrhoea, but as it is often difficult to tell it from liquid

ABDOMEN: DIGESTIVE SYSTEM

stools, it is also included under this heading.

PROBABLE
GASTROENTERITIS
IRRITABLE BOWEL SYNDROME
DIVERTICULAR DISEASE

POSSIBLE
FACTITIOUS DIARRHOEA
CROHN'S DISEASE
ULCERATIVE COLITIS
BOWEL CANCER
COELIAC DISEASE
CHRONIC PANCREATITIS
BACILLARY DYSENTERY
SPRUE
AIDS-RELATED DIARRHOEA
HYPERTHYROIDISM
KWASHIORKOR
POST-GASTRECTOMY SYNDROME

RARE
CARCINOID SYNDROME
CHOLERA
TYPHOID

PROBABLE

■ GASTROENTERITIS
* Loose, runny, watery.
See page 168.

■ IRRITABLE BOWEL SYNDROME
Slightly loose normal stool. *See page 148.*

■ DIVERTICULAR DISEASE
Normal stool, but may be blood-streaked, or with dark blood mixed in.
See page 149.

POSSIBLE

■ FACTITIOUS DIARRHOEA
Loose, but normal. *See page 152.*

■ CROHN'S DISEASE
Loose, but normal. *See page 152.*

■ ULCERATIVE COLITIS
Loose stools with blood, mucus and pus. *See page 151.*

■ BOWEL CANCER
Loose, but normal, and may be blood-streaked. *See page 149.*

■ COELIAC DISEASE
Loose, pale and bulky. *See page 146.*

■ CHRONIC PANCREATITIS
Loose pale, bulky, smelly. *See page 168.*

■ BACILLARY DYSENTERY
Loose, bloody, pus and mucus. *See page 168.*

■ SPRUE
Malabsorption that starts with an initial attack of diarrhoea.
* Persistent diarrhoea.
* Stools are bulky, pale and fatty.
* Progressive weight loss.
* Anorexia.
* Anaemia.
* Oedema.
* Inflamed tongue.

Requires antibiotics.

■ AIDS-RELATED DIARRHOEA
AIDS patients commonly have diarrhoea and abdominal pain as symptoms. Investigations are needed to decide whether these symptoms are related to AIDS alone or to bacterial infection.

■ HYPERTHYROIDISM
Loose, but normal. *See page 433.*

■ KWASHIORKOR
Loose, but normal. *See page 146.*

■ POST-GASTRECTOMY SYNDROME
After the removal of part of the stomach (a gastrectomy), diarrhoea is a common complaint. Fortunately, since the introduction of modern ulcer- curing drugs, gastrectomy is no longer as common an operation as it once was.

RARE

■ CARCINOID SYNDROME
See page 169.

■ CHOLERA
Profuse, watery. *See page 168.*

■ TYPHOID
Loose, watery. *See page 169.*

BLOOD FROM THE BACK PASSAGE

This can appear in several forms: fresh, bright red; darkish, coming from the colon; or 'tarry,' coming from even higher up the gut, say the duodenum. In general, any disease that can cause bleeding in the gut can produce either vomited blood, and/or blood passed in stools.

PROBABLE
PILES
ANAL FISSURE

POSSIBLE
POLYPS
DIVERTICULAR DISEASE
BOWEL CANCER
BLEEDING PEPTIC ULCER
DRUG-INDUCED

RARE
OESOPHAGEAL VARICES
INTUSSUSCEPTION
JEJUNAL DIVERTICULUM
MECKEL'S DIVERTICULUM

PROBABLE

■ PILES
Medical term, haemorrhoids. These are lumps of tissue that may push out from the anal canal: a very common complaint.
* Bright red bleeding after defaecation, seen in the lavatory pan and on the paper.
* Pain is not a symptom of uncomplicated haemorrhoids.
* Fleshy lumps felt protruding

ABDOMEN: DIGESTIVE SYSTEM

intermittently from the anus after defaecation, which go back inside of their own accord.
* However, some piles remain permanently protruding.

Piles are normally caused by a diet which is abnormally low in roughage; stress, leading to changes in diet; or pregnancy, which puts pressure on the veins around the rectum. You can usually cure 90 per cent of piles by increasing the amount of roughage in your diet, ideally by adding bran. Severe cases may need injection or, rarely, surgical treatment.

Piles are, in fact, rather like the blow-out of an inner tube through a slit in the outer wall of a car tyre. They are distended veins which lie underneath the lining of the rectum and anus, causing bulges which may bleed. Often the first symptom is bright red blood on lavatory paper or in the bowl.

■ ANAL FISSURE
See page 160.

POSSIBLE

■ POLYPS
Intestinal polyps (growths of the tissue lining the ileum), which are initially benign growths, may cause anaemia, or episodes of rectal bleeding. As they grow, the risk of cancerous change increases.
See also BOWEL CANCER, page 149.

■ DIVERTICULAR DISEASE
See page 149.

■ BOWEL CANCER
See page 153.

■ BLEEDING PEPTIC ULCER
This can cause a black, tarry motion, in association with other symptoms. Sometimes a black stool is the first and only sign of a significant episode of bleeding from an ulcer. The stool is black because the blood is altered by its passage through the gut.
See page 170.

■ DRUG-INDUCED
Certain drugs (particularly steroids and non-steroidal anti-inflammatory drugs, including aspirin) may cause gastric bleeding. Initial symptoms may include vomiting blood or tarry stools.

RARE

■ OESOPHAGEAL VARICES
Delicate, distended veins in the lower end of the oesophagus. They may be present with cirrhosis of the liver *(see page 150)*. They may cause massive vomiting of blood and also bleeding from the back passage or the appearance of black stools. This condition can be fatal because of sudden blood loss.

■ INTUSSUSCEPTION
This condition is extremely painful and a medical emergency. It is a bowel abnormality which tends to occur when the body tries to expel unwanted tissue such as polyps.

In children it is the commonest form of bowel obstruction, but no one knows why it occurs.

Inflamed lymph nodes may cause the gut to invaginate on, or push back into, itself.
* Severe, colicky, abdominal pain.
* Thighs and knees drawn up because of pain.
* Blood-stained stools and mucus are passed.
* Vomiting.
* Abdominal distension.

Intussusception

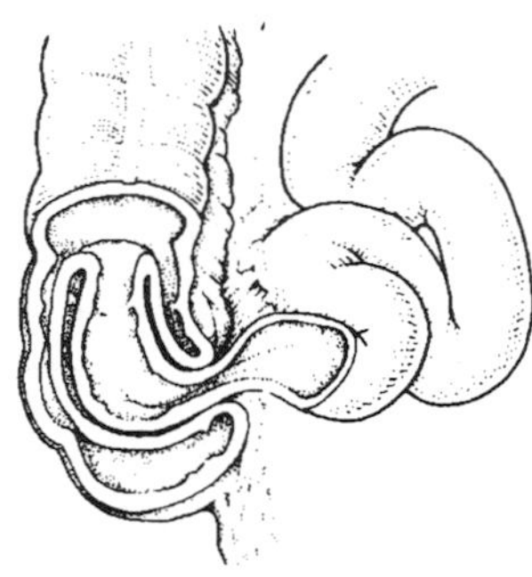

■ JEJUNAL DIVERTICULA
Like the colon, the jejunum may develop multiple diverticula. *See DIVERTICULAR DISEASE, page 149.*
* Tarry stools.
* Often pain-free.
* Sometimes diarrhoea due to altered digestion and absorption.

■ MECKEL'S DIVERTICULUM
This is like an extra appendix but originates in the ileum. Very rarely, it can cause bleeding. *See page 171.*

PAIN AROUND ANUS OR IN RECTUM

PROBABLE
ANAL FISSURE

POSSIBLE
ANAL ABSCESS

RARE
FISTULA-IN-ANO

PROBABLE

■ ANAL FISSURE
A small tear in the surface tissue of the anal canal, mainly caused by the passage of hard faeces. May have been caused by injury (perhaps during anal intercourse).
* Local pain, worse after passing a stool.
* Pain stops the individual wanting to open their bowels, and they can become constipated.
* Occasional bleeding (bright red) may be noted (in lavatory pan or on paper).

Pain-relieving creams may help healing, which will often occur spontaneously.

ABDOMEN: DIGESTIVE SYSTEM

POSSIBLE

■ ANAL ABSCESS
The anus or anal canal and rectum are common sites for infection, because of the moist environment and the many organisms present in faeces.

However, if you do develop symptoms of an abscess in or around this area, consider the possibility of underlying disease. There is an added likelihood if abscesses or infection recur. There are several different types of abscess, but all have common features, and all need surgical assessment and treatment.
* Localized throbbing pain (either around the anus or in the rectum).
* Local tender swelling.
* Reddening of the skin if near the surface.
* Often fever.
* Often malaise.
* Often a fast pulse rate.

Possible underlying diseases that should be considered are diabetes mellitus *(see page 485)* and Crohn's disease *(see page 152)*.

RARE

■ FISTULA-IN-ANO
May be the final result of an abscess which has burst through skin and bowel creating a false passage.
* Persistent faecal discharge on skin near anus.

ITCHING ANUS

Itching is usually a sign of inflammation, infection or infestation of the skin's surface. It can occur as a result of an underlying illness in the rest of the body, which makes the skin more vulnerable to this sensation in one particular area.

PROBABLE
OCCUPATIONAL HAZARD
THREADWORM
PILES
YEAST INFECTION

POSSIBLE
PRURITUS ANI
ANAL FISSURE
FISTULA-IN-ANO
PILONIDAL SINUS

RARE
DIABETES MELLITUS

PROBABLE

■ OCCUPATIONAL HAZARD
The term is a euphemism for the fact that, by its nature, the anal area, moist and subject to infective organisms, is prone to infection and irritation. People who sit all day (particularly in well-contoured car seats) and who have stressful jobs, are perhaps

especially prone to this problem.

Regular washing and proper drying will reduce itching. (*See below*.) On the other hand, overzealous washing and wiping can damage the skin surface, also causing minor irritation and itching. A mild steroid cream can be helpful; get a doctor's advice.

■ THREADWORM
See pages 153-4.

■ PILES
See page 158.

■ YEAST INFECTION
Because this area is continuously moist and damp, it is vulnerable to yeast and fungal infections such as thrush, which is caused by the yeast *candida*. Simple anti-fungal creams can cure the condition. However, it may recur.

POSSIBLE

■ PRURITUS ANI
Some people scratch the anal region as a matter of habit, or when tense. Constant scratching causes inflammation, cracking, itching and discomfort.

■ ANAL FISSURE
See page 159

Individuals with anal fissures occasionally complain of local itching or irritation.

■ FISTULA-IN-ANO
See page 160. Those with anal fistulas occasionally complain of local irritation and itching.

■ PILONIDAL SINUS
A small hole underneath the skin between the buttocks, thought to be created by a hair growing into and under the skin. It can cause recurrent infection and itching.

RARE

■ DIABETES MELLITUS
See page 485. Some diabetics complain of an itching perianal region, for which no other local cause is apparent.

CHANGE IN BOWEL HABIT

See CONSTIPATION, page 161 and DIARRHOEA, page 155 . Any change in bowel habit which does not have a simple explanation, such as a sudden change in diet, should be reported to your doctor.

CONSTIPATION

A diagnosis as well as a symptom. For details on constipation as a diagnosis, *see page 148.*

PROBABLE
INADEQUATE DIET
PREGNANCY
ANAL FISSURE
DRUG SIDE-EFFECT

ABDOMEN: DIGESTIVE SYSTEM

POSSIBLE
DIVERTICULAR DISEASE
INTESTINAL OBSTRUCTION
BOWEL CANCER
PREMATURITY
IMMOBILITY

RARE
CROHN'S DISEASE
HIRSCHSPRUNG'S DISEASE

PROBABLE

■ INADEQUATE DIET
A diet too low in fluids and/or too low in roughage will cause constipation.

■ PREGNANCY
There are two main causes for constipation in pregnancy.
* Decreased movement of the gut.
* The pressure of the growing womb on the colon.
See 148.

■ ANAL FISSURE
See page 159.

■ DRUG SIDE-EFFECT
Many painkillers, in particular codeine and morphine, contain substances which may cause constipation. Many other drugs also cause constipation as a side-effect.

POSSIBLE

■ DIVERTICULAR DISEASE
■ INTESTINAL OBSTRUCTION
See pages 149 and 151.

■ BOWEL CANCER
See page 153.

■ PREMATURITY
See page 146.

■ IMMOBILITY
Anyone relatively immobile or bedridden (for example, the elderly, or anyone who has had a head injury, stroke or progressive neurological disease) is prone to constipation.

RARE

■ CROHN'S DISEASE
See page 152.

■ HIRSCHSPRUNG'S DISEASE
See page 146.

A SWELLING FELT WITHIN THE ABDOMEN

Any organ inside the abdomen can, if diseased, appear as a swelling, a lump or a mass. You might notice this yourself, or your doctor may do so at a routine examination .

This is such a general symptom that it makes sense to list only the principal possible causes.

You must a see a doctor if you

suspect any of these problems. Pregnancy is excluded from the possibilities.

PROBABLE
INGUINAL AND FEMORAL HERNIAS
UMBILICAL HERNIA

POSSIBLE
ENLARGED BLADDER
AORTIC ANEURYSM
CANCER OF THE COLON OR RECTUM
GALL BLADDER
PROBLEMS OF THE OVARIES
STOMACH DISEASE

RARE
APPENDICITIS
KIDNEY DISEASE
LIVER DISEASE
DISEASED PANCREAS
DISEASED SPLEEN
DISEASED UTERUS

PROBABLE

■ INGUINAL AND FEMORAL HERNIAS
Hernias are protrusions of bowel through weak spots in the muscular wall of the abdomen. Although not, strictly-speaking, in the abdomen, they may be noticed as lumps in the groin. Inguinal hernias are very much more common than femoral hernias.
* May make a gurgling sound.
* Can be pushed back into the abdomen.
* May disappear at night, reappearing once you are up and about.
* In men, hernias may extend into the scrotum.

Hernias gradually enlarge.

Sometimes the bowel gets trapped in the hernia, causing intestinal obstruction *(see page 151)*. If this happens, the following may be noticed:
* The hernia becomes painful.
* It cannot be pushed back.
* Intermittent abdominal pain.
* Possibly vomiting.

Surgery may be needed.

■ UMBILICAL HERNIA
Symptoms are the same as for inguinal and femoral hernias, *above*, but are less likely to obstruct the gut. They are commonest in babies and infants, particularly if they are black. They sometimes disappear as the abdominal muscles develop.

POSSIBLE

■ ENLARGED BLADDER
Caused by *ENLARGED PROSTRATE, page 190.*
* Mid-line swelling in the lower abdomen above the pubic bone.
* Constant pain.
* Inability to pass urine.
* Possibly dribbling of urine.

ABDOMEN: DIGESTIVE SYSTEM

■ AORTIC ANEURYSM
Swelling of the body's main artery. It may burst without warning.
* Abdominal pain.
* A swelling in middle of abdomen which pulsates in time with the heart beat.
* Back pain.
* Sometimes, sudden collapse.

Often the individual is unaware of the aneurysm until the sudden onset of severe pain.

■ CANCER OF THE COLON OR RECTUM
See BOWEL CANCER, page 153.

■ GALL BLADDER
The gall bladder may become enlarged for two main reasons. If it is caused by infection:
* Upper right abdominal pain.
* May be a tender mass jut below the right rib margin.
* Pain may be made worse by breathing in.
* Fever.
* Malaise.

If it is a tumour (of the pancreas, bile ducts or gall bladder):
* Jaundice.
* Non-tender mass in right upper abdomen.
* Pale stools.
* Dark urine.
* Other signs of malignant disease may be present.

■ PROBLEMS OF THE OVARIES
Ovarian cysts (*page 171*) and cancer of the ovaries can produce abdominal swelling; in case of latter sometimes very marked and weight loss despite the swelling.

■ STOMACH DISEASE
Virtually the only reason for a palpably enlarged stomach in an adult is tumour, although even in established cases, for example stomach cancers, the enlarged stomach can only be felt in a minority of individuals, especially if the cancer is at the outlet of the stomach — the pylorus. The pylorus may be felt occasionally in babies with hypertrophic pyloric stenosis (*see below*). Other features of stomach cancer (rare under the age of 45) include:
* Anorexia.
* Indigestion and abdominal pain.
* Weight loss.
* Anaemia.
* Upper abdominal midline mass.
* Occasionally vomiting, if the pylorus in blocked.
* Even more occasionally, vomiting blood.

Sometimes the individual goes to a doctor complaining of jaundice and ascites *(see page 150)* both the result of the tumour having already spread.
* Hypertrophic pyloric stenosis. Mostly in baby boys. The stomach outlet is blocked by thickened intestinal muscle.

RARE

■ APPENDICITIS
Inflammation of the appendix. A lump is rarely a noticeable feature of appendicitis; however, if appendicitis is not diagnosed at an early stage, a lump may subsequently appear a few dys later which can be felt in the right side of the abdomen.

* Right-sided lower abdominal pain — often starts over the 'belly button' or umbilicus, and then moves down and to the right.
* Pain worse on pressing over appendix.
* There may be fever.
* Anorexia.
* Nausea and sometimes vomiting.
* Malaise.
* Sometimes other tissues wrap around the inflamed appendix for protection and a lump can be felt in the right lower abdomen; this is called an appendix mass.

■ KIDNEY DISEASE
Kidney enlargement may be noticed on the right or left sides of the abdomen and in the loin, and may be felt as a mass.

Enlargement is caused by tumour, polycystic disease or urinary obstruction *(see relevant entries in ABDOMEN: URINARY SYSTEM).*

Enlargement is one, not often very noticeable, symptom of these conditions.

■ LIVER DISEASE
The liver lies under the right rib cage but extends across the midline. The individual may feel or see the enlargement as a mass moving in and out with respiration. The main reasons for enlargement are:

Cirrhosis
See page 150.

Cancer
Several types of cancer can spread to the liver, including breast and lung. But they do not automatically do so; and in most cases, the cancer is already diagnosed and being treated. Occasionally, the liver is the original site of the tumour, known as a hepatoma; can be treated surgically.

Infection
The liver may become infected by a number of organisms and liver abscesses may develop.
* Swinging fever.
* Sweating.
* Right upper abdominal pain.
* Enlarged, tender liver.
* Sometimes jaundice.
* Malaise.

Hydatid disease
Infection from a tapeworm: causes cysts to form in the liver.
* Often, no symptoms.
* Occasionally the liver is enlarged because of a big cyst.

■ DISEASED PANCREAS
The pancreas lies at the back of the abdomen and may enlarge through inflammation or malignant disease.

Cancer of the pancreas:
* Abdominal pain.
* Wasting.
* Nausea.
* Jaundice.
* Pale stools.
* Dark urine.
* Occasional vomiting.

Pancreatitis
See page 150. Acute pancreatitis sometimes develops a complication called a pseudocyst: a large cyst which may be felt as a mass in the middle of the abdomen.

Abdomen: Digestive System

■ DISEASED SPLEEN
The spleen may be felt as a mass in the abdomen when enlarged two to three times its normal size. Its tip can be felt under the left rib margins. It may be enlarged by any viral infection, but if it is noticed as a mass; the main causes would be:

Malaria *See page 453.*

Kala-azar
An infection spread by sandflies.
* Fever.
* Sweating.
* Massive splenic enlargement.
* Liver enlargement.
* Lymph gland enlargement.
* Anaemia.

Chronic myeloid leukaemia
* Anaemia.
* Discomfort in abdomen due to large spleen.
* Night sweats.
* Fever.
* Loss of weight.
* Occasional generalized itchiness.

Myelofibrosis
Often in association with other illnesses such as cancer.
* Anaemia.
* Weakness.
* Enlarged spleen.
* Gout.

■ DISEASED UTERUS
See CANCER OF THE WOMB, page 353.

RIGID ABDOMEN

See PERFORATED VISCUS, page 149.

TENDER ABDOMEN

See all symptoms involving abdominal pain, this page and pages 167-74.

CONSTANT VERY SEVERE PAIN IN THE ABDOMEN

As a main symptom this will quite rightly send you straight to a doctor. Don't delay the visit. The causes listed here are not common, but they need immediate attention.

POSSIBLE
PERFORATED VISCUS
MESENTERIC VASCULAR OCCLUSION

RARE
ACUTE PANCREATITIS
RUPTURED AORTIC ANEURYSM

POSSIBLE

■ PERFORATED VISCUS
See page 149.

■ MESENTERIC VASCULAR OCCLUSION
The blood supply to the gut is interrupted because of blockage in the gut's main blood vessels.
* Severe pain, starting suddenly.
* Bloody stools.

* Vomiting.
* Shock.
* Occasionally, abdominal distension.

RARE

■ ACUTE PANCREATITIS
Occasionally, pancreatitis starts suddenly with very severe upper abdominal pain; *see page 150.*

■ RUPTURED AORTIC ANEURYSM
See AORTIC ANEURYSM, page 164.

SEVERE BUT INTERMITTENT ABDOMINAL PAIN

This suggests a different set of causes to those of constant severe pain, *page 166.*

PROBABLE
KIDNEY STONES

POSSIBLE
INTESTINAL OBSTRUCTION
BILIARY COLIC

PROBABLE

■ KIDNEY STONES
See page 184.

POSSIBLE

■ INTESTINAL OBSTRUCTION
See page 151.

■ BILIARY COLIC
Caused by gall stones temporarily blocking a bile duct.
* Intense pain lasting from minutes to hours.
* Pain is in upper abdomen, and may pass to shoulder tip.
* Vomiting.
* Individual is pale and clammy.
* Possibly jaundice.
* Possibly fever or shivering.

DIARRHOEA PLUS ABDOMINAL PAIN

PROBABLE
GASTROENTERITIS
IRRITABLE BOWEL SYNDROME

POSSIBLE
BOWEL CANCER
CROHN'S DISEASE
ULCERATIVE COLITIS
CHRONIC PANCREATITIS
BACILLARY DYSENTERY

ABDOMEN: DIGESTIVE SYSTEM

RARE
PERNICIOUS ANAEMIA
CHOLERA
TYPHOID
POST-GASTRECTOMY SYNDROME
CARCINOID SYNDROME

PROBABLE

■ GASTROENTERITIS
Otherwise known as food poisoning. Can also be caused by viral infections. Very common. Episodes rarely last more than 24 to 36 hours and cure themselves.
* Abdominal pain.
* Vomiting.
* Watery diarrhoea.
* Muscle/joint pains.
* Headache.
* Occasional fever.

■ IRRITABLE BOWEL SYNDROME
See page 148.

POSSIBLE

■ BOWEL CANCER
■ CROHN'S DISEASE
■ ULCERATIVE COLITIS
See pages 153, 152 and 151.

■ CHRONIC PANCREATITIS
Inflammation of the pancreas resulting in permanent and irreversible damage. Alcohol is commonly implicated: if you have the condition, you will have to stop drinking.
* Pain worsened by food and alcohol. Often very persistent.
* Malabsorption, due to lack of digestive enzymes, causes fatty diarrhoea.
* Weight loss.
* Diabetes develops; *see page 485.*
* Occasionally associated with jaundice, pale stools and dark urine.

■ BACILLARY DYSENTERY
Caused by person-to-person spread of a bacterium.
* Fever.
* Abdominal pain.
* Watery diarrhoea.
* After one to three days, bloody diarrhoea with mucus.

Most cases cure themselves, although antibiotics may help.

RARE

■ PERNICIOUS ANAEMIA
The lining of the stomach stops producing acid and other essential substances. Occurs in people over 30 years of age.
* Anaemia, slow onset.
* Sore tongue.
* Tingling and/or numbness of extremities (peripheral neuropathy)
* Fever.
* Abdominal pain.
* Diarrhoea.
* Mild jaundice.

■ CHOLERA
Common in India and some other underdeveloped countries. Caused by an organism present in water. A major problem when water supplies are contaminated.
* Initially, mild diarrhoea.
* Then large volumes of diarrhoea.
* Vomiting.

* Abdominal pain.
* Thirst.
* Muscle cramps.
* Slight fever.

Treatment aimed at minimizing dehydration.

Cholera

The World Health Organization (WHO) no longer recommends cholera immunization before overseas travel; and it has not issued cholera immunization certificates since 1989. Only 5 per cent of those infected with the cholera organism will develop symptoms. Today's infections are much less severe than those seen earlier in this century.

■ TYPHOID FEVER

Caused by one of the salmonella organisms. In the first week:
* Increasing fever.
* Abdominal pain.
* Headache.
* Cough.

In the second week:
* General malaise.
* Apathy.
* Fever.
* Abdominal distension.
* Diarrhoea.
* 'Rose' spots on abdomen.

Fatal in some cases, but antibiotics can change the course of the disease.

■ POST-GASTRECTOMY SYNDROME

Gastrectomy is surgical removal of the stomach. After a meal, within two or three hours, there may be:
* Upper abdominal distension.
* Faintness.
* Weakness.
* Palpitations.
* Sweating.
* Diarrhoea.

■ CARCINOID SYNDROME

Carcinoid tumours may appear in any part of the gut. They cause many symptoms, due to the chemicals they secrete, including:
* Facial flushing.
* Explosive, watery diarrhoea.
* Abdominal pain.
* Asthmatic wheeze.
* Pain in the abdomen and weight loss.
* Sweating.

ABDOMINAL PAIN AND PROGRESSIVE LOSS OF WEIGHT

This combination needs to be taken seriously. Your doctor will consider the following possibilities. They are not listed in order of probability: diagnosis depends upon accompanying symptoms.

CROHN'S DISEASE, *page 128.*
ULCERATIVE COLITIS, *page 151.*
CHRONIC PANCREATITIS, *page 168.*
CANCER OF THE PANCREAS, *page 165.*
CANCER OF THE STOMACH, *page 164.*
CANCER OF THE BOWEL, page 153.
SPREAD OF CANCER TO THE LIVER, *page 165.*

ABDOMEN: DIGESTIVE SYSTEM

ABDOMINAL PAIN PLUS VOMITING

PROBABLE
GASTROENTERITIS
MESENTERIC ADENITIS

POSSIBLE
PEPTIC ULCER
APPENDICITIS
KIDNEY STONES
OVARIAN CYST
SALPINGITIS (PYOSALPINX)
BILIARY COLIC
STOMACH CANCER

RARE
MECKEL'S DIVERTICULUM
ACUTE PANCREATITIS
INTESTINAL OBSTRUCTION
PORPHYRIA

PROBABLE

■ GASTROENTERITIS
See page 168.

■ MESENTERIC ADENITIS
Often mistaken for appendicitis in children; *see page 164*. This condition is caused by enlargement of lymph glands in the stomach, usually caused by a viral infection. Typically, there are common cold symptoms, plus:
* Pain and tenderness in the right lower abdomen; pain may also be present throughout the abdomen.
* Fever.
* Nausea and vomiting.

At surgery, enlarged glands are found with a normal appendix. The adenitis settles of its own accord.

POSSIBLE

■ PEPTIC ULCER
The term covers ulcers of the stomach and duodenum. There is a wide range of symptoms which vary considerably from person to person:
* Pain in the epigastrium (upper middle part of the abdomen).
* Pain is recurrent.
* Heartburn may be present.
* Pain may radiate to the back.
* Pain may be present for a few weeks at a time.
* Night waking because of pain is common.
* Possibly nausea and vomiting.
* Food can either improve or worsen the pain.

Ulcers can bleed, causing anaemia and tarry stools or haematemesis. *See BLOOD FROM THE BACK PASSAGE, page 157 and ABDOMINAL PAIN PLUS VOMITING BLOOD, page 171.*

They can also perforate — *see PERFORATED VISCUS, page 149.*

■ APPENDICITIS
See page 164.

■ KIDNEY STONES
See page 184.

■ <u>OVARIAN CYST</u>
Ovarian cysts may be attached to the ovary on a stalk. If the cyst rotates, it will tighten the stalk, causing severe pain.
* Sudden onset of lower abdominal pain.
* Vomiting.
* Cyst may bleed, causing pain and irritating the inside of the abdominal cavity.

May mimic appendicitis if on the right ovary.

■ <u>SALPINGITIS (PYOSALPINX)</u>
Abscess on a Fallopian tube — one possibility in the wider picture of *PELVIC INFECTION, page 349.*

■ <u>BILIARY COLIC</u>
See page 167.

■ <u>STOMACH CANCER</u>
See STOMACH DISEASE, page 164.

RARE

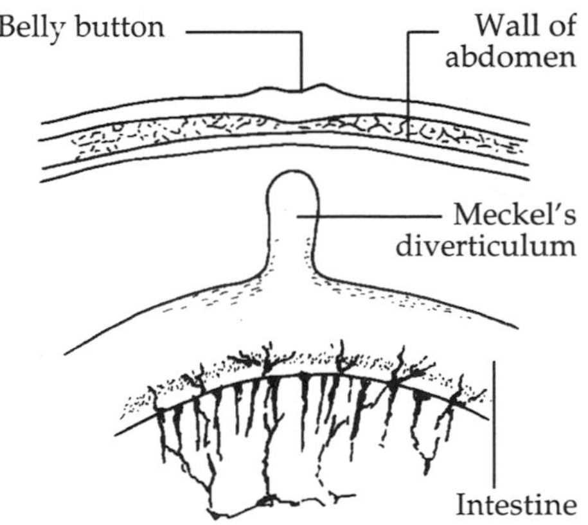

■ <u>MECKEL'S DIVERTICULUM</u>
A diverticulum (*see diagram*) is an out-pouching — a little sac; this type occurs in the ileum.

Symptoms mimic appendicitis if it becomes inflamed *(see page 164)* and may also cause:
* Anaemia.
* Intestinal obstruction.
* Rectal bleeding.

■ <u>ACUTE PANCREATITIS</u>
■ <u>INTESTINAL OBSTRUCTION</u>
See pages150 and 151.

■ <u>PORPHYRIA</u>
A group of metabolic diseases. The following are the commonest features:
* Intermittent abdominal pain.
* Vomiting.
* Constipation.
* Fever.
* Fast pulse.
* Neurological abnormalities.

ABDOMINAL PAIN PLUS VOMITING BLOOD

A rare combination, but if you have both these symptoms, you must consult your doctor. Bleeding may continue even without vomiting, putting you in danger until the source is detected and the bleeding stopped.

PROBABLE
MALLORY-WEISS TEAR
ACUTE GASTRITIS

ABDOMEN: DIGESTIVE SYSTEM

POSSIBLE
PEPTIC ULCER
DRUG-INDUCED

RARE
CANCER OF THE STOMACH
HIATUS HERNIA AND
OESOPHAGITIS

PROBABLE

■ MALLORY-WEISS TEAR
A small tear in the lining of the upper stomach caused by vomiting. First noticed in studies of alcoholics.
* Vomiting, often recurrent.
* Fresh blood may be vomited (medical term, haematemesis).
* Tarry stools.
Normally self-healing without further treatment.

■ ACUTE GASTRITIS
Inflammation of the lining of the stomach caused by food, drugs, alcohol or infection.
* Indigestion.
* Occasionally blood is vomited.
This usually looks like coffee grounds; the blood is altered by the gastric juices.

POSSIBLE

■ PEPTIC ULCER
See page 170.

■ DRUG-INDUCED
Some drugs, particularly steroids and non-steroidal anti-inflammatory drugs, including aspirin, can cause gastric bleeding. This may be experienced as vomiting up blood or passing tarry stools (melaena).

Non-steroidal anti-inflammatory drugs.
This group of drugs was originally introduced to treat arthritis, and they are now widely prescribed. Their side-effects on the intestine are significant: it is estimated that as many as 4,000 deaths per year in the U.K. may result from bleeding caused by these drugs. Elderly people who take them continuously are at greatest risk.

RARE

■ CANCER OF THE STOMACH
See STOMACH DISEASE, page 164.

■ HIATUS HERNIA AND
■ OESOPHAGITIS
Inflammation of the gullet caused by reflux of stomach contents.
* Heartburn.
* Difficulty in swallowing.
* Bitter fluid comes into mouth ('waterbrash' or 'repeating').
* Vomiting.
* Nausea.
* Occasional anaemia.
* Occasionally, if very severe, may cause melaena or haematemesis.

ABDOMINAL PAIN PLUS VOMITING AND FEVER

PROBABLE
GASTROENTERITIS
URINARY TRACT INFECTION

POSSIBLE
ACUTE PYELONEPHRITIS
PELVIC INFLAMMATORY DISEASE
APPENDICITIS
CHOLECYSTITIS

RARE
INTESTINAL OBSTRUCTION
ACUTE PANCREATITIS
MECKEL'S DIVERTICULITIS
PORPHYRIA

PROBABLE

■ GASTROENTERITIS
See page 168.

■ URINARY TRACT INFECTION
See page 183.

POSSIBLE

■ ACUTE PYELONEPHRITIS
See KIDNEY INFECTION, page 183.

■ PELVIC INFLAMMATORY DISEASE
See page 352.

■ APPENDICITIS
See page 164.

■ CHOLECYSTITIS
The gall bladder may become inflamed and infected because of gall stones, which form from fats, calcium and pigment. Many people have them, but they often remain unnoticed unless the individual develops cholecystitis.
* Upper right abdominal pain.
* Tenderness just below the right rib margin.
* Pain may be made worse by breathing in.
* Fever.
* Malaise.
* Vomiting.
* Jaundice may develop if stones block biliary tract.

See a doctor without delay.

RARE

■ INTESTINAL OBSTRUCTION
■ ACUTE PANCREATITIS
See pages 151 and 150.

■ MECKEL'S DIVERTICULUM
See page 171.

■ PORPHYRIA
See page 171.

ABDOMINAL PAIN, VOMITING AND JAUNDICE

PROBABLE
CHOLECYSTITIS
BILIARY COLIC

POSSIBLE
ACUTE PANCREATITIS

RARE
CANCER OF THE PANCREAS
CANCER OF THE STOMACH

PROBABLE

■ CHOLECYSTITIS
See page 173.

■ BILIARY COLIC
See page 167.

POSSIBLE

■ ACUTE PANCREATITIS
See page 150.

RARE

■ CANCER OF THE PANCREAS
See page 165.

■ CANCER OF THE STOMACH
See STOMACH DISEASE, page 164.

APPARENT CONSTIPATION ALTERNATING WITH DIARRHOEA

This is a possible combination, but it is best to explore the possibilities in detail by separately reading *CONSTIPATION, page 162 and DIARRHOEA, page 155 and CHANGE IN BOWEL HABIT, page 161.*

CONSTIPATION AND ABDOMINAL PAIN

Explore the full possibilities by reading *CONSTIPATION, page 162* and *ABDOMINAL PAIN, pages 166-74.*

INDIGESTION

Indigestion, heartburn, dyspepsia — these terms tend to be used interchangeably for a variety of symptoms of upper abdominal pain, flatulence, belching, acid in the mouth, and nausea.

Occasional, mild indigestion, which settles with simple, over-the-counter remedies, is of little significance. It becomes an important symptom when it recurs frequently, or becomes more persistent than usual. It is a sign of change in your normal pattern of tolerance to food and carries a clear message: seek medical advice.

Abdomen: Digestive System

Digestive system

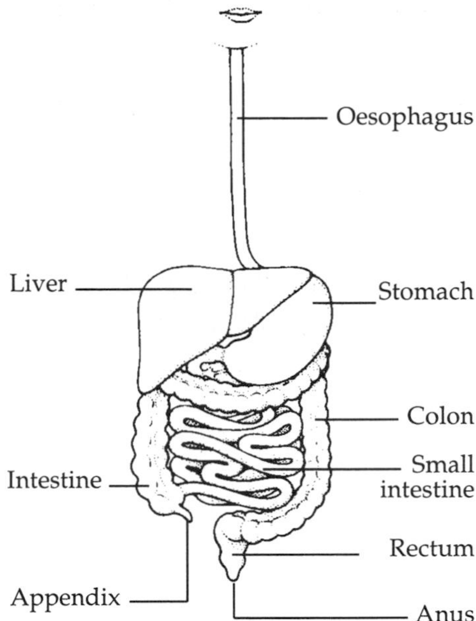

Gall stones

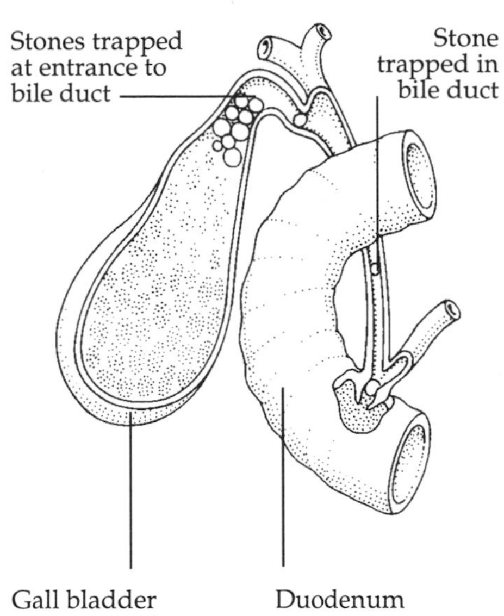

PROBABLE
NON-ULCER DYSPEPSIA
OESOPHAGITIS AND HIATUS HERNIA
PEPTIC ULCER
PREGNANCY

POSSIBLE
GALL STONES

RARE
CANCER OF THE STOMACH
CANCER OF THE OESOPHAGUS
ACHALASIA
CHRONIC PANCREATITIS

PROBABLE

■ NON-ULCER DYSPEPSIA
A term used to describe groups of symptoms such as:
* Upper abdominal pain.
* Nausea.
* Flatulence and belching when there is no evidence of an ulcer after special tests.

■ OESOPHAGITIS AND HIATUS HERNIA
See page 172.

■ PEPTIC ULCER
See page 170.

■ PREGNANCY
See page 148.

Abdomen: Digestive System

POSSIBLE

■ GALL STONES
See page 173.

RARE

■ CANCER OF THE STOMACH
See STOMACH DISEASE, page 164.

■ CANCER OF THE OESOPHAGUS
See page 121.

■ ACHALASIA
See page 120.

■ CHRONIC PANCREATITIS
See page 168.

CRAMPING PAINS IN THE ABDOMEN

See all combinations of symptoms involving ABDOMINAL PAIN, pages 166-74.

LOSS OF APPETITE

See page 474.

FLATULENCE OR BELCHING

See INDIGESTION, page 174.

DIARRHOEA, BLOODY

See DIARRHOEA, page 155 and BLOOD FROM THE BACK PASSAGE, page 157.

DIARRHOEA PLUS VOMITING

See DIARRHOEA, page 155 and*VOMITING, page 142;* also *GASTROENTERITIS, page 168,* one of the standard causes.

'STOMACH ACHE'

See all combinations of symptoms involving ABDOMINAL PAIN, pages 166-74.

NAUSEA

See VOMITING, page 142.

DYSPEPSIA

See INDIGESTION, page 174.

HEARTBURN

See INDIGESTION, page 174.

INCONTINENCE

Lack of control over the act of urination so that accidental or unplanned leakage occurs. Any irritation or inflammation may predispose to some degree of leakage. Age often worsens these problems. It is estimated that over 3,000,000 people in the UK have some degree of incontinence of faeces and urine.

PROBABLE
ENLARGED PROSTATE
BLADDER NECK OBSTRUCTION
URINARY TRACT INFECTION
IRRITABLE BLADDER
STRESS INCONTINENCE

POSSIBLE
CYSTOCELE
RECTOCELE
PROLAPSE
STROKE
EPILEPSY
MULTIPLE SCLEROSIS

RARE
SPINAL CORD INJURY
CAUDA EQUINA SYNDROME

PROBABLE

■ ENLARGED PROSTATE
See page 187.

■ BLADDER NECK OBSTRUCTION
See page 187.

■ URINARY TRACT INFECTION
See page 183. Especially in the elderly.

■ IRRITABLE BLADDER
See page 188.

■ STRESS INCONTINENCE
Often in women who have had children.
* Leakage of urine when coughing, laughing or sneezing.
* Leakage when straining.

POSSIBLE

■ CYSTOCELE AND RECTOCELE
These two conditions are common in women who also suffer from stress incontinence — above. They are caused by weakness of the vaginal wall, which allows the bladder (cystocele) or rectum (rectocele) to bulge into the vagina. This distortion of anatomy (often felt as a bulge) can cause leakage of urine.

■ PROLAPSE
The structures that keep the womb in place deteriorate after multiple childbirth and with age. In some women this allows the womb to prolapse — to drop down into the vagina — where it may often be seen or felt.
* Red lump at vagina.
* Sometimes bleeds.
* Discharge may be present.
* Associated with urinary leakage.
* May be pushed back internally.
* Comes back out on

Abdomen: Urinary System

straining/coughing/sneezing.

■ STROKE
Anyone who has suffered a stroke may develop incontinence or difficulty in urination.

Sometimes the bladder distends with urine, but because of lack of sensation no pain is felt, although the individual may appear restless and sweaty. Some overflow incontinence may develop.

■ EPILEPSY
In major epileptic fits *(see page 384)*, symptoms include:
* Jerking movements.
* Tongue biting.
* Urinary incontinence (the entire bladder empties spontaneously during the fit).

■ MULTIPLE SCLEROSIS
See page 406. Early symptoms reported to a doctor can include:
* Weakness or numbness in a limb.
* Heaviness in a limb.
* `Jumping' legs.
* Muscular spasms.
* Impaired vision.
* Hesitancy, frequency, incontinence and retention of urine may all be present.
* Altered sensation in limbs and trunk.

RARE

These diseases can be associated with very sudden loss of bladder control — together with other symptoms.

■ SPINAL CORD INJURY
* Weakness of the limbs below the level of damage.
* Sensory loss below the level of damage.
* Loss of bladder control — usually resulting in retention of urine.

Urgent medical attention is required.

■ CAUDA EQUINA SYNDROME
Meaning damage to the lowest part of the spinal cord. Can be caused by bone damage, tumour or a `slipped disc'.
* Back pain.
* Loss of sensation at the lower back and around the buttocks and anus.
* Leg weakness.
* Loss of bladder control.

Urgent medical attention is required.

NEED TO URINATE URGENTLY OR OFTEN

This symptom usually suggests that the bladder itself is irritated. The commonest cause is urine infection — cystitis. *See page 182; also PROBLEMS WITH URINATING, page 187.*

URINATING TOO MUCH, OR TOO OFTEN

The obvious cause is drinking too much tea, coffee or alcohol. These all stimulate the production of urine and can make you want to urinate during the night.

PROBABLE
URINARY TRACT INFECTION

POSSIBLE
ENLARGED PROSTATE
DIURETICS
DIABETES MELLITUS

RARE
DIABETES INSIPIDUS
CHRONIC RENAL FAILURE
ALDOSTERONISM
HYPERCALCAEMIA

PROBABLE

■ URINARY TRACT INFECTION
See page 183. Causes frequent urination, rather than excessive volume.

POSSIBLE

■ ENLARGED PROSTATE
See page 187. Again, causes frequent urination, rather than excessive volume.

■ DIURETICS
A range of drugs given to reduce high blood pressure or to treat heart failure. Their intended effect is to increase the amount of urine passed, in order to reduce the amount of fluid in the system and so lessen tension in the blood vessels. Some people taking these drugs find that they need to get up at night in order to urinate.

■ DIABETES MELLITUS
See page 485. New cases may suddenly experience:
* Increased volume of urine (polyuria).
* Increased thirst (polydipsia).
* Rapid weight loss.
* Malaise.
* Other symtoms such as vomiting, muscle cramps, abdominal pain.

If untreated, coma and death may follow. In the elderly, onset is slower and eye, nerve or kidney symptoms may be the first signs.

RARE

■ DIABETES INSIPIDUS
See page 485. Don't confuse it with diabetes mellitus, above. It may arise spontaneously or after injury to the head (typically after surgery or an accident); because of brain tumours; or because of infection. The main symptom is:
* Enormous volumes of urine — about 9 pints/5 litres passed daily.

■ CHRONIC KIDNEY FAILURE
Any disease resulting in kidney failure *(see INABILITY TO URINATE, page 189)* can cause excess urine at some stage.

■ ALDOSTERONISM
You may hear this described as Conn's Syndrome, which is one form of the disease. Caused by a

tumour of the adrenal gland. The blood chemistry becomes abnormal, leading to:
* Muscle weakness.
* Excessive urination.
* Excessive thirst.
* High blood pressure.

■ HYPERCALCAEMIA
High levels of calcium in the blood may be caused by a number of conditions and diseases including:
* Abnormalities of the parathyroid glands (*see diagram page 133*).
* Excess Vitamin D.
* Sarcoidosis: a rare illness of body tissues leading to the deposit of material, described as sarcoid, in various sites in the body.
* Malignant bone tumours (primary or secondary).
* Thyrotoxicosis: an illness caused by having too much thyroid hormone.
The symptoms of excess calcium in the blood are:
* Anorexia.
* Nausea.
* Vomiting.
* Thirst.
* Polyuria (passing urine more often than normal).
* Constipation.
* Muscle fatigue.

URINE LOOKS DARK

PROBABLE
CONCENTRATED URINE

POSSIBLE
HEPATITIS
FOOD OR DRUG

RARE
CANCER OF THE PANCREAS
HAEMAGLOBINURIA
'CRUSH' SYNDROME
MELANOMA
ALKAPTONURIA

PROBABLE

■ CONCENTRATED URINE
If you have spent a long time in a hot atmosphere, or if you have been physically very active, without also increasing your fluid intake, you may notice that your urine is a dark yellow colour, and that it is passed in small amounts. In the absence of other symptoms, this is normal. By increasing your fluid intake, or by avoiding the heat or exercise, urine will be back to normal within 24 hours.

POSSIBLE

■ HEPATITIS
Inflammation of the liver. There are several different types, some, particularly hepatitis B, are more serious than the others. If you suspect hepatitis, you must see a doctor. General symptoms may include:
* Fever.
* Malaise.
* Anorexia.

* Muscle and joint pains.
* Jaundice.
* Dark urine: it can be dark yellow, orange or brown.
* Stools become pale.

■ FOOD OR DRUG
Several foods and drugs can cause discolouration of different hues. Examples are:
* Orange — rhubarb, senna.
* Red — beetroot, blackberries.
* Green/blue — methylene blue dye.

After stopping the food or drug, urine should be back to normal within about 24 hours.

RARE

■ CANCER OF THE PANCREAS
A malignant tumour of the pancreas which blocks the bile ducts. This means that yellow bile is passed out in the urine.
* Jaundice.
* Dark yellow/orange/brown urine.
* Pale stools.
* Abdominal and back pain.
* Weight loss, anorexia.

■ HAEMAGLOBINURIA
In contrast to haematuria (which is the medical term for blood in urine, *see this page)* haemoglobinuria means broken down red blood cells in the urine. It is caused by several different diseases or conditions and the urine is often more brown than red. It appears in association with illnesses and diseases such as: haemolytic anaemias; thrombocytopaenic purpuras; cardiac disease (for example, after valve replacement); malaria; septicaemias.

Discoloured urine is unlikely to be the first or only symptom of these conditions, and in most cases the individual will already be under a doctor's care.

■ 'CRUSH' SYNDROME
See page 191.

■ MELANOMA
A melanoma is a skin cancer *(see page 244)*. In some advanced cases, the pigment melanin gets into the urine and colours it dark brown or black.

■ ALKAPTONURIA
This is an example of 'inborn errors of metabolism': in other words, the body fails to deal correctly with certain chemicals in the blood, which are then excreted in urine, which becomes progressively darker if left standing.

BLOOD IN URINE

The significance of blood in the urine varies greatly from the simple and easily treated to the severe and life-threatening. It should never be ignored as a symptom. If recurring, its significance increases. Again, do not ignore. Red blood cells in the urine (the medical term is haematuria) may come from any part of the urinary tract — the kidneys, the ureters (which connect the kidneys to the bladder), the bladder and the urethra (*see illustration, page 183*). Blood may also appear in

ABDOMEN: URINARY SYSTEM

urine because of generalized disease.

It may become apparent in several ways. The urine may appear the colour of blood (frank haematuria), or in smaller quantities it may only colour it pinkish, or give it a smoky or cloudy appearance. Occasionally clots of blood are passed with minimal colouring of the rest of the urine. Also, blood may appear only at the beginning or end of urination.

The male and female urinary tracts differ in that the male has a prostate gland and two seminal vesicles (*see illustration, page 183*). In females of child-bearing age, menstrual loss of blood may sometimes be mistaken for blood in the urine. In these cases, the bloody discolouration disappears as the period ends.

Some foods, particularly beetroot, can discolour the urine.

PROBABLE

CYSTITIS
URINARY TRACT INFECTION
KIDNEY INFECTION (PYELONEPHRITIS)

POSSIBLE

KIDNEY STONES
PROSTATITIS
BENIGN TUMOURS OF BLADDER/KIDNEY
ENLARGED PROSTATE
CANCER OF THE PROSTATE
CHRONIC NEPHRITIS
INJURY
EXERCISE

RARE

CANCER OF THE BLADDER/KIDNEY
WILM'S TUMOUR (CHILDREN)
ENDOCARDITIS
ANTICOAGULANT THERAPY
BILHARZIA

PROBABLE

■ CYSTITIS

Inflammation of the bladder lining, giving symptoms of urine infection.

* Frequent passing of urine.
* Burning or scalding as you urinate.
* Bursting to go but little result.
* Having to rush to pass urine with urgency.
* Dull ache in lower abdomen;may persist or worsen after urination.
* Fever; backache.
* Dark, cloudy or blood-stained urine.

Mild cases may clear without the use of antibiotics.

Children

Blood in the urine should always be taken seriously. Investigation will be required. While an adult may commonly suffer an infection causing blood to appear in the urine, this is not acceptable in children. Any urine infection in a child is an unusual event. It may be the first sign of an abnormality in the structure of the urinary tract. Rarely, accompanying swelling in the abdomen may be due to a Wilm's tumour.

■ URINARY TRACT INFECTION
Symptoms as for cystitis; in addition, there may be more severe symptoms such as:
* High fever.
* Pain in the back, loin, groin, front of abdomen.
* Vomiting, nausea.
* Sweating.
Will require antibiotics.

Resistance to infection
Increasingly, the bacteria causing urinary infections (and cystitis) do not respond to commonly prescribed antibiotics. This is known as bacterial resistance. Hence the importance, where possible, of sending a urine culture test to the laboratory before treatment starts.

■ KIDNEY INFECTION
Medical term: pyelonephritis. In this instance, the urine reveals infection but in addition the kidney itself is affected.
Symptoms as for cystitis, plus:
* Severe fever.
* Loin pain.
* Tenderness and sensitivity in the loin and side of abdomen.
* General feeling of being unwell.
Cystitis symptoms may not be marked, particularly in the early stages, when the symptoms may be confined largely to the upper abdomen; for example:
* Pain, vomiting, nausea.
Severe and advanced cases (also termed acute nephritis) will show diminished urine output, swelling of face and ankles, headache and other symptoms as above.

Female bladder

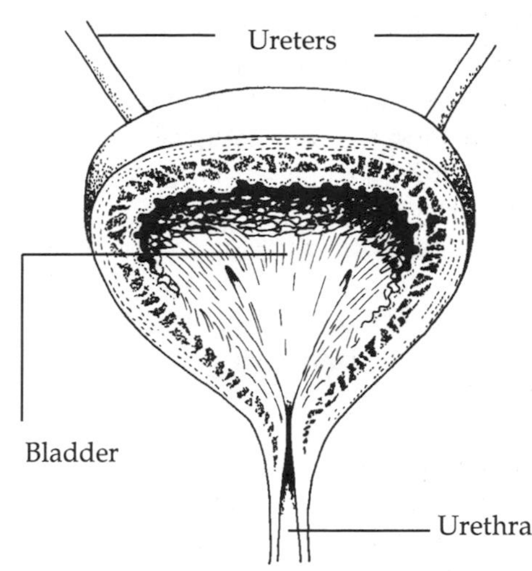

Male bladder

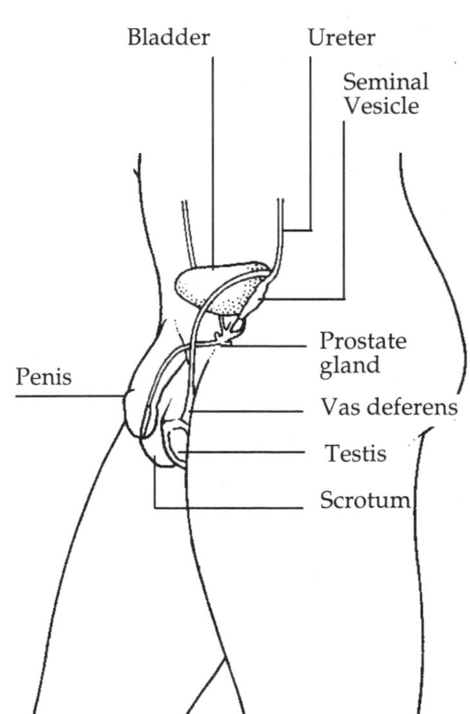

ABDOMEN: URINARY SYSTEM

Persistent symptoms
If you find symptoms persist after, or during, treatment with antibiotics, seek the result of your urine culture test. It will reveal which antibiotics can kill the bacteria. You will hear this referred to as a test to reveal bacterial sensitivity.

POSSIBLE

■ KIDNEY STONES
* Extremely severe pain, coming and going in unbearable waves, localized to one side over kidney area (loin and extreme side of abdomen).
* Vomiting.
* Sweating.

Typically, pain is said to spread from the back, around the side to the front of the abdomen and from there to the scrotum/groin area.

■ PROSTATITIS
Men only.
* Fever.
* Pain in the rectal area behind scrotum.
* Difficulty in passing urine.
* Sensation of passing hot urine.

■ BENIGN TUMOURS OF BLADDER/KIDNEY
Benign tumours of the urinary tract may cause bleeding. Symptoms may include:
* Painless haematuria (blood in urine), sometimes copious.
* General health is otherwise sound.
* Occasional obstruction of the passage of urine, due to blood clot.
* Anaemia (if there has been unrecognized bleeding for some time).

Urological assessment is required.

■ ENLARGED PROSTATE (MEN)
Difficulty in:
* Passing urine.
* Starting/stopping stream.
* Holding on to pass urine later.
* Preventing dribbling.

Inability to pass urine (retention of urine) requires medical intervention and catheterization.

■ CANCER OF PROSTATE
As for enlarged prostate. Diagnosis is frequently made only during operative intervention for enlarged prostate symptoms. After about 80 years of age, nearly every male has cancer of the prostate. It lies dormant in the gland, seldom causing severe problems at that age.

■ CHRONIC NEPHRITIS
* Nocturnal passage of large quantities of urine.
* Anaemia.
* Swelling.
* Shortness of breath.

■ INJURY
Injuries to the lower chest or pelvis (such as a blow or a stab wound) may damage underlying structures. If you have any blood in your urine after such an injury, whether in large or small quantities, you will need a full medical assessment in order to rule out serious damage to the urinary, or any other, system.

■ EXERCISE
It is now widely recognized that certain types of prolonged, repeated exercise — in particular, marathon running — may cause transient appearances of blood in the urine.

RARE

■ CANCER OF THE BLADDER/KIDNEY
Simple tests such as urine cytology, to examine the cell content of urine, can reveal the presence of malignant cells. Commonest in adults over 50.
* Painless haematuria — blood in urine.
* Pain in the loin.
* Swelling in loin or abdomen.
* Occasionally bone pain, due to spread of the tumour.
* Fever.
* Loss of weight.
* Anaemia.

■ WILM'S TUMOUR (CHILDREN)
The child has:
* One-sided, abdominal swelling.
* Painless blood in urine.
* Loss of appetite.
* Anaemia.
* Pain in late stages only.

Modern drugs and medical techniques have revolutionized the treatment of this condition. Early diagnosis is important.

■ ENDOCARDITIS
Multiple symptoms appear. The affected individual will be very ill. Symptoms include:
* Rash.
* Joint pains.
* Finger clubbing *(see page 296)*
* Fever.
* Chest pain.

■ ANTICOAGULANT THERAPY
Individuals who are taking anticoagulants (blood-thinning medication) may notice blood in their urine. They should consult their doctor, who will probably recommend reducing the dose of the drug.

■ BILHARZIA
Or schistosomiasis. Caused by an organism that inhabits water. Common in Africa, the West Indies, South America and Japan.
* Blood in urine.
* Pain on passing urine.
* Frequent passing of urine.

Cancer of the bladder can develop, as well as liver damage.

BLOOD IN URINE PLUS PAIN WHEN URINATING

The **probable** causes are: urinary tract infection; cystitis; kidney stone.

The **possible** causes are: acute pyelonephritis; prostatitis.

The **rare** cause is: bilharzia, above. All are covered under *BLOOD IN URINE, page 181.*

KIDNEY PAIN

The kidneys are situated at the side of the abdomen, towards the back. This area is known as the kidney or loin area.

The most likely cause of pain in this area is infection. There are a number of other possible causes all of which are convered in *BLOOD IN URINE, page 181 and BLOOD IN URINE PLUS PAIN WHEN URINATING, page 185.*

POSSIBLE
ACUTE PYELONEPHRITIS
PROSTATITIS
GONORHHEA

RARE
BILHARZIA

PAIN WHEN URINATING

Pain when passing urine is almost always a sign of cystitis or urine infection. Rarely, it can be one of the symptoms caused by a kidney stone or venereal infection such as NSU; *see NON-SPECIFIC URETHRITIS, page 188.* Also, the conditions listed under *BLOOD IN URINE, page 181* may all cause pain on passing urine as an early symptom, prior to the appearance of blood in the urine.

PROBABLE

- URINARY TRACT INFECTION
- CYSTITIS
- KIDNEY STONES

See BLOOD IN URINE, page 181.

POSSIBLE

- ACUTE PYELONEPHRITIS
- PROSTATITIS

See BLOOD IN URINE, page 181.

- GONORRHEA

A sexually transmitted disease. Often has no symptoms in women, although vaginal discharge, pelvic inflammatory disease and pain on passing urine may be experienced.

If a man has genital symptoms (and he may not) there will be:
* Urethral discharge.
* Discomfort on passing urine.
* Cloudy urine.
* Reddening and pain around the glans of the penis and urethra.
* Enlarged lymph nodes in the groin.

URINE LOOKS CLOUDY

A number of body products, but mainly blood, pus cells and microrganisms, can have this effect. Other symptoms may well be noticed at the same time. Urine which is concentrated but normal often goes cloudy if left standing. Cloudy appearance does not always signify illness.

PROBABLE
URINARY TRACT INFECTION
CYSTITIS
KIDNEY STONE

RARE

■ BILHARZIA *See page 185.*

PROBLEMS WITH URINATING

These include such symptoms as hesitancy or difficulty in starting to urinate; poor urine stream; and dribbling. The underlying causes tend to be either obstruction to the passage of urine; or structural abnormalities of the urinary tract; pain on urinating due to other causes such as infection; neurological defects may also affect urination.

PROBABLE
ENLARGED PROSTATE
BLADDER NECK OBSTRUCTION
URINARY TRACT INFECTION
GONORRHEA
NON-SPECIFIC URETHRITIS

POSSIBLE
IRRITABLE BLADDER
URETHRAL STRICTURE
PROSTATITIS
KIDNEY STONES
DRUGS

RARE
URETHRAL TUMOURS
SPINAL CORD DAMAGE
NEUROLOGICAL DISEASE
STROKE

PROBABLE

■ ENLARGED PROSTATE (MEN)
The gland can be enlarged as a result of benign or malignant tumours. Symptoms may be similar in both cases:
* Difficulty or hesitancy when starting to urinate.
* Poor stream.
* Terminal dribbling.
* Feeling as though the bladder has not emptied.
* Need to urinate in the night (nocturia).
* Sudden desire to pass urine.
* Some blood in the urine.
* Sometimes, leakage of urine: overflow incontinence. *See below.*
* Later in the disease, acute obstruction occurs with inability to pass urine at all. Severe abdominal pain develops because of the distended bladder.

In some cases, the obstruction develops so slowly that the bladder compensates by enlarging over a period of weeks or months. There is minimal discomfort and the urine frequently leaks out, without the individual being able to control it. The bladder does not empty properly, remaining distended, which is often seen as abdominal swelling. This type of urine loss is called overflow incontinence. Medical assessment is always needed. Cancer of the prostate may also cause:
* Back pain.
* Bone pain.

■ BLADDER NECK OBSTRUCTION
Symptoms similar to an enlarged prostate, but occurring in a

ABDOMEN: URINARY SYSTEM

younger age group and, occasionally, in women. Caused by overgrowth of the bladder muscle at its outlet to the urethra.

■ URINARY TRACT INFECTION
See page 183.

■ GONORRHEA
See page 186.

■ NON-SPECIFIC URETHRITIS
A common sexually transmitted disease caused by an organism called *Chlamydia*. Often there are no symptoms. If there are symptoms, men will have:
* Discomfort or itch on passing urine — making it difficult to urinate.
* Discharge (white, yellow) from penis.

Women will have:
* Pain/burning on passing urine.
* Occasional vaginal discharge.

The womb and Fallopian tubes can be infected; *see also PELVIC INFLAMMATORY DISEASE, page 352.*

NSU or NON-SPECIFIC URETHRITIS
It is very important to have this disease treated. Both partners must receive treatment, since, even with a total absence of symptoms, *Chlamydia* may be present. Untreated chlamydial infections can cause infertility.

POSSIBLE

■ IRRITABLE BLADDER
A term encompassing different symptoms caused by irritation of sensory or motor nerves to the bladder. Other causes (such as infection) must be excluded first. Special tests are needed to confirm the diagnosis. Symptoms can be one or more of:
* Frequent desire to pass urine (for example every 30 minutes).
* Pain over the bladder.
* Difficulty in passing urine (small volumes) and the bladder still feels full.
* Sometimes retention of urine occurs.
* Occasionally leakage of urine.

■ URETHRAL STRICTURE
Urethral stricture is a narrowing of the outflow passage from the bladder. It is commoner in men than women and may be caused by previous infection (perhaps gonorrhoea), surgery, damage by an instrument or a catheter (typically during delivery of a baby). Symptoms are progressive:
* Poor stream.
* Needing to strain hard to empty the bladder.

■ PROSTATITIS
See page 184.

■ KIDNEY STONES
See page 184.

■ DRUGS
See page 190.

RARE

■ URETHRAL TUMOURS
Benign or malignant tumours may cause progressive obstruction of

the urethra in men and women leading to:
* Poor stream.
* Need to strain harder than usual to pass urine.

■ SPINAL CORD DAMAGE
■ NEUROLOGICAL DISEASE
■ STROKE

See INCONTINENCE, page 177.

URINE DRIBBLES

Meaning either a poor stream, or dripping when trying to stop the flow of urine. Can be a form of incontinence.

The following, all dealt with in detail under *PROBLEMS WITH URINATING, pages 187-9,* can all be occasional causes of dribbling:

PROBABLE

■ ENLARGED PROSTATE

■ BLADDER NECK OBSTRUCTION

■ URINARY TRACT INFECTION

POSSIBLE

■ URETHRAL STRICTURE

■ PROSTATITIS

RARE

■ URETHRAL TUMOURS

URINATING AT NIGHT

You may often have had to get up during the night to pass urine, especially if you have had anything to drink within a few hours of going to bed. It is only abnormal if it develops as a new symptom, or if the number of times you get up increases significantly.

The commonest causes are an enlarged prostate gland (in men) and bladder irritability (in women).

Drugs are another important cause. Diuretics can often be taken once daily, in the morning, to minimize this difficulty. *See also PROBLEMS WITH URINATING, page 187 and URINATING TOO MUCH, OR TOO OFTEN, page 178.*

INABILITY TO URINATE

The medical term is anuria, and it is a serious problem. Don't confuse it with passing small volumes of concentrated urine infrequently, as in hot atmospheres or after strenuous exercise.

Urination can be arrested for three main reasons: first obstruction in the urethra *(see illustration page 183)*; second, failure of the bladder muscle to contract; and third, both kidneys may stop producing urine, because they are diseased, or because of disease elsewhere.

The first two cases are described as retention of urine. In all three

ABDOMEN: URINARY SYSTEM

cases, but particularly in the last, there may be a period of hours or days when the volume of urine gradually diminishes.

In the case of obstruction, there will be severe pain because of an increasingly distended bladder. Failure to excrete urine results in a build-up of toxic chemicals in the blood — and so it is, of course, a medical emergency.

PROBABLE
ENLARGED PROSTATE
KIDNEY STONES
URETHRAL STRICTURE

POSSIBLE
SURGERY OR INJURY
DRUGS
PYELONEPHRITIS
MALIGNANT TUMOURS
SHOCK
SEPTICAEMIA

RARE
INJURY
SPINAL CORD DAMAGE
NEUROLOGICAL DISEASE
POISONING
BLOOD TRANSFUSION
'CRUSH SYNDROME'

PROBABLE

■ ENLARGED PROSTATE
Much the most common reason (in men only) for a sudden inability to pass urine is an enlarged prostate gland causing an obstruction to the outlet from the bladder. You will feel pain as the bladder distends.

See page 187. All the other causes in this section are much less common.

■ KIDNEY STONE
See page 184. If a stone lodges in the urethra or at the neck of the bladder it will block the passage of urine. In addition to urine failure:
* Pain because of distended bladder.
* Inability to pass urine.

In men, pain may radiate to the tip of the penis.

■ URETHRAL STRICTURE
See page 188.

POSSIBLE

■ SURGERY OR INJURY
Any event that causes uncontrolled blood loss, and thus low blood pressure, can damage the kidneys and prevent them from working. The elderly, and those with chronically raised blood pressure, are vulnerable to this type of kidney damage.

■ DRUGS
A number of drugs may unexpectedly cause retention of

urine, particularly in patients with prostatic disease. Examples of are amitryptiline and imipramine.

■ PYELONEPHRITIS
See KIDNEY INFECTION, page 183.
In severe, untreated cases, the kidneys may be so badly damaged that they stop working. No urine is produced and the patient gets more and more sick, with:
* Weak pulse.
* Fever.
* Rigors.
* Vomiting.

■ MALIGNANT TUMOURS
Any malignant tumour of organs in or near the pelvis can involve parts of the urinary tract, blocking the urethra, ureters, bladder or kidneys. Cancers of the colon, uterus, ovaries, bladder and prostate can all have this effect. But it is very rare for anuria to be the first symptom, and the diagnosis has usually been made long before.

■ SHOCK
See also page 408. If shock is untreated or untreatable, the kidneys fail to produce urine and gradually urine output tails off to nothing. A grave condition, as is:

■ SEPTICAEMIA
Infection of the bloodstream and whole body from any cause. It can lead to shock *(see page 408)*, which, if untreated or severe, results in acute kidney failure.
Possibly fatal.

RARE

■ INJURY
Direct injury to the urethra (particularly in men) occurs typically in car accidents where the pelvis has been fractured. Because of the damage, urine cannot pass: a medical emergency which in most cases is promptly treated because the patient is already in hospital.
Very occasionally, a kick to the male scrotum, or crotch, may damage the urethra, or indeed the spinal cord.

■ SPINAL CORD DAMAGE
■ NEUROLOGICAL DISEASE
See page 178.

■ POISONING
A number of drugs may directly damage the kidneys, causing kidney failure. These include mercury, arsenic and bismuth.

■ BLOOD TRANSFUSION
If a patient is given blood which is incompatible with his or her own, the result may damage the kidneys and cause kidney failure. This is one reason why such care is taken when giving blood, and why it is only given when needed.

■ 'CRUSH SYNDROME'
Damaged leg muscles, sustained in a crushing injury to the lower limbs, causes toxins to enter the blood stream, resutling in direct damage to the kidneys.
Discoloured urine may be a symptom. The longer the limb is crushed, the greater the risk.

The Heart, Chest, Lungs and Breathing

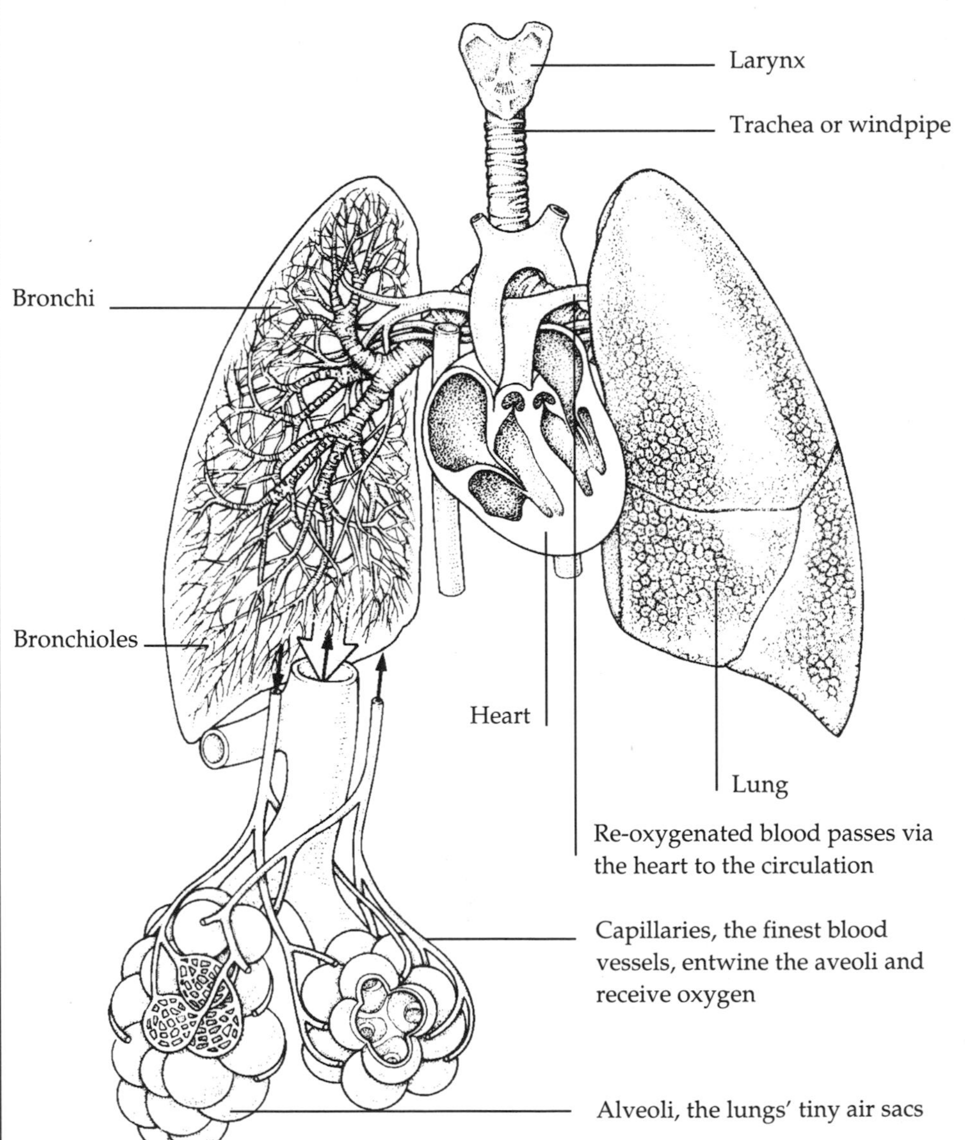

THE HEART INTRODUCTION

The heart is a superb pump: it gives years of service, responding automatically to all the varied demands of growth, activity and stress, so that we are rarely aware of its action.

How does the heart work? Two major systems, both electrical, control the heart's activity; there is also an in-built mechanism that increases the heart's muscular effort in response to high demand.

Emotion and stress are communicated to the heart by a branch of the nervous system called the autonomic system. It is this system that, for example, sets the heart beating faster when you notice a bull in the next meadow, and continues to increase both its speed and power when you realize there is no fence between you and the bull.

Next, within the heart itself there are two electrical pacemakers that control the rate of heartbeat. The main one, the sino-atrial node, normally sets the rate, transmitting a regular firing signal down an electrical pathway to the second pacemaker, a relay station called the atrio-ventricular node. From there, the signal to beat is transmitted to the rest of the heart by other electrical tracts. The atrio-ventricular node may also act as a pacemaker should the sino-atrial node fail for some reason.

Clearly there are many opportunities for malfunction in this system. If there is a problem, heart-rhythms may be too fast, too slow or irregular. These irregularities are felt in various ways: perhaps a thumping in the chest or a fluttering sensation; sometimes only skilled examination can detect a problem. This section analyses the possibilities.

It is important to realize that occasional rhythm disorders are common and are not necessarily a sign of disease. It is remarkable that there are not more of them, considering that an average heart will be making some three thousand million heart beats during a 70-year lifetime. Where irregularities decrease the pumping efficiency of the heart significantly, faintness, dizzy turns or, at worst, collapse may follow.

It is worth remembering that the diagnosis of heart irregularities, palpitations and similar disorders can be a highly technical matter; tremendous advances in research have been made in the last 25 years. The sources of electrical malfunction can now be traced to individual sections of wiring in the heart, in some cases allowing precise surgery to control the fault.

The journey from seeing the heart as a something that can break, to thinking of it as a mechanism that would do credit to a Grand Prix Formula 1 computerized fuel management system, has been long. As with so many other systems in our bodies, with a more precise understanding has come admiration of the sophistication of an activity we take for granted.

HEART MAKES EXTRA BEATS

This is a common symptom with an interesting explanation. What happens is that the heart beats twice in rapid succession. The extra beat goes unnoticed.

However, the next beat of the heart is delayed by a fraction of a second and it is this slight delay that you may be aware of. During the delay, blood continues to fill the heart, bringing into play an automatic mechanism that makes the heart beat more forcefully the fuller it gets. The next beat after the delay is, therefore, extra-powerful, and is felt as a thump in the chest.

PROBABLE
UNEXPLAINED
TOO MUCH COFFEE OR TEA
ALCOHOL
CIGARETTE SMOKING
FEVER

POSSIBLE
ANXIETY
INDIGESTION

RARE
COMPLICATIONS OF HEART ATTACK
EXCESS DIGOXIN
RHEUMATIC CARDITIS

PROBABLE

■ UNEXPLAINED
In the young or early middle-aged.
* Happens occasionally.
* Otherwise sound health.
* The extra beat causes no other symptoms: no faintness or chest pain.

■ TOO MUCH COFFEE OR TEA
The small amounts of caffeine in these drinks is responsible for the 'lift' they provide. Taken in excess — and what constitutes excess is an individual matter — the caffeine will cause:
* Rapid heart rate.
* Extra beats.
* Tremor.
* Anxiety.
* Increased output of urine.
Treatment is simply to reduce intake.

■ ALCOHOL
Alcohol has a direct effect on the heart. This increases with time and excessive use and can lead, in rare cases, to heart failure.

■ CIGARETTE SMOKING
Nicotine has a stimulant effect on the heart, increasing its rate and output. Extra beats are one reflection of this.

■ FEVER
Heart rate rises by about ten beats per 0.5 degree centigrade rise in temperature and increases the chance of extra beats. Some infections, as well as causing fever, can irritate the heart.

POSSIBLE

■ ANXIETY
Has its effect via the autonomic nervous system *(see THE HEART, INTRODUCTION , page 193)*, increasing the resting rate of the heart and the chances of extra beats. Other well-known features include:
* Tension in neck, shoulders.
* Constant feeling of pressure in the head.
* Excess sweating, tremor.
* Constantly feeling that something dreadful is about to happen.

■ INDIGESTION
It is uncertain how this affects the heart. Probably it results from a reflex action in those nerves which serve both the digestive system and the heart, though there may be direct irritation of the heart by a distended stomach. The features of indigestion are familiar.
* Bloating, belching.
* Acid, burning sensation after meals.
* Discomfort felt behind breast bone.

RARE

■ COMPLICATIONS OF HEART ATTACK
Extra beats are common in the days after a heart attack, often producing few symptoms. They have a different origin from benign extra beats, arising instead from spontaneous beating of the ventricles, the main pumping chambers of the heart. It is usual continuously to monitor the heart's electrical activity in the days after a heart attack looking for just such ventricular extra beats. They can be a warning of the sudden, uncontrolled activity of the ventricles which causes collapse and possibly sudden death.

■ EXCESS DIGOXIN
Digoxin is a drug widely used to treat heart failure. In excess it causes:
* Nausea and vomiting.
* Very slow pulse, with extra beats.
* Fatigue.
* Red or green hallucinations.
* Abdominal pains.

Mild cases can be corrected by temporarily dropping digoxin. Severe cases need intensive treatment in hospital.

■ RHEUMATIC CARDITIS
Fortunately this once-common disease in children is now a rarity in the developed world, but is still prevalent elsewhere.
* Begins two to three weeks after a bad sore throat.
* Joint pains; stiffness flitting from limb to limb.
* Fever.
* Rashes rapidly coming and going.
* Rapid pulse, extra beats.
* Sudden, fidgety movements.

There is danger of permanent damage to the heart valves leading later to heart disease.

HEART BEATS IRREGULARLY

People's sensitivity to their heartbeat varies. Some will feel that a very rapid but regular heart rhythm is an irregularity while others are able to focus precisely on the rhythm. A doctor will listen to the heartbeat through a stethoscope while feeling the pulse at the wrist: this often allows a simple rhythm to be diagnosed. Where there is doubt, an ECG recording of the heart is needed.

PROBABLE
SINUS ARRYTHMIA
SICK SINUS SYNDROME

POSSIBLE
EXTRA BEATS

RARE
PULMONARY EMBOLUS

PROBABLE

■ SINUS ARRHYTHMIA
Careful observation of your own pulse will reveal a change in rhythm as you breathe. The autonomic pathways mentioned elsewhere slow the heart as you breathe out and let it run faster as you breathe in. In some people this is particularly noticeable and may cause alarm. It is not a disease but an exaggeration of a normal reflex. The reflex is especially noticeable in children.
* Otherwise well.
* Clear relationship to breathing.
* Rhythm changes by about ten beats per minute faster or slower.

■ SICK SINUS SYNDROME
The sino-atrial node is the trigger in the heart that fires the electrical signal which causes the heart to beat *(see THE HEART, INTRODUCTION, page 193)*. So vital is this area of the heart that it has its own blood supply, but with age that blood supply can become diseased, resulting in erratic functioning of the trigger.
* Pulse may vary between very fast or very slow.
* Symptoms vary from none at all to fainting to loss of consciousness.

Treatment is usually a pacemaker.

POSSIBLE

■ EXTRA BEATS
Extra beats happening frequently will give the impression of an irregular heart beat. It is difficult to diagnose this situation without an ECG. Treatment aims to cure the underlying cause. *See HEART MAKES EXTRA BEATS, page 194.*

RARE

■ PULMONARY EMBOLUS
A blood clot blocking the circulation to part of the lung and usually

arising from a clot in a vein in the calf.
* Sudden feeling of pressure in the chest.
* Breathlessness.
* Possibly sharp chest pain and coughing blood.
* Heart rhythms varying from fast but regular to irregular.

PALPITATIONS (INCLUDING RAPID REGULAR HEART RATE)

Strictly speaking, 'palpitations' simply means an awareness of the beating of the heart but most people use it to mean not just awareness of the heart, but an awareness of some abnormality in the beat. So this symptom is subdivided into: **1** an awareness of a rapid but regular heartbeat; **2** irregular heartbeats; **3** rapid and irregular heartbeat. Extra heart beats (see the previous section) may also cause palpitations. There is much overlap between causes, so it is best to check in all relevant sections.

RAPID BUT REGULAR HEART RATE

PROBABLE
FEVER
EXERCISE
EMOTION
PAROXYSMAL TACHYCARDIA

POSSIBLE
PREGNANCY
ANAEMIA
HEART FAILURE
HYPERTHYROIDISM
DRUGS

RARE
ELECTRICAL CONDUCTION DISORDERS
BERI-BERI
BLEEDING
MYOCARDITIS
CARDIOMYOPATHY

PROBABLE

■ FEVER
Heart rate rises by ten beats per minute per 0.5 degree centigrade rise in temperature so that very high fevers will be accompanied by correspondingly high pulse rates. There is no specific treatment. Relief comes with the disappearance of fever.

■ EXERCISE
Any but the gentlest exercise will cause a modest rise in heart rate as the heart responds to the increased demand from the muscles and the lungs for larger quantities of oxygen-rich blood. Pulse rates above 120-130 per minute should be viewed with suspicion as a sign of over-exertion, under-fitness or some combination of the two. Chest pain appearing on exertion should always be checked *(see below)*.

THE HEART

■ EMOTION
Heart rate increases with excitement or acute emotional turmoil through the mechanism of the autonomic nervous system. Accompanying features include:
* Dry mouth.
* Rapid breathing.
* Tremor.

Such a response is normal in many circumstances such as fear, sexual arousal, sudden emotional shock. It is part of a co-ordinated system that prepares the body for exertion and to cope with stress. The response becomes abnormal if the individual begins to suffer from chronic anxiety, keeping his or her body in a constant state of increased arousal.

■ PAROXYSMAL TACHYCARDIA
A term used to cover all those otherwise unexplained episodes of rapid heart beat. There may be underlying causes such as an excess of stimulants such as coffee, alcohol, cigarettes *(see HEART MAKES EXTRA BEATS, page 194)*; or from heart disease *(see below)* or conduction disorders *(see below)*. Modern investigation involves wearing a recording device to capture the rapid rhythm on tape so that its nature can be analysed. Treatment can then be directed appropriately.
* Abrupt onset of rapid heart rate.
* Entirely regular rhythm.
* If rate is fast enough, faintness, lightheadedness.
* Stops as abruptly as it began.

Occasionally the rhythm is so fast or so prolonged that the heart becomes exhausted, causing breathlessness. This requires medical intervention to correct the rhythm.

POSSIBLE

■ PREGNANCY
There is a slight but sustained rise in heart rate during pregnancy, by about ten beats per minute. So if your usual rate is 70 per minute it can be expected to rise to 80 per minute. In this way the heart copes with the demands of the growing womb, placenta and baby.

■ ANAEMIA
In the anaemic state there is less capacity to transport oxygen around the body. The heart compensates by increasing its speed of pumping. This will only be a noticeable feature in cases of severe anaemia. Other symptoms are:
* Pallor.
* Slight breathlessness.
* Fatigue.

Anaemia alone is not a complete diagnosis. Further investigation is needed to find the cause.

■ HEART FAILURE
The early symptoms can be quite undramatic.
* Tiredness.
* Breathlessness on modest exertion.
* Increased heart rate.
* Swelling of ankles.
* Breathlessness lying flat.

Further tests are needed to determine the reason for the heart failure. *See also page 208.*

■ HYPERTHYROIDISM
The over-active gland can cause extra beats or a sustained rapid pulse. *See page 201.*

■ DRUGS
There are several over-the-counter drugs which can cause rapid heart rates in a few individuals, including cold remedies containing pseudoephedrine or phenylpropanolamine. Certain anti-asthmatic drugs such as salbutamol may have a similar effect.

RARE

■ ELECTRICAL CONDUCTION DISORDERS
These can be thought of as short circuits in the heart which disrupt the usually smoooth control of heartbeat *(see THE HEART, INTRODUCTION, page 193)*. Though relatively rare, there is much interest in these conditions for the light they shed on the electrical circuitry of the heart. There are surgical treatments available to cut the abnormal electrical circuits responsible for the disorder; otherwise they are controlled by medication. One of the least rare of the rare is the Wolff-Parkinson-White syndrome, which strikes most commonly at young adults:
* Recurrent bursts of rapid heart rate.
* Characteristic changes on the electrocardiograph.

■ BERI-BERI
A deficiency of vitamin B1, common in Third World countries where polished rice is a staple diet. In the developed world it occurs not infrequently in alcoholics with diets deficient in vitamins.
* Tender muscles.
* Rapid, bounding pulse.
* Often swollen ankles.
* Dementia, unsteady gait.

Rapid recovery is possible if it is recognized and treated early enough.

■ BLEEDING
Serious external bleeding is obvious, but internal bleeding can continue for several hours with few symptoms apart from:
* Increases in pulse rate.
* Thirst.
* Faintness on standing.

Eventually there will be:
* Pallor.
* Cold extremities.
* Confusion, collapse.

■ MYOCARDITIS
Inflammation of the heart muscle, due to a variety of causes most of which are infections. Some possibilities are influenza, trypanosomiasis, diptheria.
* Sudden onset of a feverish illness.
* Breathlessness, swelling of ankles.
* Breathlessness when lying flat.
* Rapid pulse.

The diagnosis requires blood tests, ECG recordings and, in difficult cases, biopsy of heart muscle.

■ CARDIOMYOPATHY
Another wide group of disorders where there is an non-inflammatory disturbance of the

heart muscle. Many cases are congenital or else related to alcoholism, or due to coronary artery disease.
* Heart failure, tiredness, breathlessness.
* In young people, fainting episodes during exercise.
* Rapid heart rates which may be both regular and irregular.

Diagnosis is by ECG and heart biopsy. These disorders need drug treatment to reduce the risk of sudden serious heart rhythm disturbance.

RAPID, IRREGULAR HEARTBEATS

Most such rhythms are either atrial fibrillations or atrial flutters. Atrial fibrillation is extremely common in old people. It may be the result of diseased coronary arteries, but frequently there are no other symptoms and life expectancy is little changed. The condition occasionally occurs in bursts in young people, when it is known as paroxysmal atrial fibrillation.

The basic defect is uncontrolled contraction of the atria, the small antechambers where blood first arrives in the heart. In fibrillation, the atria beat at rates upwards of 400 per minute, every one of those contractions sending off to the ventricles, the main pumping chambers, a signal to beat. Fortunately, only a fraction of these signals get through, but still enough to give a heart rate of between 100 to 150 beats per minute. The resulting heart rhythm is totally irregular, as felt at the pulse or as heard over the heart.

Not surprisingly, atrial fibrillation reduces the pumping efficiency of the heart and therefore causes breathlessness and swollen ankles. It also carries a small risk of sending off a blood clot which may cause a stroke or block arteries in the limbs. It is usual to treat fibrillation with digoxin, which both slows the rhythm and strengthens the heart. If there has been a previous blood clot, consideration would be given to reducing clotting of the blood by giving the anti-coagulant warfarin.

Atrial flutter is a less common condition in which the atria beat at a regular rate of between 240-360 beats per minute. This is still too fast to trigger regular contractions of the ventricles, which beat at half or a quarter of the atrial rate (90-180 per minute). Though strictly speaking this is a *regular* rapid heart rhythm, frequently the rate keeps changing abruptly, going from 180 to 120 to 90 and back again, giving an impression of irregularity. Atrial flutter is a symptom of serious heart disease and needs hospital treatment.

Episodes lasting longer than a few minutes can exhaust the heart, sending the individual into rapid heart failure, of which increasing breathlessness is a symptom.

The causes below relate mainly to atrial fibrillation.

PROBABLE
ISCHAEMIC HEART DISEASE
HYPERTHYROIDISM

POSSIBLE
MITRAL STENOSIS
ALCOHOL ABUSE
COMPLICATIONS OF HEART ATTACK

RARE
PNEUMONIA
ENDOCARDITIS
PERICARDITIS
ATRIAL SEPTAL DEFECT

PROBABLE

■ ISCHAEMIC HEART DISEASE
Blockage or 'furring up' of the blood supply to the heart. This may produce no symptoms other than fibrillation but frequently there will also be angina; *see page* 233.

■ HYPERTHYROIDISM
Atrial fibrillation may be the only sign of an over-active thyroid gland, especially in the elderly. Thus it is routine to check for this condition, whose other symptoms include:
* Sweating.
* Tremor.
* Increased appetite.
* Protruding eyes.

POSSIBLE

■ MITRAL STENOSIS
The mitral valve separates the left ventricle from the left atrium. Stenosis means that the valve has become narrowed and stiff. The most common reason for this was rheumatic fever, which is now rare in developed countries; the process of ageing is the usual reason nowadays. The condition gradually strains the heart, eventually causing heart failure.
* History of rheumatic fever years before.
* Mildest symptoms are just fibrillation.
* As the condition worsens, breathlessness, cough with bloodstained phlegm.
* Eventually swelling of ankles.
* There may be a permanent purple flush over the cheek bones.

Digoxin is used to treat mild cases, with surgery to the valve being reserved for more severe cases.

■ ALCOHOL ABUSE
Long-term alcohol abuse weakens the muscle of the heart, allowing various rhythm disorders to result.

■ COMPLICATIONS OF HEART ATTACK
In the hours and days after a heart attack the injured heart can produce a variety of disordered rhythms. The most worrying are ventricular tachychardias, where the ventricles go off into bursts of rapid beating which have the potential to turn into totally irregular, life-threatening beating.

THE HEART

Monitoring and dealing with these ventricular rhythms is one major reason for observation in a coronary care unit after a heart attack.
* Rapid thumping in the chest.
* Faintness.
* As the condition worsens, loss of consciousness.

RARE

■ PNEUMONIA
This severe chest infection can occasionally set off atrial fibrillation, which disappears after recovery. *See page 214.*

■ ENDOCARDITIS
An infection of the valves of the heart which usually attacks valves that are already abnormal, for example, after rheumatic fever. Fibrillation is just one of a variety of symptoms.
* Night sweats.
* Malaise.
* Clubbed fingernails.
* Splinter-like lines under the nails.
* Anaemia.

Aggressive long-term antibiotic treatment is needed to eradicate the infection.

■ PERICARDITIS
Constriction of the heart by fluid or by fibrous material can give rise to fibrillation.

See PERIODICAL EFFUSION, page 219.

■ ATRIAL SEPTAL DEFECT
There is a hole between the right and left sides of the baby's heart while it is in the womb. This hole should close at birth, but occasionally remains open. Symptoms can take years to develop, or a murmur may be detected on examination.
* Increased susceptibility to chest infections.
* Breathlessness.
* Palpitations including fibrillation are common.

HEART BEATS SLOWLY

By convention, this is taken as a rate of less than 60 beats per minute. Frequently it is an incidental finding in someone without symptoms, but very slow rates below 40 per minute are likely to cause dizziness, fainting and, in the elderly, confusion. There are two main causes of very slow rates. The pacemaker of the heart may be sending out a slow rhythm, or there is a block to the pacemaker rhythm so that the ventricles beat at a much slower rate than the signals sent from the pacemaker. An ECG is needed to diagnose these conditions properly.

PROBABLE
FITNESS
DRUG-INDUCED
HEART BLOCK

POSSIBLE
HYPOTHYROIDISM
SICK SINUS SYNDROME
CONGENITAL

RARE
CARDIOMYOPATHY

PROBABLE

■ FITNESS
A slow pulse is common in athletes and others who take regular physical exercise.

■ DRUG-INDUCED
Digoxin is one drug which causes a very slow pulse if given to excess. Another widely-used class of drugs called beta blockers slows the pulse to around 60 beats per minute but this is an intentional effect and is a sign of correct dosage. Beta blockers are used to treat high blood pressure and angina.

Beta-blockers are recognized as increasingly useful drugs. Sometimes they are used to quell the symptoms of anxiety. Due to their ability to stop palpitations and sweats, they are frequently taken by musicians and actors before performances. Olympic competitors in rifle shooting have been disqualified for using beta blockers to steady their aim.

■ HEART BLOCK
Heart block comes from disease of the conducting pathways that transmit the pacemaker signal to the rest of the heart. The ventricles have their own pacemaker which triggers them at 30 to 40 beats per minute, so there may be no dramatic symptoms, even with complete heart block. The usual reason for this problem is ageing or poor blood supply to the heart. It can also happen after a heart attack. Symptoms, in increasing order of severity, include:
* None at all, but noticed on an ECG tracing.
* Awareness of a slow thudding heart beat.
* Tiredness.
* Dizzy spells.
* Recurrent abrupt loss of consciousness.

Treatment is with an artificial pacemaker to maintain regular contraction.

POSSIBLE

■ HYPOTHYROIDSM
An under-active thyroid gland, whose other symptoms include:
* Coarse dry skin.
* Sensitivity to the cold.
* Slow thought, tiredness.
* Gruff voice.

Treatment with thyroid hormone has to be life-long.

■ SICK SINUS SYNDROME
Caused by the effects of ageing on the pacemaking area of the heart. This can cause rhythms from slow to fast and any combination in between.
* Palpitations.
* Dizzy spells.
* Tiredness.

See also page 196.

■ CONGENITAL
Some people are born with a slow pulse, but doctors would judge it prudent to search for other signs of heart disease such as heart murmurs or abnormal ECG traces.

RARE

■ CARDIOMYOPATHY
A general term for diseases of the heart muscle. The effect is to cause the rapid appearance of heart failure with either slow or rapid heart rates. *See also page 199.*

BREATHING INTRODUCTION

Why do we breathe? In order to provide the body's cells with the oxygen essential to their function. Also, to discharge carbon dioxide produced as a waste product of metabolism. Seen this way, breath is like the Olympic Flame, handed on from generation to generation. It is no surprise that breathing is affected by all sorts of bodily disorders. Commonest of these are simple obstructions of the airways; heart disease is also significant.

Breathing also helps to regulate the body's acid-alkaline balance. Because the brain controls breathing, disease — and also drugs — can affect those parts of it which, day in and day out, keep us breathing.

This section begins with causes of sudden breathlessness, then continues with breathlessness appearing over relatively long periods.

Causes tend to overlap, so you will see the same diagnoses coming up repeatedly. We make no apology for this: breathlessness is an alarming symptom, and some repetition is helpful.

HEIMLICH'S MANOEUVRE
There are references to this first-aid technique at several points in this section. It is named after the American physician who has promoted this simple, life-saving procedure, to be used on someone who is choking as a result of inhaling food or other solid objects.
* Stand behind the person choking.
* Extend your arms in a hug around their upper abdomen.
* With clenched fists make a hard, fast squeeze just under the breast bone.

The manoeuvre forces a blast of air out of the lungs, sufficient to dislodge something stuck in the upper airway. For full details see any modern manual of first aid.

See illustration on page 235.

RASPING, SNORING BREATHING

Also described as stertorous breathing. It is only occasionally a symptom of disease, usually just a nuisance.

Snoring is the result of vibration of the soft palate, which is at the back of the roof of the mouth. The cure is simply a matter of trying out different sleeping postures, or changing the number or firmness of your pillows.

PROBABLE
SNORING

POSSIBLE
ADENOIDS
STROKE
ALCOHOLIC STUPOR

RARE
PICKWICKIAN SYNDROME

PROBABLE

■ SNORING — *see above.*

POSSIBLE

■ ADENOIDS
These are pads of tissue at the back of the nose, similar to tonsils. They are probably intended to counter infection which might enter through the mouth and nose. In childhood, adenoids can grow so large that they obstruct nasal breathing. The child exhibits:
* Nasal speech.
* Snoring.
* Mouth breathing.
* Recurrent ear infections.

Treatment is surgical removal of the adenoids, if there is no sign of a natural decrease in their size.

■ STROKE
A blood clot or bleeding in the brain causing:
* One-sided paralysis.
* Coma.
* Stertorous breathing, typically if the individual goes into a deep coma.

■ ALCOHOLIC STUPOR
Drinking to the point of collapse frequently gives this symptom.

RARE

■ PICKWICKIAN SYNDROME
A good example of how something that was long thought to be merely a humorous observation has proved to be truly an abnormality. Charles Dickens' sleepy fat man is now understood to have suffered from partial obstruction of the trachea (a major airway), during sleep. This causes partial suffocation until the individual briefly awakes, snorts to relieve the obstruction, and goes back to sleep again. The typical picture is:
* Greatly overweight.
* Very large collar size a pointer.
* Daytime drowsiness.

Occasionally people with this condition benefit from oxygen masks during sleep. With the emphasis on scientific respectability, the imprecise but wholly apt name 'Pickwickian syndrome' is being replaced by the accurate but boring name, Sleep Apnoea Syndrome.

CHEST

HOARSE, 'WHEEZY' INTAKE OF BREATH

This is probably a stridor: *see FOREIGN BODY, PAGE 227.*

CHEST ABNORMALLY SHAPED

PROBABLE
CONGENITAL
ASTHMA

POSSIBLE
CHRONIC OBSTRUCTIVE AIRWAYS DISEASE

RARE
RICKETS

PROBABLE

■ CONGENITAL
Twists of the spine can gradually produce a mis-shapen chest. These can be treated if spotted early enough.
* Seen from behind, the spine is curved.
* Curve becomes more prominent on bending forward.

Another congenital abnormality gives a funnel-shaped chest with a depressed breastbone. This too can be corrected by surgery, which is recommended if there is a risk of the depression pressing on the heart.

■ ASTHMA
Chronic, severe asthma which is inadequately treated can result in a young adult who has:
* A broad, over-inflated chest.
* Prominent rib margins.
* Prominent breastbone, which gives a pointed appearance to the front of the chest.

The reason is thought to be years of extra effort by the muscles between the ribs, which have to work harder in asthma. They gradually pull the lower ribs into a prominent shape. This is seen less and less as asthma treatment improves. The condition rarely causes anything other than cosmetic problems and can be corrected surgically.

POSSIBLE

■ CHRONIC OBSTRUCTIVE AIRWAYS DISEASE
A general term covering chronic bronchitis and emphysema. The continual effort of breathing in these conditions can eventually, in adult life, cause a barrel-shaped chest. *See page 222.*

RARE

■ RICKETS
This disease, due to lack of vitamin D, can give rise to unsightly prominent joints where the ribs join the breast bone. Now a rarity in developed countries.

BREATHLESSNESS, RAPID ONSET

Considered here are attacks of breathlessness which happen rapidly, yet fall short of abrupt suffocation or asphyxia. There should be little difficulty in recognizing the seriousness of the situation, except perhaps with babies and children: you should be alert to drowsiness and breathlessness which interferes with feeding.

PROBABLE
ASTHMA
BRONCHIOLITIS
CHEST INFECTION

POSSIBLE
HEART FAILURE
ACUTE OR CHRONIC BRONCHITIS

RARE
ALLERGIC ALVEOLITIS

PROBABLE

■ ASTHMA

This common illness is more of a nuisance than a disability for most asthmatics most of the time. However, asthma can turn suddenly and unpredictably into a life-threatening condition.

Muscle surrounds the airways right down into the lungs. Asthma results from excessive constriction of that muscle, which narrows the airways and increases the effort required to shift air into the lungs. As a cause of chronic breathlessness *ASTHMA* is covered in detail under *BREATHLESSNESS AND WHEEZE, page 212*. Severe, acute asthma is a potential killer. There is danger for the known asthmatic who underestimates the severity of an attack. There is also danger for someone whose first attack of asthma is severe, unrecognized and who has no standard treatment at hand.

* Poor response to usual medication.
* Wheeze, especially breathing out.
* The chest feels 'tight'.
* Sweating, breathlessness, rapid pulse.
* Neck muscles strain in an attempt to increase breathing.
* As attack worsens, cyanosis, tiredness, pallor, drowsiness.
* Confusion, coma.
* Deterioration can take several hours or just a few minutes.

Known asthmatics must seek, or be given, help if their regular treatment becomes ineffective.

■ BRONCHIOLITIS

This is an infantile equivalent of asthma. It is a winter disease, caused by a particular virus. It occurs in epidemics.

* Initially the baby is snuffly, with a slight cough indistinguishable from a common cold.
* Wheezing begins and worsens over a few hours.
* Breathing produces a crackling sound, also felt through the chest.

Chest

* Breathlessness interferes with feeding.
* Breathing becomes rapid, often with grunting.
* At worst, pallor, cyanosis of lips.

First aid: put the child in a steamy atmosphere, which can improve the situation dramatically. Subsequent treatment in hospital includes the use of oxygen and humidity. Babies with this condition have an increased chance of being asthmatic later in life.

Children whose parents smoke are three times more likely to enter hospital in their first year with a chest condition than infants of non-smokers.

■ CHEST INFECTION

A severe chest infection or pneumonia can rapidly progress to difficulty in breathing.
* Wet cough, with coloured phlegm.
* High temperature.
* Flaring nostrils.
* Rapid breathing.
* Pain over the affected part of the chest.
* Cyanosis of lips and tongue.
* Sometimes bloodstained phlegm.
* Confusion.

This is more likely in the elderly or in those who are debilitated for other reasons.

POSSIBLE

■ HEART FAILURE

Predominantly a disease occurring later in life. There is often a history of heart trouble, perhaps heart attack, high blood pressure.
* Early symptoms are tiredness, breathlessness on exertion.
* Swelling of ankles
* Breathlessness worse on attempting to lie flat.
* You need to stack up pillows in order to sleep.
* In more advanced cases you may wake from sleep with a feeling of suffocation.
* Copious, frothy, pinkish phlegm.
* Relief gained from sitting upright for a few minutes.

This situation may need urgent medical help.

■ ACUTE OR CHRONIC BRONCHITIS

A chest infection can be the minor, extra stress that pushes the individual with chronic bronchitis into respiratory failure. The already limited effort that someone can put into breathing becomes too little to expel waste carbon dioxide, or to take in fresh oxygen. The result is the equivalent of suffocation over a short period.
* Severe headache.
* Warm, blue hands; rapid pulse; twitching of muscles.
* Agitation, confusion worsening to coma.

This situation needs urgent help.

RARE

■ ALLERGIC ALVEOLITIS
The alveoli are the sacs in the lung where carbon dioxide is exchanged for oxygen. An allergic reaction causes inflammation in these sacs. The consequent swelling interferes with efficient gas transfer. The commonest cause is an allergy to mouldy hay, known as farmer's lung, and is widespread in areas of non-mechanized farming.
* Breathlessness, wheezing within a few hours of exposure.
* Fever, cough and malaise, joint pains.
* Symptoms take a few days to disappear. The chronic condition shows:
* Recurrent difficulty in breathing.
* Clubbed (highly curved) fingernails *(see illustration on page 296)*.Treatment is to avoid exposure to the cause of the allergy.

BREATHLESSNESS OVER DAYS, WEEKS OR MONTHS

This type of breathlessness does not have particularly prominent secondary symptoms, at least not at first. And there are no hard and fast distinctions between all the conditions which share these symptoms, so read this section right through before drawing any conclusions.

Breathlessness that sets in over only a few days or weeks clearly needs investigation.

Breathlessness that appears more gradually can be more puzzling. It should be related to your usual level of exercise. If your principal form of physical activity is opening the garage door, do not be too surprised at your breathlessness if you have to change a tyre. Remember also that your ability to cope with sudden effort can decline completely unnoticed as long as you are still able to perform your regular activities. For example: shopping trips and gentle strolls may present no problem, but you may be alarmed at how breathless you become climbing stairs. This does not in itself suggest disease, just being out of training.

But there is a pitfall in this: while it is natural to limit exertion to the level you know you can tolerate, that level may actually be abnormally low. The best guide is to compare yourself with others of your age and general fitness. If you are the one who has to rest half-way round a golf course you may have a problem.

Bear this in mind before you jump to conclusions. Ask yourself a few questions. How long since you last did any exercise that made you sweat? Have you gained weight recently? Do you smoke heavily?

Honest answers to these questions may be illuminating.

CHEST

To improve your fitness, aim to achieve shortness of breath and sweating, over a period of 20 minutes, at least twice a week.

There are other, everyday circumstances in which breathlessness is normal. Excitement, fear and anger all generate a high breathing rate and may make you feel breathless. Only after you have excuded all these possibilities is it reasonable to wonder whether your breathlessness is a symptom of illness:

PROBABLE
HEART FAILURE
PSYCHOLOGICAL

POSSIBLE
PREGNANCY
ANAEMIA
LUNG EFFUSION
LUNG CANCER

RARE
SKELETAL ABNORMALITIES
PNEUMONCONIOSIS
MOUNTAIN SICKNESS
FIBROSING ALVEOLITIS

PROBABLE

■ HEART FAILURE
Mainly a problem for older people. The symptoms of heart failure can mistakenly be put down to ageing unless a dramatic or sudden deterioration occurs. There will often be a history of high blood pressure, angina or heart attack. Early symptoms are:
* Tiredness, decreased tolerance of exercise.
* Swelling of ankles.
* Loss of appetite.
* Later, breathlessness while lying flat in bed.
* You sleep stacked up on pillows.
* Breathlessness wakes you at night, with a frothy cough; symptoms pass off after you have sat upright for a while.

In the elderly, tiredness alone can be the only symptom of heart failure. Treatment is currently undergoing a great change for the better, so that most people can be helped considerably.

■ PSYCHOLOGICAL
A possibility in a younger person: friends or colleagues may notice over-breathing — often the individual leads a stressful life.
* Describes an inability to breathe in deeply enough.
* Otherwise sound health.
Reassurance, and thorough investigations, revealing nothing, generally help these cases.

POSSIBLE

■ PREGNANCY
A common feature of middle to late pregnancy, when the womb is enlarged and presses against the diaphragm
.

■ ANAEMIA
Blood carries oxygen around the body, so that if the volume of blood in one's body drops significantly, breathlessness ensues, together with:
* Tiredness, easy fatigue.
* Pallor on the under-surfaces of eyelids, nail beds.

Symptoms of the disorder which causes the anaemia may also be apparent, for example blood loss, poor diet. Simple investigations should quickly confirm the diagnosis.

■ LUNG EFFUSION
The lungs react to irritation in the same way that the skin reacts to a minor burn. Tissue fluid seeps out, collecting in a pool at the base of the lungs. If this pool grows large enough, it compresses the lung above, reducing its ability to function and causing breathlessness. There are no specific symptoms to indicate an effusion: it has to be detected by medical examination or chest X-ray. There is nearly always some predisposing condition. The commonest are severe heart failure, pneumonia, pulmonary embolus and lung cancer. These cause symptoms considered under *HEART FAILURE, page 208, and on pages 214, 218 and 224.*

■ LUNG CANCER
A tumour may block off a major airway, thereby putting out of action all or part of a lung, and causing breathlessness. This is not a common way for a growth to show itself. More frequent is a cough with blood or chest pain. Considered in detail on *page 224*.

RARE

■ SKELETAL ABNORMALITIES
Gross distortions of the chest wall cause the ribs to squash the lungs and heart so that their expansion is restricted. These deformities, called *KYPHOSIS or KYPHOSCOLIOSIS*, are discussed on *page 288.*

■ PNEUMOCONIOSIS
A group of occupational lung diseases caused by years of exposure to dust. Common ones are silicosis (miners, pottery workers) and pneumoconiosis and asbestosis (coal miners). The symptoms are:
* Progressive breathlessness on exertion.
* Cough.

Dust control and masks reduce the risks for workers in hazardous industries.

■ MOUNTAIN SICKNESS
The direct effect of the lack of oxygen at altitudes of about 3,500 metres or higher. The young and fit are at risk just as much as the unfit or elderly; in fact, possibly more at risk because the young will be climbing faster. This is a dangerous condition. Early

symptoms are:
* Breathlessness.
* Headache, tiredness.
If ignored these will progress to:
* Profuse bloodstained cough.
* Nausea, confusion.
* Coma.

All cases need descent to lower altitudes; serious cases may also require resuscitation.

■ FIBROSING ALVEOLITIS
The final stage of *ALLERGIC ALVEOLITIS* *(see page 209)*, or sometimes of unknown origin.
* Chronic breathlessness.
* Clubbed fingernails *(see page 296).*
* Cough, cyanosis.

BREATHLESSNESS AND WHEEZE

Excluding acute chest infection, considered *on page 224,* this extremely common combination points to narrowing of airways, producing obstructed air flow. Often there is an allergic factor: many asthmatics, sensitive to dust and fumes, exhibit these symptoms for hours, even days on end.

PROBABLE
ASTHMA
CHRONIC BRONCHITIS
EMPHYSEMA

POSSIBLE
OCCUPATIONAL ASTHMA

RARE
DRUG REACTION
ASPERGILLOSIS

PROBABLE

■ ASTHMA
Some 10 per cent of the population suffer from asthma, and the number is believed to be rising. The classic features are:
* Recurrent breathlessness.
* Wheeze and cough.
* In children, persistent night-time cough.
* Common colds that regularly go to the chest.

Doctors are often disinclined to label a child as asthmatic until there is no doubt: it can be a disservice to the child. Helpful treatment is available. *See also page 220.*

■ CHRONIC BRONCHITIS
Believed to result from years of exposure to fumes, chemicals and smoke, of which cigarette smoke is the main avoidable culprit. The prime features are the gradual manifestation of:
* Increasingly persistent cough.
* Wheeze.
* Breathlessness.
* Large amounts of phlegm ('smoker's cough').

Chronic bronchitis does not have the same reputation as lung cancer, yet quality of life can be considerably reduced. Perpetual breathlessness, in severe cases, is every bit as miserable as the final stages of cancer.

■ EMPHYSEMA
Whereas normal lungs look like sponges with millions of tiny bubbles, in emphysemic lungs, large holes replace many of the small bubbles. This is much less efficient as a means of gas exchange, hence the breathlessness. Emphysema and chronic bronchitis nearly always co-exist, the symptoms emerging over several years.
* Breathlessness and wheeze on increasingly modest exertion.
* A barrel chest.
* Lips pursed to breathe out.
* Eventual cyanosis (blueness) of hands and tongue.

The damage to the structure of the lungs cannot be reversed.

Treatment aims to prevent further damage by discouraging smoking, preventing exposure to fumes and treating associated bronchitis.

POSSIBLE

■ OCCUPATIONAL ASTHMA
This includes many conditions associated with specific industries, in particular those producing flax, sisal, hemp or cotton. Bysinnosis is one of the commonest of these problems. It produces an asthma-like condition through allergy to cotton dust. Rare now in developed countries, but still seen frequently in India and other developing countries.
* A hazard in cotton mills.
* 'Monday morning breathlessness' on re-exposure to cotton dust.
* Wheeze, breathlessness.

RARE

■ DRUG REACTION
The drugs in widest use that can produce this reaction are beta-blockers, used to control high blood pressure or angina; aspirin and similar anti-rheumatic drugs, and a few anti-cancer drugs such as methotrexate, may also be responsible.

■ ASPERGILLOSIS
An infection caused by a fungus called aspergillus, commonly found in rotting and decaying vegetation. For most people, aspergillus is harmless. If the lungs are damaged by previous infection (such as tuberculosis) or asthma, the fungus may cause the following symptoms:
* Recurrent wheeze, cough.
* Feverish episodes.

The diagnosis is determined by blood tests and allergy testing.

BREATHLESSNESS AND COUGH

PROBABLE
CHEST INFECTION

POSSIBLE
CHRONIC BRONCHITIS
EMPHYSEMA
PNEUMONIA

CHEST

RARE
BRONCHIECTASIS
LUNG CANCER
TUBERCULOSIS

PROBABLE

■ CHEST INFECTION
Recognized by the combination of:
* Cough with yellow or green phlegm.
* Fever, modest degree of malaise.
* Breathlessness plus wheeze.

All these appear in only a couple of days, often preceded by a sore throat and a common cold.

Antibiotic treatment is usual for these common and not very serious infections.

POSSIBLE

■ CHRONIC BRONCHITIS
The strict medical definition is:
* A cough productive of phlegm for at least three months of the year for at least two consecutive years.

It is well known that smokers and workers in dusty environments risk developing the condition, but it also has an association with cold damp climates. The excessive production of phlegm amounts to an exaggeration of the lungs' defence mechanism against infection and dust: the gooey mucus 'traps' the foreign matter, which the lungs then try to expel by coughing. In permanent overdrive, the lungs begin losing their efficiency. Individuals are at risk of frequent chest infections and, in the long run, progressive shortness of breath.

Though the disease cannot be reversed, further deterioration can be delayed by giving up smoking and by avoiding dust and fumes.

■ EMPHYSEMA
Often co-exists with chronic bronchitis, but can only be diagnosed by chest X-ray in combination with lung function tests. However, it is suggested by:
* A barrel chest.
* Lips pursed to breathe out.
* At worst, cyanosis (blueness) of lips and nail beds.

■ PNEUMONIA
A serious chest infection, usually of rapid onset with:
* High fever, chills.
* Rapid breathing and cough.
* Phlegm may be rust-coloured or obviously contain blood.
* Aching, or severe sharp pain, in the chest.

Occasionally, especially in the elderly, pneumonia exhibits less clear-cut symptoms, and is suggested by abrupt weakness and fever. Aggressive antibiotic therapy means that pneumonia is no longer the feared killer it once was, though it is still a worry in the elderly or those with pre-existing problems such as heart disease, chronic bronchitis and diabetes. *See also page 222.*

RARE

■ <u>BRONCHIECTASIS</u>
In this disease, once far more common than it is today, the lung structure breaks down, making the lungs susceptible to pockets of chronic infection.
* Initially, frequent chest infections.
* Constant production of large amounts of coloured phlegm.
* Phlegm often bloodstained.
* As it worsens, breathlessness, clubbed (highly curved) finger-nails.
* Poor growth in children; fatigue.

■ <u>LUNG CANCER</u>
This diagnosis must be considered not only for a cough with breath-lessness but for any persistent breathing problem. Adult smokers are particularly vulnerable. *See page 224.*

■ <u>TUBERCULOSIS</u>
Now uncommon in developed countries, except in the poor, immigrants from the Third World, and those who neglect themselves, such as alcoholics. The usual features are:
* Malaise, weight loss.
* Cough, often bloodstained.
* Breathlessness resulting from complications.

Treatment, though prolonged, cures the disease.

BREATHLESSNESS AND FEELING TIRED/EXHAUSTED

Though lung disease is usually the cause of breathlessness, it can arise from subtle changes in the condition of the heart, blood or metabolism. Fatigue will then be a prominent symptom, before breathlessness is noticeable. Breathlessness in these situations may result from an imbalance between acid and alkaline chemicals in the body. Major disturbances of regular body functions, such as diabetes and kidney failure, generates excess acid which the body tries to reduce by blowing off more carbon dioxide with heavy deep breathing.

Remember that prolonged or severe breathlessness, for any reason, will eventually cause fatigue simply through exhaustion and a chronic lack of oxygen.

PROBABLE
ANAEMIA
HEART FAILURE

POSSIBLE
HEART DISEASE

RARE
DIABETIC COMPLICATIONS
KIDNEY FAILURE

CHEST

PROBABLE

■ ANAEMIA
Blood carries oxygen around the body so that if the volume of blood drops significantly breathlessness ensues, together with:
* Tiredness, easy fatigue.
* Pallor, particularly the undersurfaces of eyelids, nail beds.

Symptoms of the disorder which causes the anaemia may be evident, for example blood loss, poor diet. Simple investigations indicate the diagnosis. *See pages 417 and 419.*

■ HEART FAILURE
Breathlessness is a frequent symptom in the middle-aged; in the elderly an early indication of heart failure can be unusual tiredness. Once this is recognized, look for other symptoms of heart failure:
* Swollen ankles.
* Breathlessness when lying flat.

See page 208.

POSSIBLE

■ HEART DISEASE
Disturbance of heartbeat with rhythms either too fast or too slow, felt as a flutter in the chest, or as palpitations. These are inefficient rhythms producing breathlessness with fatigue. *See pages 193-204.*

Other heart diseases, for instance valve problems, cause breathlessness by decreasing the efficiency of the heart. Those with a history of rheumatic fever may find this a problem. In general, these disorders can only be detected by medical examination.

RARE

■ DIABETIC COMPLICATIONS
Diabetes is the condition that produces a high blood sugar level. The early symptoms are:
* Passing large amounts of urine.
* Thirst.
* Weight loss.

In young people, onset tends to be rapid, over a couple of weeks. In older people it may go unnoticed, apart from slightly increased urine output and a vague sense of tiredness.

Diabetes is caused by a lack of insulin, needed by the body's cells to make use of sugar. Thus, there are high levels of sugar in the bloodstream, yet the cells are unable to use it. But life must go on: the cells' metabolism turns to alternative means of generating energy. The trouble with these is their tendency to generate large amounts of acidic waste products. The body tries to compensate by blowing off large amounts of carbon dioxide, hence heavy breathing.

Meanwhile, sugar in the bloodstream spills out through the kidneys, dragging water with it. The final result is the dangerous state called diabetic ketoacidosis, and is a major medical emergency.
* Dehydration, dry mouth, intense thirst.
* Deep, sighing breathing.
* Sweet smell on breath.
* Confusion, nausea.

Rapid treatment is life-saving.

Known diabetics may fall into this state during other stressful illnesses.

■ KIDNEY FAILURE
Early symptoms are only:
* Increased passage of urine.
* Tiredness.

Blood tests at this stage allow diagnosis and consequent changes in diet which may give years of reasonable health. If eventually the kidneys fail there is an array of symptoms, including:
* Tiredness, developing into confusion.
* Deep, gasping breathing.
* Dry, furred tongue.
* Nausea, hiccups.
* Itching, anaemia.

The development of kidney transplantation has revolutionized the treatment of this condition.

BREATHLESSNESS AND CHEST PAIN

Symptoms of this kind are often caused by serious disruption of the output from the heart, or by lung malfunction. If breathlessness is the most prominent symptom, *see ASPHYXIA, page 226, or BREATHLESSNESS, RAPID ONSET, page 207,* as well as reading this section. If chest pain is most prominent, look at the sections on heart beat. In view of the importance of these symptoms, some of the information found there is repeated here.

PROBABLE
CHEST INFECTION
HEART ATTACK
PLEURISY
PNEUMOTHORAX

POSSIBLE
PNEUMONIA
PULMONARY EMBOLUS
LUNG CANCER
IRREGULAR HEARTBEAT

RARE
PERICARDIAL EFFUSION
HEART TAMPONADE

PROBABLE

■ CHEST INFECTION
The gradual appearance of fever, cough and phlegm is often accompanied by a slight ache over both lungs. *See page 208.*

■ HEART ATTACK
See also page 229.

In a middle-aged person, suspect a heart attack if there is:
* Sudden central chest pain.
* Sweating.
* Pain radiating up to the jaws or into the left arm.
* Breathlessness.

These are the classic symptoms, but in quite a few cases the heart attack is 'silent', meaning that chest pain is not the most obvious

CHEST

feature or may be absent. Instead, a heart attack may be suspected on the basis of:
* Sudden general tiredness.
* Breathlessness as a new symptom.
* Sudden worsening of existing breathlessness.
* Symptoms of heart failure: swollen ankles, breathlessness when lying flat, breathlessness during the night, tiredness.

Recently, there have been major advances in treatment so that early recognition of the problem means a much-improved chance of recovery. It is, therefore, essential to establish the diagnosis as soon as possible. Heart attacks are most common in old people, but are possible at any age; so always take dramatic chest pain seriously.

■ PLEURISY

The pleurae are the thin membranes that surround the lungs. They become inflamed for a variety of reasons, particularly infection, when you can feel a typical pain.
* Knife-like pain over a small area of the chest.
* Pain worse on breathing in.
* Breathlessness as a consequence of avoiding deep breathing.

Pleurisy commonly accompanies a chest infection. In this case, it sets in gradually over a few hours. A *PNEUMOTHORAX (see below)* causes sudden pleuritic pain.

Treatment aims both to relieve the pain and to cure the underlying condition.

■ PNEUMOTHORAX

Collapse of part of a lung, sometimes the whole lung. Quite common and needing appropriate treatment. However, pneumothorax is rarely a serious problem, though the pain may be disabling.

POSSIBLE

■ PNEUMONIA

Suggested by a combination of:
* High fever.
* Rapid breathing.
* Painful cough.

See also page 214.

■ PULMONARY EMBOLUS

A blood clot which lodges in the blood supply to a lung. Sudden breathlessness follows the reduction in the lung's efficiency. Pain in the chest is not always a symptom, but will certainly be felt if the affected part of the lung begins to die from lack of oxygen. A particular risk after a heart attack, major surgery, thrombosis in leg.

■ LUNG CANCER

This diagnosis should always be borne in mind when unusual breathlessness and chest pain are the symptoms in elderly individuals, particularly those who smoke. *See page 224.*

■ IRREGULAR HEART BEAT

Very rapid or very slow heart rates can cause chest pain, with breathlessness a result of low output from the heart. *See sections on heartbeat, pages 193-204.*

RARE

■ PERICARDIAL EFFUSION
The heart is surrounded by a lining which can become inflamed. This is known as pericarditis. The fluid released from inflammation collects around the heart, interfering with its ability to pump blood effectively. Most often, this condition follows a heart attack. Viral infections, trauma and kidney failure are other causes.
* At first, the sharp central chest pain of pericarditis.
* Pain seems to radiate to shoulders.
* Often relieved by bending forward; worse lying down.
* Breathlessness, worsening as fluid builds up.

This is not an easy diagnosis, but may be the reason for breathlessness after certain diseases. X-rays and irregular readings recorded by ECG machines help confirm the diagnosis.

■ HEART TAMPONADE
This is the most severe effect of a pericardial effusion. The condition may begin with pericarditis *(above)*, or perhaps an injury to the heart, such as a stab wound. Fluid or blood gathers around the heart until it is squashed and unable to pump. There are no straightforward or obvious symptoms apart from rapidly increasing breathlessness after the illness or injury which caused the pericarditis; occasionally distended veins in the neck may also be observed.

Diagnosis is by ECG recording and chest X-ray. Treatment is to drain off the fluid.

CHEST SYMPTOMS, COUGH INTRODUCTION

Cough is generally a reflex action of irritated lungs or voice box, or lungs trying to expel phlegm or a foreign body. Most coughs are easily recognizable for the minor problem they are, but sometimes need to be taken more seriously because of duration, pain or associated symptoms. In the very young and the elderly, coughs can be a sign of more serious illness and need more attention.

DRY COUGH WITHOUT PHLEGM

Few of us pass a year without suffering this sort of cough. It nearly always reflects minor irritation of the lungs rather than more serious disease. It passes in a week or so of using simple remedies, such as aspirin or plenty of fluid and avoiding dry atmospheres.

If there are other symptoms of illness, such as raised temperature lasting more than 48 hours, or if the cough becomes chronic, it would be sensible to see a doctor.

CHEST

PROBABLE
COMMON COLD OR UPPER RESPIRATORY TRACT INFECTION (URTI)
IRRITANT ATMOSPHERE
POST NASAL DRIP

POSSIBLE
LARYNGITIS
TRACHEITIS
ASTHMA
HABIT
WHOOPING COUGH

RARE
LUNG CANCER
ASBESTOSIS, ALLERGY, FIBROSING ALVEOLITIS
DRUG SIDE EFFECT
DISEASE OF LARYNX

PROBABLE

■ COMMON COLD OR URTI
Cough, commonly accompanied by other common cold symptoms such as:
* Rapid onset of sneezing and aches.
* Usually cures itself.

■ IRRITANT ATMOSPHERE
* Dry, dusty conditions.
* Cough is relieved in normal atmosphere.
* Not otherwise ill.

■ POST NASAL DRIP
Secretions from the nose or from the sinuses run to the back of throat and provoke cough. Treatment is aimed at the underlying condition, the commonest being chronic sinusitus, hay fever and (in children) adenoid trouble.

POSSIBLE

■ LARYNGITIS
A common winter illness causing many of the symptoms of the common cold but also:
* Raw feeling in the throat.
* Hoarseness or loss of voice.
* Often develops into chest infection.

■ TRACHEITIS
Rather similar to laryngitis, but:
* Raw feeling more in lower neck/upper chest.
* Often 'goes to the chest.'
* Rasping feeling behind breastbone.

■ ASTHMA
One of the commonest causes of chronic cough at all ages. The diagnosis, often difficult to make because cough can be caused by so many factors, is suggested by:
* Recurrent wheeze and breathlessness, particularly after exertion. However:
* A frequent, dry, night-time cough may be the first symptom, especially in children.
* Close relative(s) are very often asthmatic, too.
* Associated with eczema and hay fever.

■ HABIT
* Not otherwise unwell.
* Worsens if attention given, goes when distracted.
* Worse if nervous.

■ WHOOPING COUGH
* Causes paroxysms of cough to the point of breathlessness, followed by a whoop as air is breathed in eagerly. Mainly a disease of childhood, now increasingly rare, thanks to immunization.
* In adults, repeated, milder paroxysms can occur for weeks.
* Typically in epidemics.

RARE

■ LUNG CANCER
See page 224.

■ ASBESTOSIS, ALLERGIC, FIBROSING ALVEOLITIS
These are chronic conditions of progressive cough, breathlessness and wheezing.
* Associated with working in dusty industries such as coal, silica, cotton, farming.
* Cough, breathlessness, wheeze progressive over months and years.
* Finger clubbing *(see illustration page 296)*. The precise cause is unknown.

■ DRUG SIDE EFFECT
An unpredictable side effect of so-called ACE inhibitors, increasingly used to treat high blood pressure.

■ TUMOUR OR INFECTION OF LARYNX
* Persitent hoarseness, pain in neck, enlarged glands in neck. *See page 125.*

Three other conditions — MEDIASTINAL COMPRESSION, IRRITATION OF THE DIAPHRAGM and POLYARTERITIS NODOSA — have cough as a symptom.

The first occurs when organs inside the chest are squeezed by tumours. The second is caused by a liver abscess or an abscess beneath the diaphragm and the third is a disease causing generalized inflammation of the blood vessels.

These conditions are not only exceptionally rare but have an array of other symptoms — including breathlessness and progressive weight-loss (cancer); rashes and joint pains (polyarteritis nodosa); sweats and breathlessness (abscess). Among these, *cough is relatively minor.*

Some or all of these symptoms in combination require early medical attention.

COUGH PLUS PHLEGM

Most likely to be caused by a minor infection of the lungs, which in most people will settle rapidly. Those with other serious conditions such as heart disease or diabetes may need antibiotics to control the infection.

CHEST

PROBABLE
COMMON COLD — UPPER RESPIRATORY TRACT INFECTION (URTI)
BRONCHITIS
CHEST INFECTION

POSSIBLE
CHRONIC BRONCHITIS
EMPHYSEMA
PNEUMONIA

RARE
BRONCHIECTASIS
TUBERCULOSIS
LUNG ABSCESS
INHALED FOREIGN BODY
PNEUMOCONIOSIS
CYSTIC FIBROSIS
AIDS

PROBABLE

■ COMMON COLD OR URTI
* After first few days, a 'wet' cough with coloured phlegm, but otherwise feeling well.

■ BRONCHITIS
* Cough, phlegm and wheeze.
* Feeling mildly unwell.
* Some breathlessness.

■ CHEST INFECTION
* Copious cough, phlegm, fever.
* Sweats and feeling unwell.
* Onset over a day or two.
* May be accompanied by pleurisy — a knife-like pain between the ribs when breathing in.

POSSIBLE

■ CHRONIC BRONCHITIS
* Cough, phlegm and wheeze for weeks on end, possibly for most of the year. A disease especially of smokers, long-term exposure to dusty atmospheres and of people who live in damp, northern climates such as Britain's. Don't dismiss the morning 'smoker's cough'; this is your lungs telling you that they are being killed by fumes — their reaction is to push out large amounts of phlegm.
* Frequent episodes of bronchitis, summer and winter.
* Chronic cough.
* Breathlessness eventually becomes a constant feature.

It is essential to give up smoking.

■ EMPHYSEMA
* A late development of chronic bronchitis or asthma, giving breathlessness and constant wheezing.
* Ability to breathe deeply decreases.
* Barrel-shaped chest may be a later sign.

Chest X-ray needed to confirm diagnosis.

■ PNEUMONIA
A serious infection of part or all of one lung. You feel very ill.
* Rapid onset.
* Breathlessness or fast breathing.
* General aching, tiredness, cough.
* Sweats — sometimes drenching,

especially at night.
* Pain over affected part of lung.

RARE

■ BRONCHIECTASIS
A disease in which the structure of the lungs breaks down, reducing their efficiency.
* Gradual appearance of chronic cough, with copious phlegm.
* Bad breath.

Chest X-ray needed to confirm diagnosis.

■ TUBERCULOSIS
* Chronic fatigue, malaise, weight loss, anorexia *(see page 424)*.
* Groups especially at risk are those with low incomes, poor/overcrowded housing; immigrants; alcoholics.

■ LUNG ABSCESS
See under COUGH PLUS BLOODY PHLEGM.

■ INHALED FOREIGN BODY
* Typically in children. A child can (unnoticed) inhale a peanut or similar small object. A coughing fit probably follows — which the parent overlooks. Chest infection plus typical symptoms *(see page 224)* then develops, and never really clears. If these symptoms are neglected, the child becomes listless and run-down after several weeks. Inhaling a foreign body sometimes creates stridor; *see ASPHYXIA, page 276.*

Chest X-ray needed to confirm diagnosis.

■ PNEUMOCONIOSIS
A group of diseases in which the lungs become stiffer and stiffer, unable to expand properly.
* Associated with dusty industries such as coal, silica, cotton and farming.
* Cough, breathlessness, wheeze progressive over months and years.
* Finger clubbing: *see page 296.*

■ CYSTIC FIBROSIS
A childhood disease, caused by inherited genetic abnormality.
* Repeated chest infections, failure to grow.
* Diarrhoea, weight loss.

■ AIDS
Groups especially at risk are intravenous drug users, homosexuals and bisexuals.
* Weeks of malaise, weight loss, fatigue, fevers.

Diagnosis confirmed by blood tests. Sputum culture will show unusual organisms.

COUGH PLUS BLOODY PHLEGM

One of nature's day-glo symptoms: never ignore it. In older people (50 plus) and especially in smokers it calls for careful investigation. In younger people there is more likely to be a relatively innocent cause. Even so, they should have an immediate check-up.

Remember that many cases of cough plus bloody phlegm are

eventually diagnosed as 'cause unknown' — the symptom simply goes away.

PROBABLE
CHEST INFECTION

POSSIBLE
PNEUMONIA
LUNG CANCER
BRONCHIECTASIS
CAUSE UNKNOWN

RARE
HEART FAILURE
MITRAL STENOSIS

PROBABLE

■ CHEST INFECTION
* Yellowish or greenish plegm which contains streaks or blobs of blood, possibly red, possibly rust-coloured. Not an uncommon symptom.
* Mildly unwell with raised temperature and aches.

POSSIBLE

■ PNEUMONIA
See page 214. The infection causes so much inflammation that blood oozes into the lungs where it mixes with phlegm.

■ LUNG CANCER
There is now little doubt that smoking causes most cases of this, one of the commonest forms of cancer. Smokers in particular, and especially smokers in the 50-plus age range, should be alert to the early warning signs because the sooner the disease is diagnosed, the better the results of treatment, and the outlook of treatment is slowly improving.

None of these symptoms on their own is absolutely diagnostic of lung cancer, indeed they often prove to be false alarms. However, this is a situation when over-caution is to be encouraged, particularly if you are in the risk group. Combinations of two or more symptoms should arouse increased suspicion.
* A persistent cough, whether dry or with phlegm. Smokers get used to smokers' coughs, making it all the more important to be aware if the cough worsens. An early lung tumour causes this symptom by irritating the lining of the air passages.
* Frequent or unusually persistent chest infections. This can mean that a small tumour is acting as a focus for repeated infection.
* Coughing blood. Even small amounts mixed with phlegm should be investigated and all the more so if the cough produces pure blood. A small tumour can have this effect by oozing blood from its surface.
* Breathlessness — because a tumour has caused collapse of part of a lung.
* Persistent pain or ache in the chest, due to inflammation from a tumour.
* Loss of appetite and weight. For

reasons not clearly understood, many cancers cause loss of weight and appetite before the cancer has otherwise shown itself.

Ninty five per cent of lung cancer cases are due to smoking. It is increasingly recognized that the remaining five per cent may largely be caused by passive smoking.

■ BRONCHIECTASIS
See page 223.

■ CAUSE UNKNOWN
* Despite thorough investigation, in some cases the cause remains unknown.

RARE

■ HEART FAILURE
* Gradual onset of breathlessness, swollen ankles, inability to lie flat.
* Frothy pink sputum, rather than pure blood.

■ MITRAL STENOSIS
* History of rheumatic fever — *see page 448.*
* Gradual development of breathlessness, fatigue, dilated veins on cheekbones, giving a 'flushed' appearance, breathlessness when lying flat.

COUGH, BLOODY PHLEGM and CHEST PAIN

Pain in the lungs points to inflammation or injury of the pleura the thin outer 'skin' that covers the lungs. Inflammation of the pleura frequently accompanies chest infections, when it is called pleurisy.

PROBABLE
CHEST INFECTION

POSSIBLE
PNEUMONIA
PULMONARY EMBOLUS
CHEST INJURY

RARE
LUNG CANCER WITH BONE SPREAD

PROBABLE

■ CHEST INFECTION
See page 224.

POSSIBLE

■ PNEUMONIA
See page 214.

The phlegm is typically rust-coloured (that is bloodstained) rather than containing pure blood and is otherwise green or yellow due to the underlying infection.

■ PULMONARY EMBOLUS
This is a blood clot blocking blood flow to part of a lung. Symptoms may range from mild, knife-like chest pain to collapse.
* Increased risk after surgery, in

the obese, in those recovering from a heart attack, in women on the contraceptive pill and during pregnancy.
* Coughing blood.
* Pain worse on breathing in.
* If the embolus is large, faintness and sweating, collapse.
* If also a swollen calf, suggests a leg thrombosis *(see page 310)* as reason.

■ CHEST INJURY
Caused by an injury severe enough to damage the lungs directly, or to break a rib, which then punctures a lung.
* Knife-like pains.
* Worse on breathing in.

RARE

■ LUNG CANCER WITH SECONDARY SPREAD TO BONES
In the later stages of lung cancer, a patient might experience this combination of symptoms.

Cancer of the lung can spread to other parts of the body, for example the bones. If a rib is involved, there will be persistent chest pain, especially at night; a specific tender spot on the rib; and other signs of the disease; *see page 224.*

ASPHYXIA (SUFFOCATION)

Obstruction to the flow of air through the mouth, down the trachea or into the lungs. Always look for some simple reversable cause, typically something stuck in the throat. The symptoms of asphyxia are:
* Rapid or abrupt onset.
* Sudden cough, choking and spluttering.
* Rapid cyanosis (bluish colouring) of lips, tongue.
* Panic.
* Stridor, a low- to middle-pitched sound from the larynx, mainly on breathing in. It is also caused by viral infection and is common in children: the child may wake with loud, frightening breathing noises — a highly distinctive coarse wheezing intake of breath, plus cough and fever. Steam inhalation relieves the symptoms.

Of course, your first move, if you suspect something trapped in the throat, will be to try to dislodge it. Then call for help. Then, if you know how, give artificial respiration until help arrives. Usually these situations call for emergency attention as quickly as possible.

PROBABLE
FOREIGN BODY
SWELLING OF LARYNX
LARYNGO-TRACHEITIS

POSSIBLE
PNEUMOTHORAX
PULMONARY EMBOLUS

RARE
EPIGLOTTITIS
DIPHTHERIA
TRACHEO-OESOPHAGEAL FISTULA
TUMOURS AND CYSTS

PROBABLE

■ FOREIGN BODY
A piece of meat or a similar chunk of firm food is the usual culprit in adults. In children, food can be to blame, but consider also small toys, pen tops, beads, peanuts. The prime signs are:
* Choking.
* Acute stridor: noisy, hoarse, 'wheezing' intake of breath.
* Clutching at throat.

First aid: try to dislodge any easily accessible foreign body, or else perform *HEIMLICH'S MANOEUVRE, see page 204.*

If the foreign body gets past the larynx and makes its way down into the lungs, the coughing and stridor will pass off. In the lungs it will act as a focus for chronic infection, or even a lung abscess. Cough and recurrent infection after a choking fit should be viewed with suspicion because of this possibility.

■ SWELLING OF LARYNX
An acute, severe allergic reaction causes widespread swelling of soft tissues, including the larynx.

Commonest after insect stings or injections. Some people are hypersensitive to specific foods: nuts are commonly to blame.
* Swelling of lips, limbs and throat
* Acute wheezing.
* Collapse.

■ LARYNGO-TRACHEITIS
A simple laryngitis may occasionally develop into severe swelling. Children whose airways are narrow, and will become obstructed on modest swelling of the soft tissues, are most at risk.
* Hoarseness developing into stridor *(see page 226).*
* Laboured breathing, cyanosis (bluish tinge to skin, especially lips).

POSSIBLE

■ PNEUMOTHORAX
Lungs are like balloons in some ways, and, just like a balloon, sometimes part of a lung bursts and collapses. Small collapses go unnoticed. Large ones will cause noticeable symptoms and if air continues to leak out from the puncture into the chest, rapid breathlessness will become a problem.
* Sudden, knife-like chest pain.
* Worse breathing in.
* Breathlessness worsening over a few minutes.

Treatment of a large pneumothorax will require emergency treatment: a needle will be inserted through the chest wall to let out the air compressed inside the chest. The lung gradually reinflates over a few days with the help of a chest drain — a tube leading out of the lung.

■ PULMONARY EMBOLUS
A blood clot obstructing blood flow through the lung.
* Sudden chest pain, often knife-like.
* Coughing blood.

See page 218.

CHEST

RARE

■ EPIGLOTTITIS
The epiglottis lies just out of sight at the very back of the throat. Infection can cause it to swell until it obstructs the back of the throat. This is an illness found in young children, whose airways are still narrow.
* Begins as a simple sore throat.
* Child develops a very high temperature.
* Begins to drool saliva because swallowing is painful.
* Laboured breathing, cyanosis.

If you suspect that your child has epiglottitis it is important *not* to try to peer down the throat as that can cause complete obstruction. An examination should only be performed in hospital where an emergency tracheostomy can be undertaken.

■ DIPHTHERIA
A terrible illness which routine vaccination has virtually eliminated from developed countries. A membrane forms at the back of the throat which obstructs breathing. In addition, the germ responsible produces toxic substances that affect the heart and nervous system.
* Begins as a simple sore throat.
* A grey membrane forms at the back of the throat.
* Dramatic enlargement of lymph nodes in the neck.
*Breathlessness, cyanosis.

Although there is specific treatment, diphtheria is still a most serious illness.

■ TRACHEO-OESOPHAGEAL FISTULA
An abnormality of new-born babies. During embryonic life, the airways and the gullet develop in close proximity to each other. If the trachea opens into the gullet rather than the back of the mouth, food will travel straight from the gullet into the lungs.
* Cough, asphyxia each time the baby feeds.
* Chest infection develops rapidly.

Once recognized, the problem is cured by surgery.

■ TUMOURS AND CYSTS
Although these diseases of the larynx or thyroid gland grow quite slowly, they can rapidly increase in size if they start to bleed. The swelling causes obstruction.

The diagnosis might be considered in an adult who is known to have a growth and who suddenly becomes breathless.

CHEST PAIN

Though chest pain is commonly and understandably taken as a sign of heart disease, there are many other causes to be considered, not all of them involving the heart. So many vital structures pass through the chest that the list of possibilities is long. There are the gullet, the great vessels coming from the heart, the windpipe and the airways going down into the lungs. Pain may stem from the ribs themselves, the muscles between the ribs or from the nerves. The lungs can ache and inflammation from within the abdomen may give rise to pain in the chest. And certainly, some chest pains, particularly perhaps in born worriers, are psychological. Finally there are pains which remain totally unexplained, even after extensive investigation.

That said, sudden severe chest pain must be taken seriously and needs urgent medical assessment to exclude a heart attack. Recent advances in the treatment of heart attacks require medical attention to be given within a very few hours of the attack. It is therefore all the more important to get help as soon as possible. It is one area of medicine where doctors, given a classic picture, will back their hunches and treat first, diagnose later, even if immediate test results are negative.

This section is divided as follows:

A heart attack.

Sudden chest pain.

Persistent or recurrent chest pain.

A HEART ATTACK

Everyone should be aware of the classic symptoms of a heart attack because early treatment is vital.

* Sudden, severe central chest pain.
* Begins at rest.
* Worse on exertion.
* Pain is crushing, vice-like, gripping.
* May radiate up to the jaws or down the arms, usually the left.
* Breathlessness.
* Sweating.
* Cyanosis (blueness) of lips.

A heart attack occurs when the blood supply to part of the heart is blocked off. Pain comes from the heart muscle in much the same way that cramp occurs in other muscles in other circumstances.

For many years, the treatment was to deal with the complications that can arise, such as heart failure or rhythm disorders *(see pages 193-204)*. Nowadays, treatment aims to limit the amount of damage to the heart that occurs during the attack, but this calls for treatment within hours. This makes it all the more important to get an early diagnosis in hospital.

Not all heart attacks will show all of the features above: pain is not always a prominent feature, especially in the elderly; sometimes there is just:

* Sudden onset of tiredness.
* Irregular pulse.
* Heart failure, with breathlessness and swollen ankles.

In these circumstances, much can still be done to help.

Keep this picture in mind when referring to the sections dealing with other causes of chest pain.

Your doctor does.

SUDDEN CHEST PAIN, POSSIBLY A HEART ATTACK

Sudden chest pain is always worrying, but just how worrying depends on associated features. The classical symptoms of a heart attack have been given, but subtleties may help sway the diagnosis. Did the pain come on very suddenly, or over a few minutes? Is breathlessness a feature? Do you feel ill? Does movement make a difference? Were there previous symptoms?

Diagnostic possibilities are different at different ages. Heart disease would not be the first diagnosis for a young person, whereas in an older person it is often difficult to rule out heart disease completely, so tests will commonly be ordered although the symptoms are not completely typical. It is generally safest for a layperson to regard severe chest pain in an adult as a disorder of the heart until proven otherwise.

Doctors will make additional judgements based on the individual's overall condition, including skin colour, pulse, blood pressure or signs of heart disease such as fluid on the lungs or abnormal heart rhythms. An electrocardiogram recording of the heart can be helpful; so are blood tests, but these take time, so doctors will often make a diagnosis based on history and examination while awaiting the outcome of investigations.

PROBABLE
HEART ATTACK

POSSIBLE
OESOPHAGITIS
NERVE IRRITATION
PEPTIC ULCER
PNEUMOTHORAX

RARE
PULMONARY EMBOLUS
DISSECTING AORTIC ANEURYSM
PERICARDITIS
PANCREATITIS

PROBABLE

■ HEART ATTACK
See page 229. Should be suspected on the basis of
* Sudden onset of severe central chest pain.
* Onset at rest.
* Prolonged and crushing in nature.

POSSIBLE

■ OESOPHAGITIS
Inflammation of the gullet can be extremely painful, with many features resembling a heart attack:
* Central chest pain.
* Spreads up to neck, down arms.
* Sweating.

Can be difficult to distinguish from heart pain. There may be a

previous history of:
* Indigestion, belching.
* Burning pain after food.
* Taking drugs which irritate the gullet such as aspirin.
* Relief with antacids.

However, if occurring for the first time in the middle-aged or elderly, heart disease must be carefully considered.

■ NERVE IRRITATION
Nerves run in bands between the ribs, encircling the chest. It is quite common for one of these nerves to become irritated, causing pain.
* Sharp chest pain.
* Radiates from the back towards the front of the chest.
* Worse on movement.
* No breathlessness or sweating.
* Pain comes and goes from minute to minute.
* Often one small part of the chest wall is tender.

This condition can be dramatic when it appears but is entirely benign, needing no more than painkillers and rest.

■ PEPTIC ULCER
Ulceration in the stomach or upper small bowel (duodenum). The pain from a peptic ulcer tends to be:
* Confined to the upper abdomen.
* Burning in nature.
* Worse at night.
* Appears to radiate into the back.
* Preceded by weeks or months of indigestion.
* Possibly blood in vomit.
* Upper abdominal pain on pressure.

Treatment is totally different from that for a heart attack, consisting of intensive anti-acid treatment.

One in ten people will have an ulcer at some time in their lives. This condition used to be commonest in men; now it is almost as common in women. Smoking, family history and taking certain painkillers all increase the risk of developing a peptic ulcer.

■ PNEUMOTHORAX
Sudden collapse of part of a lung.
* Sudden, knife-like chest pain.
* Localized usually to the side of the chest, not central.
* Breathlessness is a possibility.

RARE

■ PULMONARY EMBOLUS
A blood clot lodging in the lungs causing:
* Sudden pressure in chest.
* Discomfort rather than pain.
* Pain, if present, is knife-like.
* Breathlessness.
* Sudden cough with bloodstained phlegm.

Pulmonary embolus is associated with thrombosis of leg veins, giving a painful swollen calf. It can occur after surgical operations.

■ DISSECTING AORTIC ANEURYSM
The aorta is the great artery which carries blood away from the heart. If diseased, the walls can weaken, bulge and eventually start to leak. In the days or weeks before this stage there may be warning signs

such as:
* Vague upper chest pain.
* Pulsation (feeling of strong, throbbing pulse) in the upper chest.
* Breathlessness through obstruction of part of the lung.
* Hoarseness.
If the aneurysm begins to leak there will be:
* Pain similar to heart attack.
* Possibly vomiting blood.
* Collapse through blood loss.

This condition is very difficult to distinguish from a heart attack by examination alone. The diagnosis is usually made on the result of a chest X-ray. Surgery is possible, depending on the site of the leakage. Frequently fatal.

■ PERICARDITIS
Inflammation of the lining around the heart giving rise to:
* Sharp central chest pain.
* Worse on movement.
* Worse on breathing.

Pericarditis may be caused by a viral infection. It can usually be treated and a full recovery is possible.

■ PANCREATITIS
The pancreas lies at the back of the upper abdomen. It is the gland that produces insulin and other substances that digest food. If the pancreas becomes inflamed, these substances are released and start to 'digest' the internal organs with which they come into contact. Inflammation of the pancreas is most common in alcoholics or in those with gallstones. The very severe pain of pancreatitis can appear to spread up into the chest.
* Pain radiates into the back.
* Nausea and vomiting.

There will be upper abdominal tenderness on examination. This is a serious condition which calls for intensive treatment in hospital.

RECURRENT OR PERSISTENT CHEST PAIN

This means symptoms that come and go over days, weeks or months. Again, the possibilities depend on the person's age, previous medical history and any associated features of disease.

Recurrent chest pain is common and is not always explainable. In young people, the reason often remains obscure, even after intensive investigation.

PROBABLE
ANGINA
HIATUS HERNIA

POSSIBLE
CHONDRITIS
DA COSTA'S SYNDROME
HEART RHYTHM DISORDERS
LUNG DISEASE
GALL BLADDER DISEASE

RARE
AORTIC VALVE DISEASE
SEVERE ANAEMIA
AORTIC ANEURYSM
PERICARDITIS

PROBABLE

■ ANGINA
Angina is pain arising from the heart. The reason is nearly always coronary artery disease: that is, 'furring up' of the blood vessels that carry blood to the heart itself. This causes a *partial* blockage of blood flow, and gives no symptoms until you exert yourself. Then, the heart's increased demand for blood cannot be met, resulting in angina:
* Central chest pain.
* Often radiates to neck or down left arm.
* Comes on with exertion.
* Goes after only a few minutes of rest.
* Worse in cold weather, after meals, emotional stress.

It is common to investigate angina with X-rays which highlight the blood flow around the heart, a technique known as angiography. The information gathered from this test will help the doctor to decide whether to replace the blood vessels to the heart, done in an operation known as coronary artery bypass grafting.

Angina is an important warning sign of heart disease, but in itself it is not dangerous and is *not* a warning of an imminent heart attack. Most individuals who experience angina enjoy years of active life with no more inconvenience than it takes to keep in a supply of anti-angina medication.

■ HIATUS HERNIA
A common condition in which part of the stomach moves up into the chest. As a result the diaphragm — which normally creates a valve-type mechanism — allows gastric acid to cause pain in the upper part of the stomach and the gullet.

Symptoms may be noticed for the first time during pregnancy, or be made worse by it; this is also so if you are obese.
* Pain worse on lying flat or bending over.
* Pain which is burning or searing in nature.
* May appear to radiate up to the neck.
* Burping or belching.
* Relieved by antacids.

Treatment varies from simply avoiding tight clothing and raising the head of the bed, to a range of drugs or, very rarely, an operation to tighten up the muscles.

A new range of drugs, called proton pump inhibitors, has revolutionized the treatment of hiatus hernia. They can bring remarkable and rapid relief.

POSSIBLE

■ CHONDRITIS
Where the ribs meet the breastbone there are joints made up of cartilage which can become inflamed. This may occur after injury, out of the blue or sometimes in epidemics of a viral infection called Bornholm disease (named after the Baltic island where an epidemic was documented).

CHEST

* Onset over a few hours.
* Aching on either side of the breastbone.
* Individual joints may be swollen and tender.
* Worse on breathing, or with changes of posture.
* Sometimes a mild fever.

This condition is not dangerous, but may be extremely painful and alarming at the start and can last for several weeks.

■ DA COSTA'S SYNDROME
A kind of cardiac neurosis: a psychological problem of anxiety showing itself as:
* Recurrent pains over the heart.
* Breathlessness out of proportion to effort.
* Nervousness.
* Palpitations.

There is no doubt that individuals are genuinely distressed by their symptoms, which are treated by psychological support once heart disease has been ruled out.

■ HEART RHYTHM DISORDERS
Very rapid or very slow heart rates can bring on angina, even in individuals with no other heart disease.
* Palpitations.
* Breathlessness.
* Abrupt onset, abrupt finish.

For details, *see pages 193-204.*

■ LUNG DISEASE
Many disorders can give rise to chest pain which may be mistaken for heart disease, including severe infections and cancer. *See pages 219-26.*

■ GALL BLADDER DISEASE
Lying high up in the right side of the abdomen, a diseased gall bladder can give rise to pain which appears to be in the chest. It is commonest in middle-aged women. There is usually little difficulty in distinguishing this as a cause.
* Pain builds up over a few minutes.
* Lasts for several hours.
* Pain and tenderness mainly under the ribs on the right side.
* May appear to radiate into the chest or to the tip of the shoulder.
* Nausea, vomiting is common.
* Restlessness.

A first attack may be puzzling, but usually a pattern emerges: pain provoked by certain foods, especially fatty ones, with episodes of niggling pain in between major attacks. The usual reason is gallstones, for which there is a variety of treatments, mainly surgical.

RARE

■ AORTIC VALVE DISEASE
This valve controls blood flow between the heart and the aorta, the major artery from the heart. The valve can become stiff and inefficient; this is known as aortic stenosis, usually a result of ageing, though rheumatic heart disease was once a common cause.

Occasionally, children are born with an abnormal valve. As the valve is so stiff, it has to beat harder to force blood out and this puts a strain on it. For years there may be no symptoms, but with

increasing stiffness there will be some combination of:
* Angina.
* Heart rhythm irregularities.
* Breathlessness.
* Fainting on exertion.

The condition produces a characteristic heart murmur that a doctor can detect. The treatment is by heart valve replacement, though other treatments are used in childhood or in the elderly and infirm.

■ SEVERE ANAEMIA

It is unusual for anaemia to become so severe without other symptoms, but it does happen occasionally, especially with pernicious anaemia. This starves the heart of oxygen, and angina is the result.
* Pallor or yellowish tinge in pernicious anaemia.
* Sore tongue.
* Tiredness, breathlessness.

Most forms of anaemia respond rapidly to treatment.

■ AORTIC ANEURYSM

In the days or weeks before this ruptures, there may be intermittent chest pain. See page 231.

■ PERICARDITIS

May account for several days of chest pain. See page 232.

HEIMLICH'S MANOEUVRE
* Stand behind the person choking.
* Extend your arms in a hug around their upper abdomen.
* With clenched fists make a hard, fast squeeze just under the breast bone.

The manoeuvre forces a blast of air out of the lungs, sufficient to dislodge something stuck in the upper airway. For full details see any modern manual of first aid.

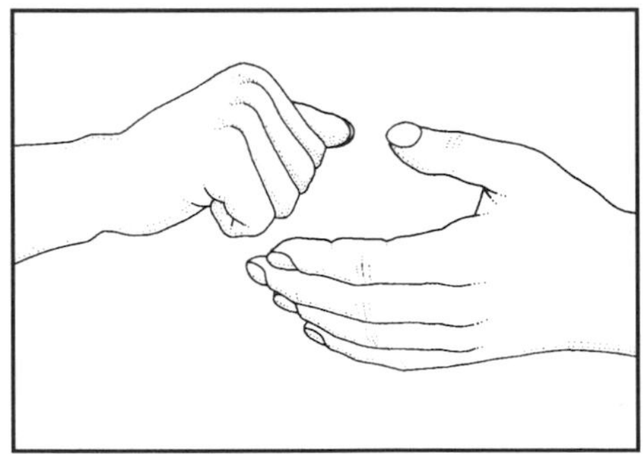

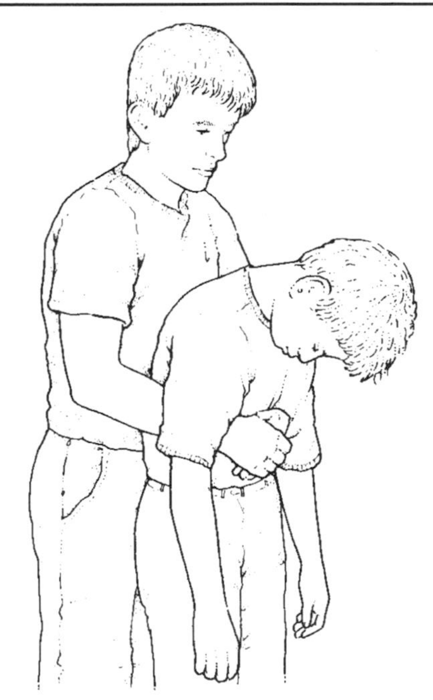

THE SKIN AND HAIR

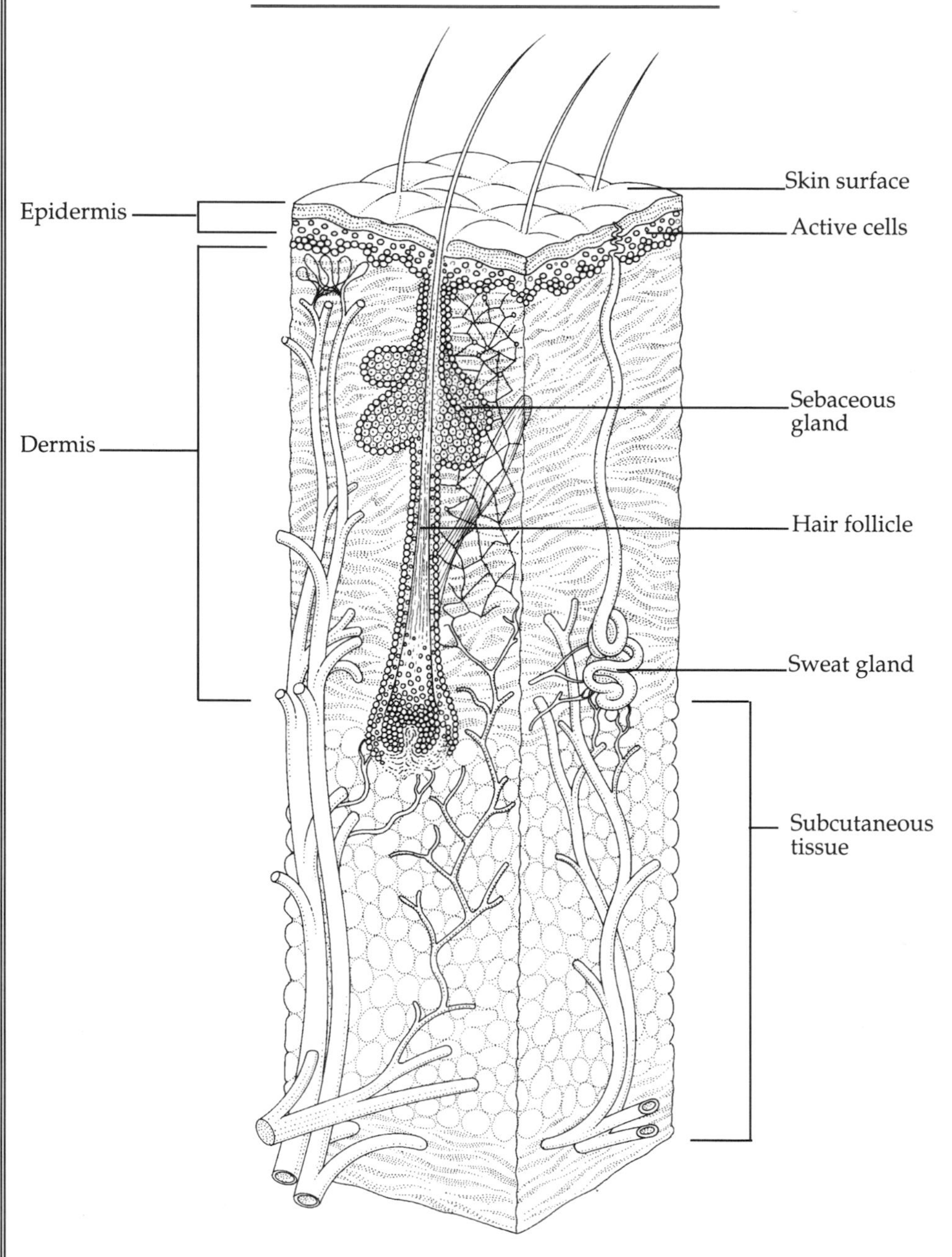

THE SKIN INTRODUCTION

When it comes to diagnosis, your skin (largest of the body's organs) has unique advantages: it can be seen and felt; and the changes it undergoes when diseased, or when there is underlying disease elsewhere in the body, are often highly significant.

However, many people are, understandably, reticent when it comes to discussing changes in their skin — particularly in those areas normally hidden by clothes. Doctors *never* regard such changes as embarrassing: they think of them *only* as essential clues to diagnosis.

RASHES

Are analysed here into four key different types, with cross-references to pages where they are covered in detail.

RASHES DEVELOPING BLISTERS

- CHICKEN POX
- ECZEMA
- HERPES SIMPLEX
- HERPES ZOSTER
- IMPETIGO

See pages 242,239 and 240.

- PUSTULAR PSORIASIS

See under PSORIASIS, page 242.

- DERMATITIS HERPETIFORMIS

See page 240.

RASHES OF RED/PURPLE OR BLACK/DARK SPOTS

See BLEEDING 'UNDER' THE SKIN, page 253.

RASHES EXTENDING OVER MOST OF THE BODY

- CHICKEN POX

See page 242.

- DERMATITIS HERPETIFORMIS

See page 240.

- DRUG REACTIONS

See page 245 under BLUE — GENERAL.

- ECZEMA

See page 239.

- GERMAN MEASLES

Rubella. *See page 138.*

- MEASLES

See pages 444-5.

- PORPHYRIA CUTANEA TARDA

See page 240.

- PSORIASIS

See page 242.

- SCALDED SKIN SYNDROME

See page 241.

- TINEA VERSICOLOR

See page 248.

- URTICARIA

See page 258.

- VITAMIN A DEFICIENCY

See HARD SKIN, page 257.

■ VITILIGO
■ VIRAL INFECTIONS
See page 248, and PAPILLOMA or WART, page 251.
(Smallpox is now considered to be eradicated worldwide.)

RASHES IN A LOCALIZED AREA
See section covering that part of body.

WHITEHEADS

See BLACKHEADS AND WHITEHEADS/ACNE, below.

PIMPLES

Are covered under *BLACKHEADS AND WHITEHEADS/ACNE, below.*

BLACKHEADS AND WHITEHEADS/ACNE

Most people have a number of blackheads at any one time and they are not necessarily a sign of any skin abnormality.

They will develop whenever the skin's pores become blocked. If long-standing, or infected, they may become whiteheads, or even become *Acne vulgaris*, commonly known as acne or teenage pimples. The exact cause of acne is unclear to doctors. The changes it makes to the skin are the visible effects of infection and inflammation.

Over-activity of the sebaceous, or oil-producing, glands in the skin is one factor. Undoubtedly, hormones also play a part. Diet plays less of a role than was once thought.

■ ACNE VULGARIS
* Starts at puberty.
* Blackheads — pinpricks of black matter — can be seen blocking the entrance to sebaceous glands. Otherwise known as comedones.
* Most commonly affects face, upper chest and back.
* Skin may appear greasy.
* Skin bacteria infect the matter in the blocked duct causing local redness, pain and swelling (papules).
* Pus develops, forming pustules (whiteheads).
* This process can continue for years.

If untreated, it can scar the skin. Modern treaments may not cure it, but they can improve matters considerably. All individuals with severe acne should be offered antibiotic treatment, either as tablets or in a lotion to apply to the skin.

BLISTERS

Collections of fluid trapped between different layers of skin. They come in different shapes and sizes. Larger than $^{2}/_{10}$in/5mm, they are described here as bullae; smaller, as vesicles.

PROBABLE
INJURY
ECZEMA
HERPES SIMPLEX
IMPETIGO

POSSIBLE
CHICKEN POX
SHINGLES
ERYTHEMA MULTIFORME

RARE
PEMPHIGOID
PUSTULAR PSORIASIS
DERMATITIS HERPETIFORMIS
PEMPHIGUS VULGARIS
PORPHYRIA CUTANEA TARDA
EPIDERMOLYSIS BULLOSA
SCALDED SKIN SYNDROME

PROBABLE

■ INJURY
Extremes of heat or cold; friction; caustic chemicals; certain plants; some animals; jelly fish; insect bites: all can cause blisters.
* Localized to the site of injury.
* Surrounding skin may be reddened.

■ ECZEMA
* Often most marked in the skin 'flexures', for example the creases at the elbows, or behind the knees.
* Itching.
* Redness.
* Raised red areas.
* Vesicles.
* Weeping.
* Scaling.
* Crusting.

■ HERPES SIMPLEX
This can causes blisters anywhere on the body. the commonest form is that known as a 'cold sore', affecting the lips. After the first infection, recurrences may occur at times of debility or after exposure to hot sun or cold.
* Skin is locally irritable.
* Then reddening and painful.
* Small lumps appear to form vesicles.
* The vesicles burst and crust over.
* The whole cycle takes 10 to 14 days to subside.

See also LIPS — CRACKED etc, page 84.

■ IMPETIGO
A skin infection which is passed on easily by contact.
* Redness.
* Vesicles and bullae form.
* Bursting and dirty brown/black crusting occurs.
* Common around mouth, face and ears.

See also page 84.

The Skin

POSSIBLE

■ CHICKEN POX
See page 242.

■ SHINGLES
Herpes zoster. Arises when the chicken pox virus is reactivated after lying dormant for years in the nerves of the area affected.
* Initially, an itchy, localized area of skin on one half of the body.
* Pain develops.
* Reddening occurs; small lumps appear.
* Vesicles form.
* Crusting, followed by healing, sometimes taking up to a month.
* Pain (post-herpetic neuralgia) may be persistent and difficult to treat.

■ ERYTHEMA MULTIFORME
See page 87.
Vesicles and bullae may occur with this disease, which arises from an infection or a reaction to a drug or medicine.

RARE

■ PEMPHIGOID
In the elderly.
* Sudden onset of bullae on limbs and trunk. They may arise from reddened or swollen skin.
* Bullae may be filled with blood-stained fluid.
* Unlike the blisters of pemphigus, these are intensely itchy.

■ PSORIASIS (PUSTULAR)
See page 242.

■ DERMATITIS HERPETIFORMIS
An auto-immune disease.
* Itchy rash on the extensor (outer) aspect of elbows, knees and buttocks.
* Multiple small blisters appear in these areas.
* Almost always associated with coeliac disease *(see page 146)*. As the coeliac disease inproves with treatment, so will the skin condition.
Treated with dapsone; *see under METHAEMOGLOBINAEMIA, page 245.*

■ PEMPHIGUS VULGARIS
A serious condition commonly affecting people between 40 and 60 years old.
* Crops of widespread bullae (skin and mucous membranes), often starting in the mouth.
* Skin may blister after simple pressure.
* Bullae burst, leaving weeping, reddened and painful skin, which may become infected.
Cannot be cured, but treatment with steroids and antibiotics considerably improves matters.

■ PORPHYRIA CUTANEA TARDA
* Associated with liver damage — often alcohol induced.
* Exposed skin blisters, scars and becomes pigmented.
* Excess hair may grow on face and eyebrows.
Treatment includes giving up alcohol.

■ EPIDERMOLYSIS BULLOSA
Several different types of this inherited disease exist. Bullae develop after minimal injury — typically minor friction — and

become infected.

■ SCALDED SKIN SYNDROME
Caused by infection in children, and drug sensitivities in adults.
* Sudden onset of malaise.
* Raised temperature.
* Widespread redness.
* Multiple vesicles and bullae.
* Vesicles and bullae join, causing large areas of skin to lift off, like a severe scald.

May be fatal.

SCARRED OR PITTED SKIN

In theory, any repeated inflammation or disease process will leave the skin scarred and pitted. In practice, the commonest culprit is acne, the universal plague of adolescence; *see page 238.* The worst cases leave permanent marks on the face and shoulders.

SCALY SKIN

True scaling is limited to just a few conditions and diseases.

Excluding the commonest of them, dandruff *(see page265)*, this leaves:

PROBABLE
FUNGAL INFECTIONS
ECZEMA

POSSIBLE
PSORIASIS

RARE
PELLAGRA
ICHTHYOSIS

PROBABLE

■ FUNGAL INFECTIONS
See page 252.

■ ECZEMA
See page 239.

POSSIBLE

■ PSORIASIS
See page 242.

RARE

■ PELLAGRA
Vitamin B3 (niacin) deficiency.
* Dementia.
* Severe diarrhoea.
* Scaly changes (dermatitis) of exposed skin.

■ ICHTHYOSIS
See page 262.

THE SKIN

SCABS

If the skin surface is damaged and fluid (serum, pus, blood) leaks out (either directly or into blisters which subsequently burst) then golden brown or black crusts — scabs — form on the surface or at the edges of the damaged skin. *See also BLISTERS, pages 239-41.*

PROBABLE
IMPETIGO
ECZEMA
INJURY
HERPES SIMPLEX

POSSIBLE
CHICKEN POX
HERPES ZOSTER

RARE
PEMPHIGUS VULGARIS
PSORIASIS
DERMATITIS ARTEFACTA

PROBABLE

■ IMPETIGO
■ ECZEMA
■ INJURY
■ HERPES SIMPLEX
See pages 239-41.

POSSIBLE

■ CHICKEN POX
An infectious disease caused by the same virus that causes shingles *(see HERPES ZOSTER).*
* Crops of spots at different stages.
* Spots are red, raised, form vesicles then pustules (vesicles filled with pus).
* Pustules burst and crust over.
* Fever.
* Malaise.

■ HERPES ZOSTER
See page 240.

RARE

■ PEMPHIGUS
See page 240.

■ PSORIASIS
A skin disorder of unknown cause.
* Multiple red lesions of varying size.
* The red areas are covered with thick silver scales.
* If the scales are scraped off, the underlying skin may bleed.
* May occur on any part of the body, but frequently on knees, elbows and scalp.
* Some individuals develop arthritis *(see page 301)* in association with the psoriasis.

Pustular psoriasis is an uncommon form of the condition in which pus-filled vesicles (pustules) arise from the affected skin. When these break down some crusting may occur.

■ DERMATITIS ARTEFACTA
Some people suffering from psychological disorders deliberately harm themselves, for example by burning, scratching or even applying caustic fluids. The resulting injuries may well include extensive scabs and crusts, for which there is no clear explanation.

Sometimes child abusers cause similar injuries to children. To specialists' eyes these patterns can appear quite distinctive.

PEELING OR FLAKING SKIN

Occurs in association with many skin diseases, but typically BLISTERS and RASHES, whose other symptoms are just as, if not more, noticeable, and which are listed under those headings.

And, of course, peeling skin is the eventual and unfortunate outcome of sunburn.

Some skin diseases benefit from sunlight: psoriasis and vitamin deficiencies are obvious examples. However, it is now established beyond much doubt that sunbathing predisposes to skin cancer. No sunbathing can be considered entirely safe. You increase your risk considerably if:

– You have fair skin and sunbathe (redheads with freckles should avoid the sun);
– You expose yourself to the sun around the middle of the day;
– If you develop any redness of the skin. This means you are burnt.

Burnt skin means a higher risk of skin cancer.

It is wise to keep to the following rules when you are on holiday, or during sunny spells:

• Increase your exposure to the sun very gradually.
• Wear T-shirts and hats.
• Use a high-factor sun protection cream.
• Cover children well.
• Reapply sun blocks after bathing.
• Avoid the midday sun.

Protective creams *are* effective and should be used.

SKIN APPEARS PALE

See pages 417-24.

SKIN APPEARS BLUISH

See pages 424-5.

SKIN APPEARS BLACKENED

See DISCOLOURATION OF THE SKIN, page 244.

YELLOW SKIN

See YELLOWISH SKIN — JAUNDICE, page 245.

LOCALIZED YELLOW AREAS IN THE SKIN

■ XANTHOMATA
Localized, well-defined deposits of fatty material just below the skin surface. May occasionally be a sign of excess lipids (fats) in the blood, which in turn may predispose to arterial disease. Most commonly seen around the eyes, when the deposits are called xanthelasma.

■ GOUTY TOPHI
See GOUT, page 279.

YELLOWISH SKIN — JAUNDICE

See page 247; also pages 150, 154, 155, 174, 434.

DISCOLOURATION OF THE SKIN

Meaning any abnormal change in the colour of your skin. This can happen because of a local problem, or because of a general ('systemic') disease of one or more of the body's organs or systems. There are several conditions where changed skin colour is a major feature.

Well-known types of skin discolouration are listed here by the type of colour change and by whether the change is local or general. Obviously, colour changes will usually be more obvious in people with light skins than in those with dark skins.

Not listed here are spots and rashes, which are covered on *pages 237-8.*

BLACK — LOCAL

■ MOLE
Common in adults, a millimetre or two in diameter, or much larger. Typically brown/black in colour. Some have hairs growing from them. They are harmless, but see immediately below.

■ MALIGNANT MELANOMA
A general term for the several different forms of skin cancers, commonest in fair-skinned individuals who have had lengthy, frequent exposure to the sun. They are increasingly common, very probably because more people take holidays in the sun. The role of ozone-depletion in the atmosphere is less certain, but may be an important factor. Some malignant melanomas are extremely aggressive.

Malignant melanomas start as small black areas and are often difficult to tell from moles. Even a vague suspicion that you may have one is reason enough to show it to a doctor without delay: early diagnosis improves the chances of successful treatment. Once treated, you may need to be followed up for several years. The warning signs are:

* Bleeding.
* Itching.
* Colour change.
* Pain.

* Change in size or shape.
* Appearance of smaller lesions nearby.
* Ulceration.

Any one of these warning signs should prompt you to visit your doctor.

■ ACANTHOSIS NIGRICANS
Black linear pigmentation in the armpit, the groin, on the face and neck. Most commonly occurs in association with an underlying malignant tumour. Rare, and untreatable.

■ DRY GANGRENE
See also ITCHING OR NUMBNESS OF THE FINGERS AND TOES, page 321.
Gradual loss of blood supply to a toe or a foot, or any extremity, may cause this condition. The affected part becomes withered and black and may drop off — typically a frost-bitten toe.

BLUE — LOCAL
■ CYANOSIS *See BLUISH SKIN, page 424.*

■ MONGOLIAN BLUE SPOT
A blue/black area typically seen on the buttocks and sacral region in West Indian and Asian children. May often be mistaken for a bruise; can be several centimetres across.

■ BLUE NAEVUS
Similar to *MONGOLIAN BLUE SPOT*, above, but occurs elsewhere on the body. May be only a few millimetres in size.

■ LIVIDO RETICULARIS
An exaggeration of the body's normal response to heat and cold: white areas of skin surrounded by a 'chicken wire' pattern of bluish blood vessels.

BLUE — GENERAL
■ CYANOSIS *See page 424.*

■ AMIODARONE
This drug, for treating heart irregularities, may rarely cause a bluish-grey, slaty discolouration of the skin.

■ METHAEMOGLOBINAEMIA
Can occur through exposure to certain drugs, for example dapsone, for treating leprosy or dermatitis herpetiformis, or certain chemicals. Some people inherit the condition, which affects the oxygen-carrying capacity of the haemoglobin in red blood cells.

■ OCHRONOSIS
Affects cartilage and other connective tissue, for example the whites of the eyes. The cartilage underlying the skin looks bluish or blue-black, whereas normally the overlying skin colour would predominate. Caused by an abnormality of amino-acid metabolism called alkaptonuria.

BROWN — LOCAL
■ PREGNANCY
As pregnancy progresses, the nipples, the genitalia and a line down the centre of the abdomen become progressively darker - turning from pinkish to brownish — *See also CHLOASMA, page 246..*

The Skin

■ CHLOASMA
A brownish pigmentation of the face that occurs in some pregnant women.

■ VENOUS ULCERATION
Long-standing varicose veins in the legs *(see page 310)* cause brownish pigmentation of the lower legs and feet. Sometimes there is ulceration, too, particularly on the inner side of the ankle.

■ ERYTHEMA AB IGNE
A reddish-brown irregular discolouration which appears after long exposure of skin to heat. May well be noticed on the shins of an elderly person who spends hours in an armchair close to an open fire.

■ SEBORRHOEIC WART
A flattish, brownish wart, slightly raised above the surrounding skin. Sometimes they occur in considerable numbers. Also known as senile warts because they appear during middle-age and later.
Harmless.

■ CAFE-AU-LAIT SPOTS
Like large freckles; may be multiple. Occasionally associated with 'neurofibromatosis.'

■ ADDISON'S DISEASE
Caused by long-standing underactivity of the adrenal glands.
* Brownish/dark pigmentation of skin, especially skin creases, nipples, genitalia, old scars and gums (in the last, may appear grey).
* Weakness, fatigue.
* Weight loss, anorexia.
* Craving for salt.
* Nausea, vomiting, diarrhoea.
* Low blood pressure.
* Hair loss — occasionally.
* Vitiligo — occasionally. *See page 248.*

BROWN — GENERAL
■ FRECKLES
May occur naturally or may appear in increased numbers after exposure to the sun. May grow darker than usual and may coalesce, if exposed to sun. Mostly on face, shoulders and arms, but may cover the entire body. Commonest on redheads.
Avoid the sun if you have freckles; *see PEELING OR FLAKING SKIN, page 243.*

■ HAEMOCHROMATOSIS
Also called bronze diabetes. An abnormality of metabolism of iron from birth causes:
* Diabetes mellitus *(page 485)*.
* Bronze skin.
* Cirrhosis.
* Joint inflammation.
* Heart abnormalities.
* Shrunken testes, reduced libido.

ORANGE — GENERAL
■ CAROTENAEMIA
Eating too much food containing carotene, typically carrots and tomato juice, causes an orange discoloration of skin. Carotene is the active ingredient of some 'sun-tan' tablets.

PINK — LOCAL
■ SALMON PATCH NAEVUS
A salmon-pink birthmark. Can occur anywhere, but often on the neck. Some persist, but most disappear after a few years.

PURPLE — LOCAL

■ PORT-WINE STAIN

A permanent birth mark caused by an abnormality of the capillary blood vessels producing an often extensive discoloured area on the face and neck. Permanent, but can be disguised with make-up.

■ KAPOSI'S SARCOMA

Bluish-red areas appear on the skin. This is a malignant tumour that used to be seen mainly in Africa, but is now encountered all over the world as one of the complications of AIDS.

PURPLE — GENERAL

Likely to be cyanosis; *see page 424. See also BLUE — GENERAL, page 245.*

REDNESS — LOCAL

Described as erythema.

■ FLUSHING

As a response to heat, or embarass-ment; and in association with the menopause, *page 328.*

■ ERYTHEMA AB IGNE

See BROWN, above.

■ PALMAR ERYTHEMA

Redness of the palms of the hands. Seen in alcoholics and in others suffering from liver disease.

■ ERYTHRASMA

Reddish-brown discolouration of the skin, particularly near skin folds (breasts, armpits, groin). The skin is dry and the areas are irreg-ular and slightly scaly. Caused by bacterial infection.

■ PAGET'S DISEASE OF THE NIPPLE

Localized redness with scaling and inflammation, mimicking eczema. If you notice such changes on the nipple or areola (the pink area around the nipple), see your doctor immediately: don't be over-concerned — however, the possibility of an underlying breast cancer must be excluded. *See also pages 336-8.*

REDNESS — GENERAL

■ VIRAL INFECTION

Many viruses will cause non-specific reddening of the skin. As soon as the infection subsides, so does the rash.

■ DRUG REACTION

A diffuse reddening of the skin associated with taking new tablets or other medication. The reddening may be patchy or blotchy, or widespread. Itching (medical term, pruritus) often accompanies these reactions. Penicillin and aspirin commonly cause this reaction.

YELLOWNESS — GENERAL

This is never a local condition.

■ JAUNDICE

Yellowish whites of the eyes, and yellow skin gradually progressing to a deeper, browner colour. There may also be itching (with resulting scratch marks), pale stools and dark urine.

■ URAEMIA

See pages 260-1.

THE SKIN

■ MEPACRINE
This anti-malarial drug can cause yellowing of the skin.

WHITENESS OR PALENESS — LOCAL

■ VITILIGO
Destruction of pigment-producing cells (melanocytes) in the skin, giving white patches. In the dark-skinned, these can be quite disfiguring. *See also ADDISON'S DISEASE, page 246.*

■ HALO NAEVUS
Some moles *(see BLACK, above)* become pale and the area round them loses pigment. Mole and surrounding area are known as halo naevi. Vitiligo *(above)* may also develop.

■ TINEA VERSICOLOUR
A fungal infection of the skin.
* Initially, areas of irregular brown colouration.
* Predominantly upper body, arms and neck.
* Later, these patches lose their pigment, giving pale areas.

Treatable with anti-fungal creams.

■ POST-INFLAMMATORY
Any inflamed or damaged skin — say from a graze, a burn, a herpes sore — may lose its usual colour after healing. Normal pigmentation may return after a few months.

■ LEPROSY
See page 318.

■ ARTERIAL BLOCKAGE
See PERIPHERAL VASCULAR DISEASE, page 318.

■ PHLEGMASIA ALBA DOLENS
This means blockage of the principal veins draining blood from the leg. Typically after being bed-ridden.
* Initially, malaise.
* Pain in groin and thigh.
* Leg-swelling follows.
* Leg is pale and feels cold.

■ RAYNAUD'S PHENOMENON AND DISEASE
See page 488.

WHITENESS OR PALENESS — GENERAL

■ ANAEMIA
See page 419.

■ LEUKAEMIA
See pages 424 and 490-1.

■ ALBINISM
An inherited abnormality of metabolism that results in absence of pigment in body tissues.
* Fair skin.
* White hair.
* Pink irises of the eyes.
* Problems with sight.

■ PHENYLKETONURIA
Caused by an error of metabolism resulting in an accumulation of chemicals which affect the brain. Children are screened at birth. Treatment involves avoiding foods containing phenylalanine.
* Blond hair.
* Blue eyes.
* Mental deficiency and aggression if untreated.

■ HYPOPITUITARISM
See page 265.

■ SHOCK
See page 408.

PARASITES

Scabies and lice are the principal visible parasites of the human skin and body. *See pages 259-60.*

LINEAR MARKS ON THE SKIN

These are the causes worth considering of clear, isolated, linear marks on the skin. There are others, but they are extremely rare.

■ LYMPHANGITIS
Infection in a limb can track up the lymphatic pathways to the lymph glands. May be seen on the arm and forearm after a simple injury, even a cat scratch to the hand, for example.
* Site of wound may be apparent.
* A red line extends directly from the region of the wound, continuing up towards the armpit.
* Tender lymph nodes may be felt in the armpit.

Antibiotic treatment is advised, to stop the infection.

■ SCABIES
Fine grey lines a few millimetres long. *See page 259.*

■ ACANTHOSIS NIGRICANS
See page 245.

WHITE PATCHES

PROBABLE
VITILIGO

POSSIBLE
HALO NAEVUS
TINEA VERSICOLOUR
POST- INFLAMMATORY

RARE
LICHEN SCLEROSIS ET ATROPHICUS
LEPROSY
MORPHOEA
RAYNAUD'S PHENOMENON AND DISEASE

PROBABLE

■ VITILIGO
See page 248.

POSSIBLE

■ HALO NAEVUS
■ TINEA VERSICOLOUR
■ POST-INFLAMMATORY
See page 248.

RARE

■ LICHEN SCLEROSIS ET ATROPHICUS
See page 259.

THE SKIN

■ LEPROSY
See page 318.

■ MORPHOEA
See page 257.

■ RAYNAUD'S PHENOMENON AND DISEASE
See page 488.

MINIATURE RED SPOTS

There are two causes worth considering:

■ CAMPBELL DE MORGAN SPOTS
* Tiny and bright red, often raised above the surrounding skin surface.
* Present on the chest and abdomen.

Commonest in elderly people. Of little significance.

■ SPIDER NAEVI
These are essentially red spots with several tiny vessels emanating from the centre. They can appear in children and in adults. Multiple naevi may be a feature of pregnancy, and of liver disease; also of hereditary haemorrhagic telangiectasia; *see page 86.*

SORES OR ULCERS

Are described elsewhere in the book in relation to the part of the body on which they occur.

VESICLES

Are small blisters. *See page 239.*

WHEALS

A term describing raised marks on the skin. *See URTICARIA, page 258.*

WARTS

See LUMPS IN THE SKIN, below.

LUMPS IN THE SKIN

It is best to play safe and report any lump in the skin to a doctor: most are innocent, but some need expert evaluation to rule out the possibility of malignant disease.

The earlier the diagnosis and treatment, the better the outlook. If a lump is pigmented, bleeding, irregular, ulcerated or growing rapidly, all the more reason to see a doctor without delay.

Covered here are lumps that may appear in skin anywhere on the body. Lumps specific to certain parts of the body are covered in the appropriate sections.

PROBABLE
SEBACEOUS CYST
DERMOID CYST
PAPILLOMA
WART
VERRUCA

POSSIBLE
LIPOMA
PYOGENIC GRANULOMA
GANGLION
MOLLUSCUM CONTAGIOSUM
VASCULAR MALFORMATIONS
BASAL CELL CARCINOMA

RARE
SQUAMOUS CELL CARCINOMA
MALIGNANT MELANOMA
SECONDARY TUMOUR
LYMPHOMA

PROBABLE

■ SEBACEOUS CYST
Sometimes called a wen. A harmless lump caused by build-up of sebaceous material — solidified, waxy, body fluid — in a sweat gland near the surface of the skin. May well start as an unsqueezed zit: which, if it does not become infected, can develop, over many years, into a sebaceous cyst. No relation to cancer.
* Smooth; not tender.
* Frequently multiple on scalp, neck or scrotum.
* Size ranges from a few milli–metres to several centimetres.
* A small black mark in the centre, the punctum, marks the entrance to the gland.

■ DERMOID CYSTS
These are congenital cysts which develop on the head and neck, and are commonest at the outside end of the eyebrow. They may also occur as benign tumours elsewhere on the body.

■ PAPILLOMA
■ WART
Caused by a viral infection of the skin. Small, often multiple, pain-free thickening of skin with rough skin on the surface, growing proud of the normal skin.

■ VERRUCA
A wart on the base of the foot. Because the foot is weight-bearing, the wart is pushed into the sole of the foot and can be painful.

POSSIBLE

■ LIPOMA
A benign, fatty tumour that may appear as a smooth, often soft, lump in or beneath the skin.

■ PYOGENIC GRANULOMA
Possibly caused by minor injury. A soft, red, fleshy benign tumour which bleeds easily when knocked. Often sited near a finger– or toenail.

■ GANGLION
A local degeneration of fibrous tissue. Appears as a small, firm lump, near tendons or joints. Commonly seen on the back of the wrist. Used to be treated by a blow from the family bible — to disperse the lump. Now a ganglion is either left alone or removed surgically.

THE SKIN

■ MOLLUSCUM CONTAGIOSUM
Caused by a virus.
* Crops of small pink lumps.
* Often on trunk or face.
* Each lump has a depression in the middle.

They clear up of their own accord.

■ VASCULAR MALFORMATIONS
There are many different types: spider naevus, salmon patch (also known as strawberry naevus), port wine stain, Campbell de Morgan spots, hereditary haemorrhagic telangiectasis are examples. These are rarely seen as lumps, but a cavernous haemangioma may develop as a lump. It may be extensive, covering part of the face. Often present at birth. Normally clears by about six years.

■ BASAL CELL CARCINOMA
Commonly called a rodent ulcer. *See page 103.*

RARE

■ SQUAMOUS CELL CARCINOMA
A malignant tumour, commonest in the elderly.
* Often on the head or neck.
* May be a an irregular lump.
* May bleed.
* May ulcerate.
* Local lymph nodes may be enlarged.

■ MALIGNANT MELANOMA
See page 244.

■ SECONDARY TUMOUR
Technical term, metastasis. This is cancer that has spread from a primary site to create tumours elsewhere in the body. Irregular, hard, fleshy nodule(s) or plaque(s) seen or felt in the skin of someone known to have a primary cancer raise the suspicion of metastases. It is rare for skin metastases to be the first symptom you notice of internal primary cancer, but it is possible.

■ LYMPHOMA
One particular type of lymphoma starts in the skin. It is noted as an irregular thickening. Diagnosis can only be made by taking a sample and examining it under the microscope. *See also page 490.*

SKIN TENDS TO CRACK

This is a feature of inflammation or infection of the skin. The most common causes are fungal infection and eczema.

■ FUNGAL INFECTION
Different fungal infections may affect all parts of the body, but commonly hands, feet *(see also ATHLETE'S FOOT, page 320)* and groin.
* Discrete, dry, reddened, itchy, painful areas of skin.
* Skin macerates and rubs off.
* Sometimes, associated blisters.
* Some fissuring, cracking and thickening of the skin.
* There may be an unpleasant smell.

Easily treated with anti-fungal creams and ointments.

■ ECZEMA

The term is often used interchangeably with dermatitis. May be confused with fungal infections, and vice-versa.

* Diffuse patchy redness.
* Red lumps.
* Weeping, crusting.
* Fissuring, scaling.

See page 239.

MOLES

See page 244.

BUBBLES FROM A SKIN WOUND

Bubbles and fluid oozing from a wound, or surrounding skin that feels 'crackly' when pressure is applied, suggests a very severe infection known as 'gas gangrene'. Pain, malaise and discolouration will almost always be present. Get medical help immediately.

BLEEDING 'UNDER' THE SKIN

Medical term, purpura. In fact, the skin has several layers and the term properly describes blood leaking into surrounding surface tissue. The cause is either an injury which did not pierce the skin surface; or an abnormality of blood vessels, or of blood.

When blood leaks into surrounding tissue, it is broken down and undergoes several changes of colour, from red/purple/black to brown, green and yellow.

The significance of purpura ranges from the minimal to an indication of life-threatening disorders.

PROBABLE
BRUISE
SENILE PURPURA

POSSIBLE
DRUG-RELATED
HENOCH SCHÖNLEIN PURPURA
MENINGOCOCCAL SEPTICAEMIA

RARE
BLOOD DISORDERS
SCURVY
EHLERS-DANLOS SYNDROME
DISSEMINATED INTRAVASCULAR COAGULATION

PROBABLE

■ BRUISE

Bruises can be divided (in order of size) into petechiae, or ecchymosis. If there is also a visible or palpable swelling, the term haematoma is used. Bruising may be caused by direct injury — say a blow with a hammer, or indirect pressure — for example, strangulation.

The Skin

■ SENILE PURPURA
* Blotchy, well demarcated purple patches.
* Often seen on legs or arms.
* Part of the ageing process.

POSSIBLE

■ DRUG-RELATED
May be associated with taking steroids.
* Well-demarcated red and purple blotches.

Stop the medication and see your doctor if purpura develops.

■ HENOCH SCHÖNLEIN PURPURA
Cause unknown. In adults and children.
* Purpura.
* Urticarial rash.
* Painful joints.
* Abdominal pain.
* Bloody diarrhoea.
* Blood in the urine.

Normally resolves of its own accord, although steroids may be advised. Complications may affect the kidney.

■ MENINGOCOCCAL SEPTICAEMIA
See also MENINGITIS, pages 444 and 453. A life-threatening condition occurring with or without meningitis. Affects pre-school children most severely.
* Sudden onset of purpuric rash, which may be extensive or minimal.
* Malaise.
* Fever.
* Rapid deterioration and collapse.
* Death may occur within hours.

If suspected, and certainly if the child has had contact with another case of meningitis, see a doctor urgently.

RARE

■ BLOOD DISORDERS
Blood disorders such as leukaemia or aplastic anaemia often show themselves with sudden onset of widespread bruising. *See also page 416.*

■ SCURVY
See page 426.

■ EHLERS-DANLOS SYNDROME
An inherited disease in which the body cannot make normal supporting tissue.
* Markedly 'double-jointed' joints.
* Skin scars easily.
* Bruising is common.
* Skin is soft and velvety in texture.

■ DISSEMINATED INTRAVASCULAR COAGULATION
A potentially fatal condition caused by failure of the blood clotting mechanism. Often associated with severe infection. Rarely seen outside hospitals.

BOILS AND CARBUNCLES

■ A BOIL
Is an abscess in a hair follicle. Also known as a furuncle.
* Prime sites are the neck, armpit

and buttocks.
* Local redness.
* Swelling.
* Pain.
* Develops a point and discharges yellow/green pus.

■ CARBUNCLE
Is a collection of boils that may interconnect under the skin.

Recurrent boils or carbuncles suggest the possibility of underlying disease, particularly diabetes mellitus, *see page 485*. Urine can be tested for sugar as a quick screening method. Another cause of recurrent boils may be poor personal hygiene. Occasionally, the diagnosis of acne vulgaris *(see page 238)* may have been missed.

Boils and carbuncles will normally come to a head, discharge their fluid naturally and disappear. However, this may take so long or be so painful that it is tempting to lance the boil at an early stage. **Don't.**

It is important that this is done when the boil is 'ripe'. See your doctor or practice nurse to have a boil lanced — if it is done inexpertly, the result may be severe scarring.

Nowadays, antibiotics can often clear boils either before they become too painful or before they discharge.

BULLAE

Medical term for a large blister. *See page 239*.

CORNS AND CALLUSES

Both words describe harmless thickening of the skin, which develops as a protective measure.

■ A CORN
Typically appears on the upper surface of the little toe, where the toe rubs against shoes.

■ A CALLUS
Plural, callosities, is a thickening of the skin of the hands or feet. People who go habitually barefoot develop callosities on the pressure-bearing areas of the sole.

Likewise, manual workers develop callosities on the palms of the hands, typically at the base of the fingers.

FLAB

Apart from obvious folds of fatty tissue that go with obesity, flab is sometimes used to describe skin which has lost elasticity: you can pick it up in folds, and it fails to return immediately to its original contours. There are three main causes:

■ AGEING
With age, skin loses its elasticity.

The Skin

Wrinkles, skin creases and sagging jaw lines are part of the process — and provide limitless work for cosmetic surgeons.

■ DEHYDRATION
The body needs a certain amount of water in order to function properly. Severe loss of fluid can arise because of reduced intake (for example when someone is in a coma) or increased output (for example with diarrhoea or vomiting).

The result is flabby, turgid skin, which will not unwrinkle when pinched. Naturally, this effect of fluid loss does not happen overnight.

■ MASSIVE WEIGHT LOSS
If you are obese, and manage, with a commendable spurt of willpower, to lose a large proportion of your weight very rapidly, you may be unjustly repaid with a new problem. The skin needs time to compensate for the loss of fat; meanwhile, huge lax folds of skin develop, particularly on the abdomen, buttocks, thighs and upper arms. Cosmetic surgery may be helpful in some cases.

HARD SKIN, LOCAL OR GENERAL

The obvious diagnosis is a corn or callus, covered separately on *page 255*. Here are the less self-evident causes.

PROBABLE
KELOID

POSSIBLE
LYMPHOEDEMA
POST-PHLEBITIC LIMB
MYXOEDEMA

RARE
VITAMIN A DEFICIENCY
MORPHOEA
SCLERODERMA
CANCER

PROBABLE

■ KELOID
Describes excessive scarring after cuts or injury and is seen most commonly in black people. The site of the injury hardens, with an overgrowth of hard scar tissue above the level of the surrounding skin. Why some people develop keloid scarring and others don't is a mystery. It is harmless, but severe cases sometimes require treatment for the scar tissue, either by injection or by further surgery. There is no guarantee that this will lead to a more satisfactory appearance.

POSSIBLE

■ LYMPHOEDEMA
■ POST-PHLEBITIC LIMB
See SWOLLEN ANKLE, page 309.

■ MYXOEDEMA
Puffy swelling of the skin, particularly on hands, feet and ankles and around eyes. May be seen with hypothyroidism, *page 461.*

RARE

■ VITAMIN A DEFICIENCY
* Night blindness.
* Abnormality of the cornea leading to inflammation, scarring and blindness.
* Rough, dry skin.

■ MORPHOEA
A localized variant of scleroderma *see below.*
* Well-defined, pale areas.
* The skin in these areas is smooth and hard.
* Loss of hair at these sites may occur.
* Ulceration may occur.

■ SCLERODERMA
An auto-immune disease.
* Hard, rigid skin develops.
* Tiny red spots (telangiectasia) are evident.
* Skin becomes shiny and smooth.
* Hands become stiff.
* Joints may become stiff.
* Skin of face is affected, making the mouth appear small.
* Face lacks expression.
* Raynaud's phenomenon *(see page 488)* develops.
* Swallowing is impaired and weight loss follows.

See also PROBLEMS WITH SWALLOWING PLUS WEIGHT LOSS, page 122.

■ CANCER
Secondary or metastatic cancer deposits (having spread from a primary site elsewhere) can arise in the skin, giving small areas which are hard to the touch. They may be single or multiple. A somewhat specialized example is a secondary deposit in the navel, called Sister Mary's nodule, after the nun who first observed it.

AN ITCHY RASH

PROBABLE
ECZEMA
URTICARIA (HIVES)
SCABIES
LICE
INSECT BITES
FUNGAL INFECTION

POSSIBLE
PITYRIASIS ROSEA
LICHEN SIMPLEX
PRURITUS ANI
VULVAL ITCH
DRUG REACTION

RARE
NODULAR PRURIGO
LICHEN SCLEROSIS ET ATROPHICUS

The Skin

PROBABLE

■ ECZEMA
See page 239.

■ URTICARIA
Commonly called hives. A type of allergic reaction, triggered by various different agents. Typically, urticaria appears suddenly and dramatically. The wheal may come and go quite quickly, clearing in one area, only to reappear in another.
* Red, blotchy areas with puffy, paler patches in the middle.
* Some swelling.
* Itchy, often intensely so.

There are several types, grouped according to cause or appearance. One form, dermatographia, is particularly severe: just stroking the skin firmly raises a wheal — you can even draw a picture on the skin.

The most common form is allergic urticaria. Common causes include: plants, chemicals, food, medicine colourants.

■ SCABIES
■ LICE
■ INSECT BITES
Can occur as an itchy rash, or with no obvious rash. Details, *pages 259-60.*

■ FUNGAL INFECTION
See page 252.

POSSIBLE

■ PITYRIASIS ROSEA
Commonest in young people, and may be associated with a viral infection.
* A single, itchy red lesion may appear anywhere on the trunk — the herald patch.
* After a few days, scattered patches of pinkish elevated areas develop. They characteristically lie along the line of the ribs.
* The rash persists for about six weeks.

Usually no treatment is required. Calamine lotion or, in severe cases, antihistamine drugs, may help.

■ LICHEN SIMPLEX
You scratch an itchy place. The itchiness goes for a while, but as soon it comes back, you scratch again. A vicious cycle of scratching and itching develops, causing local inflammation. The inflammation causes thickening of the skin, with furrows or lines developing in the chronic case.

■ PRURITUS ANI
■ VULVAL ITCH
These conditions are often characterized by itching plus rash. *See pages 161 and 360.*

■ DRUG REACTION
If you are allergic to a drug, the classic reaction is:
* Widespread rash, but predominating on trunk.
* Patchy reddening.
* Some local swelling.
* Intense itching.

Reactions to drugs can occur

even after long-term use.

RARE

■ NODULAR PRURIGO
* Multiple warty areas.
* Intensely itchy.
Cause unknown, but possibly initiated by scratching.

■ LICHEN SCLEROSIS ET ATROPHICUS
* Involves skin around the vulva.
* White, pale skin.
* Clearly delineated.
* Reddened areas within the affected skin.
* Itchy.
When seen on children this may wrongly be attributed to abuse.

ITCHING - WITHOUT A RASH

Covered here is persistent, severe itching that has become a nuisance. The medical term is pruritus.

Close inspection with a magnifying glass may reveal either of the common causes — scabies and lice. Scratch marks are the obvious evidence of severe itching, and of course they also reveal to the doctor where the symptom is at its worst. Excluded here are an itching scalp caused by a bad bout of dandruff, covered separately on *page 265*; and itching in the anal area, covered separately on *page 161*.

PROBABLE
SCABIES
LICE
INSECT BITES, INCLUDING FLEAS
FIBREGLASS
SENILE PRURITUS
THREADWORM

POSSIBLE
PREGNANCY
LIVER DISEASE
JAUNDICE
DRUGS
PSYCHOLOGICAL

RARE
DERMATITIS HERPETIFORMIS
URAEMIA
BLOOD DISORDERS

PROBABLE

■ SCABIES
Infestation with the scabies mite, which burrows under the skin.
* Severe itching is noted.
* Mite burrows may be seen as grey lines a couple of millimetres long.
* Burrows are often between fingers or front of wrists.
* Eventually, raised, reddened areas may appear all over the body.
* Scabs may develop because of scratching.

THE SKIN

■ LICE
Commonly known as nits. There are three main types: head lice, body lice and pubic lice.
* Persistent itching.
* Local lymph nodes may enlarge.
* Eggs may be seen on the bases of hairs; or you may see lice themselves: they are quite elusive.
* Spread by direct contact with other infected hairs or skin.
* The pubic louse may cause itching in the anal or vulval regions.

■ INSECT BITES, INCLUDING FLEAS
* Itching at the site of the bite.
* Reddened, hard nodules at the site of the bite appear later.
Fleas are commonly the culprits; commonest in homes with cats.

■ FIBREGLASS
Glass fibres can become invisibly embedded in skin, causing itching. Protective clothing should be worn.

■ SENILE PRURITUS
The elderly sometimes complain of itching for which no cause can be found: it may be the result of the ageing process.

■ THREADWORM
See WORMS, page 153.
* Itching and irritation around the anus.
Most children have this common complaint at some time. Treatment is simple, and available either directly from the chemist or from a doctor.

POSSIBLE

■ PREGNANCY
Many women complain of itching in the last months of pregnancy. Local causes such as thrush need to be excluded.

■ LIVER DISEASE
■ JAUNDICE
Any condition, and typically liver disease, which causes *JAUNDICE,* may also cause intense itching. The itching may arise before the yellow skin colour is noticed.

■ DRUGS
Some drugs, for instance, penicillin and aspirin, can cause severe allergic reactions, with itching. And some of the narcotic drugs, including cocaine and heroin, may cause itching, sometimes related to impurities.

■ PSYCHOLOGICAL
Itching without any cause found after full examination and investigation may be a sign of underlying psychological problems.

RARE

■ DERMATITIS HERPETIFORMIS
See page 240.

■ URAEMIA
High levels of urea in the blood are one of the end results of untreated renal (kidney) failure. A number of symptoms may be present:
* Dry, coated tongue.
* Breath smelling of urine.

* Hiccups.
* Nausea and vomiting.
* Dry, yellow-brown skin with a whitish 'frost'.
* Marked itching.
* Anaemia.

■ BLOOD DISORDERS
A number of blood and related diseases may cause severe itching. They include: *Polycythemia rubra vera*; lymphoma; Hodgkin's disease; leukaemias.

PRURITUS

The medical term for itching. *See pages 257-61.*

SKIN FEELS CLAMMY

See page 472, also 408. If associated with coldness, look at ITCHING OR NUMBNESS etc, page 320.

DRY SKIN

The two simple explanations are inflammation, or failure of the sweat glands to work normally.

PROBABLE
ECZEMA
FUNGAL INFECTIONS

POSSIBLE
HEAT (SUN) STROKE
HYPOTHYROIDISM

RARE
URAEMIA
VITAMIN A DEFICIENCY
ICHTHYOSIS

PROBABLE

■ ECZEMA
See page 239. When not in a phase of acute inflammation, patches of skin affected by eczema may feel dry and rough to the touch.

■ FUNGAL INFECTIONS
See page 352.

POSSIBLE

■ HEAT (SUN) STROKE
Prolonged physical work in hot conditions or staying too long in the sun puts anyone, even the fit athlete, at risk of heat stroke.

Commonest in the very young and the elderly. Symptoms may develop rapidly.
* Dry skin, hot to the touch.
* High temperature.
* Weakness.
* Thirst.
* Headache.
* Confusion.

If untreated, can be fatal. It is important to protect yourself against the sun:

• wear hat, shirt; apply sun block; maintain a high fluid intake (no alcohol);
• keep cool by taking frequent showers or swimming;
avoid exposure to the midday sun.

If you supect this condition, seek medical help urgently.

■ HYPOTHYROIDISM
See page 461.

RARE

■ URAEMIA
See page 260.

■ VITAMIN A DEFICIENCY
See page 257.

■ ICHTHYOSIS
A group of inherited disorders of the skin, in which the skin is thickened, dry and flaky. Often the inner aspect of skin overlying joints (typically armpits and elbow creases) is spared.

Very occasionally, these changes, appearing in later life, may be associated with underlying malignant disease.

BODY ODOUR

This is possibly the vaguest and most subjective symptom of all. Doctors and dentists see many people who believe that they smell, or that some part of them smells, even though no one else has commented.

Some people seem to be abnormally sensitive to smells. And some people, notably small children, have a virtually non-existent sense of smell.

Serious underlying disease is *very* rarely the reason for offensive body odour. If you put aside obvious cases of body odour caused by stale sweat, and if you also exclude psychological cases, where the smell is a belief rather than a physical fact, body odour usually comes down to three relatively common possibilities:

■ ATHLETE'S FOOT: a fungal infection of the feet with reddened, itchy, painful areas between the toes, fissuring and cracking. The feet and shoes give off a characteristic cheesy odour, which is sometimes strong enough for others to smell, even if the shoes are on.

■ BAD BREATH *See page 88.*

■ OFFENSIVE DISCHARGES, for example vaginal discharge.

...and one rare possibility:

■ FISH ODOUR SYNDROME
One of several rare metabolic diseases.

The first three are easily remedied by self-help and commonsense use of over-the-counter medications. The last needs specialist treatment and advice on odour-concealment.

LIFELESS HAIR

Loss of 'body' or 'life' in the hair is to some extent inevitable with advancing years. It is also seen in association with the medical conditions that cause baldness. Severe stress, such as that caused by major, prolonged illness, can also affect the quality and thickness of hair. Vitamin deficiency and severe undernourishment will also affect hair quality.

LOSS OF HAIR OR BALDNESS

Normal baldness (also described as alopecia) — part of the male ageing process — is characterized by:

* Recession of the hairline at the forehead and temples.
* Thinning of the hair on the crown. It becomes dry and lifeless; loses 'body'.
* A gradual meeting of the hairless areas so that hair remains only on the sides and back of the head.

Women do not have a hereditary tendency to baldness. Although dramatic hair loss may be experienced by women (*see below*) total baldness is not seen.

Female hair does, however, thin with age. While some thinning is inevitable, occasionally families notice a marked trend towards thin hair, again associated with ageing, passed from mother to daughter.

Abnormal hair loss can of course be a sign (in women as well is in men) of scalp disease, or more generalized disease. Most such cases, as this section shows, are fairly easy to distinguish from normal baldness.

Stages of male baldness

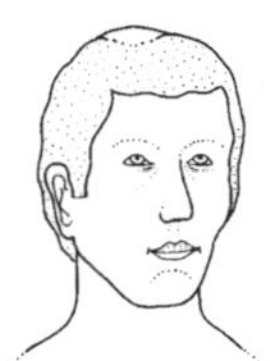

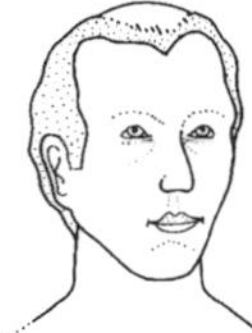

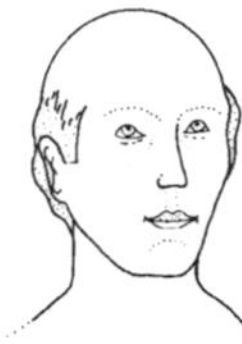

PROBABLE
ECZEMA OR DERMATITIS
ALOPECIA AREATA
CHILDBIRTH

POSSIBLE
INJURY
PSORIASIS
IRON DEFICIENCY
HYPOTHYROIDISM
POST-MENOPAUSAL CHANGE
RINGWORM
TELOGEN ALOPECIA

RARE
AIDS
HYPOPITUITARISM
ANOGEN ALOPECIA

Hair

PROBABLE

■ ECZEMA OR DERMATITIS
Any inflammatory skin inflammation may cause loss of hair in the areas affected.
* Complete patches of hair loss.
* Skin is inflamed, weeping and crusting.
* Scales may be seen.
* There may well be dermatitis or eczema elsewhere on the body.

■ ALOPECIA AREATA
The commonest cause of patchy baldness.
* Local areas of total baldness.
* Normal skin.
* Several patches may occur together.
* Regrowth normally occurs spontaneously after a few months.

This is often seen at a time of stress, such as bereavement.

■ CHILDBIRTH
Many women notice changes in hair substance and texture before and after childbirth: it tends to be generally thinner and finer.

After childbirth, or even in pregnancy, it is not unusual for there to be dramatic hair loss. Large quantities of hair seen in the bath or basin at this time should not cause alarm. Normally hair growth recovers with time. In rare cases, the original texture of the hair is never restored.

POSSIBLE

■ INJURY
Burns, skin loss or even deep cuts can damage hair-bearing skin, so that hair may never re-grow.

Generally speaking, hair does not grow on scar tissue. The only solution is to hide such areas by expert combing and styling.

■ PSORIASIS
* Hair loss in areas of psoriasis on the scalp.
* Silvery, scaly red patches seen in scalp.
* Other signs of psoriasis seen elsewhere on body; *see page 242.*

■ IRON DEFICIENCY
* Generalized hair loss or thinning.
* May improve after taking iron supplements.

See also IRON DEFICIENCY ANAEMIA, page 422.

■ HYPOTHYROIDISM
See page 461.
* Hair is sparse.
* Hair may be dry and thin.

■ POST-MENOPAUSAL CHANGE
Hair texture may change in and around the menopause due to alterations in hormone balance. The role of hormone replacement therapy in protecting against or reversing the effects of the menopause is a subject of continuing research.

■ RINGWORM
Medical term *tinea capitis*. A fungal infection of the skin of the scalp.
* Circular bald patches.
* Scaling of the skin.
* Brittle hair stumps remain.

Treated with anti-fungal creams.

■ TELOGEN ALOPECIA
A term describing diffuse loss of hair which is in the resting stage of its life-cycle. A number of causes have been identified, unrelated to local scalp disease, including: childbirth (*see above*); emotional stress; any illness with fever; loss of blood; any major illness.

Except in some *very* rare cases, the hair commonly grows again after a few months.

RARE

■ AIDS
Hair loss may be noted in the later stages of AIDS.

■ HYPOPITUITARISM
Under-activity of the pituitary gland may show itself in many ways, including:

* Absence of sexual function (absence of libido).
* Absence of periods in females.
* Pale skin.
* Hair loss.
* Visual defects.
* Weight gain and fatigue.

See also page 000.

■ ANOGEN ALOPECIA
Some drugs affect hair during their growth phase, notably anti-cancer 'cell poisons' given as courses of 'chemotherapy'.

Vitamin A toxicity is another example. After stopping the drug, hair will eventually grow again, but the texture of the hair may be quite different to what it was before.

Site of pituitary gland

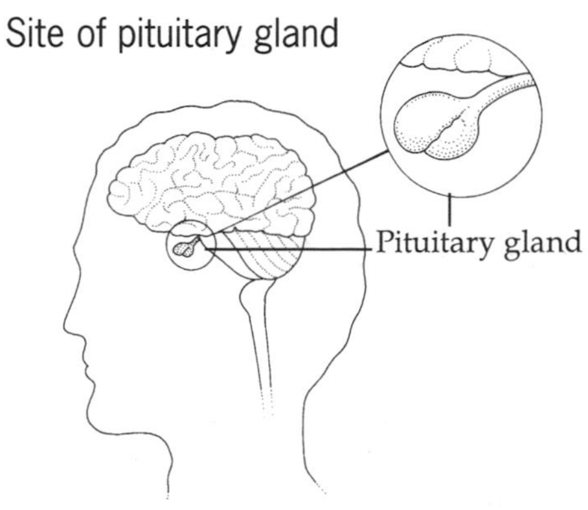

DANDRUFF

The causes of this almost universal condition are unclear, although some research suggests that it may occasionally be due to underlying infection, or to a generalized skin disease such as psoriasis, *page 242.* For most, dandruff arises from time to time because of the skin's natural tendency to flake — to shed its topmost layer — so that it can be renewed from below. General ill-health may make it worse, but dandruff is so natural and common that it is unhelpful to try to explain it away as a sign of poor physical condition.

The worst cases are accompanied by itching of the scalp.

Use of anti-dandruff shampoos really does help. Persist with the treatment as long as the dandruff remains. If this does not improve the situation, it is worth discussing the problem with your doctor. He or she can prescribe a variety of treatments, ranging from strong, tar-based shampoos to special shampoos containing ketoconazole. This is extremely effective.

Steroid scalp lotions may also be helpful in some circumstances.

UNWANTED BODY HAIR

It is one of nature's many ironies that while baldness is almost universally an unwanted male symptom, unwanted body hair is almost exclusively a female symptom. Covered here is hirsutism in its specific sense of a male pattern of hair distribution on a woman.

PROBABLE
NORMAL PATTERN

POSSIBLE
POLYCYSTIC OVARIES
MENOPAUSE

RARE
DRUGS
ACROMEGALY
CUSHING'S SYNDROME
TURNER'S SYNDROME
CONGENITAL ADRENAL HYPERPLASIA

PROBABLE

■ NORMAL PATTERN
Patterns of hair growth on face, limbs and body vary according to country or region of origin. Individuals should compare themselves with others from a similar ethnic background before deciding that they have abnormally hairy bodies. For example, Japanese and Chinese women have very little body hair, whereas Mediterranean people may have much more.

POSSIBLE

■ POLYCYSTIC OVARIES
Otherwise known as the Stein-Leventhal syndrome.
* Hairiness.
* Obesity.
* Often absent periods.
* Ovaries have multiple cysts.

■ MENOPAUSE
Women going through the menopause may note increased amounts of hair, typically fine hair that appears on the face.

RARE

■ DRUGS
A number of drugs may increase either fine hair on the face or body hair elsewhere. They include:
* Some steroid preparations.
* Hormone treatments, including the pill.
* Minoxidil, used to treat raised blood pressure, but now also used as a hair restorer.
* Some anti-epileptic drugs.

■ ACROMEGALY
In addition to its other features *(see page 275)* women with acromegaly may have increased body hair.

HAIR

Site of adrenal gland

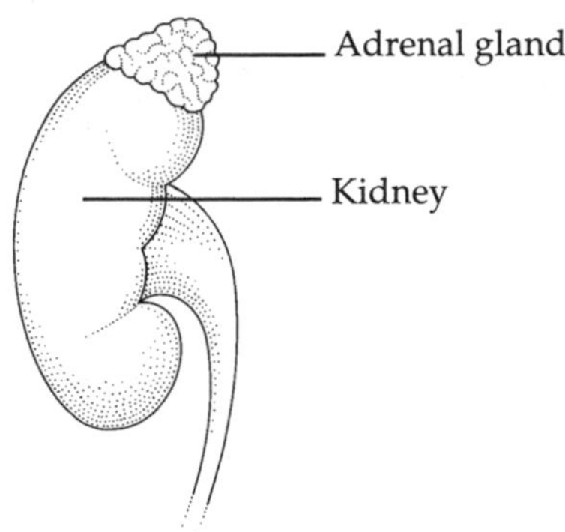

■ CUSHING'S SYNDROME

May be caused by a disorder of the adrenal gland, or by taking steroids.
* Round, 'moon' face.
* Fat deposited on back (buffalo-hump).
* Fat deposited on body (not legs).
* Muscle fatigue.
* Easily bruised skin.
* Stretch marks.
* Bone pain.

Women also note:
* Increased body hair.
* Periods stop.
* Enlarged clitoris.

Men may suffer from:
* Impotence.
* Acne.

■ TURNER'S SYNDROME

A chromosomal abnormality. The individual is genetically male, but has female characteristics, including:
* Short stature.
* No secondary sexual characteristics.
* Hardly any neck (that is, very short).
* Broad chest with widely separated nipples.
* Deafness.
* Hirsutism.

■ CONGENITAL ADRENAL HYPERPLASIA

Excessive growth of the adrenal glands from birth.
* Mild hirsutism.
* Enlarged clitoris.
* Fused labia.

May appear at a later age with:
* Acne.
* Early false puberty.
* Enlarged clitoris.
* Absent or scanty periods.

The Skeletal and Muscular Symptoms

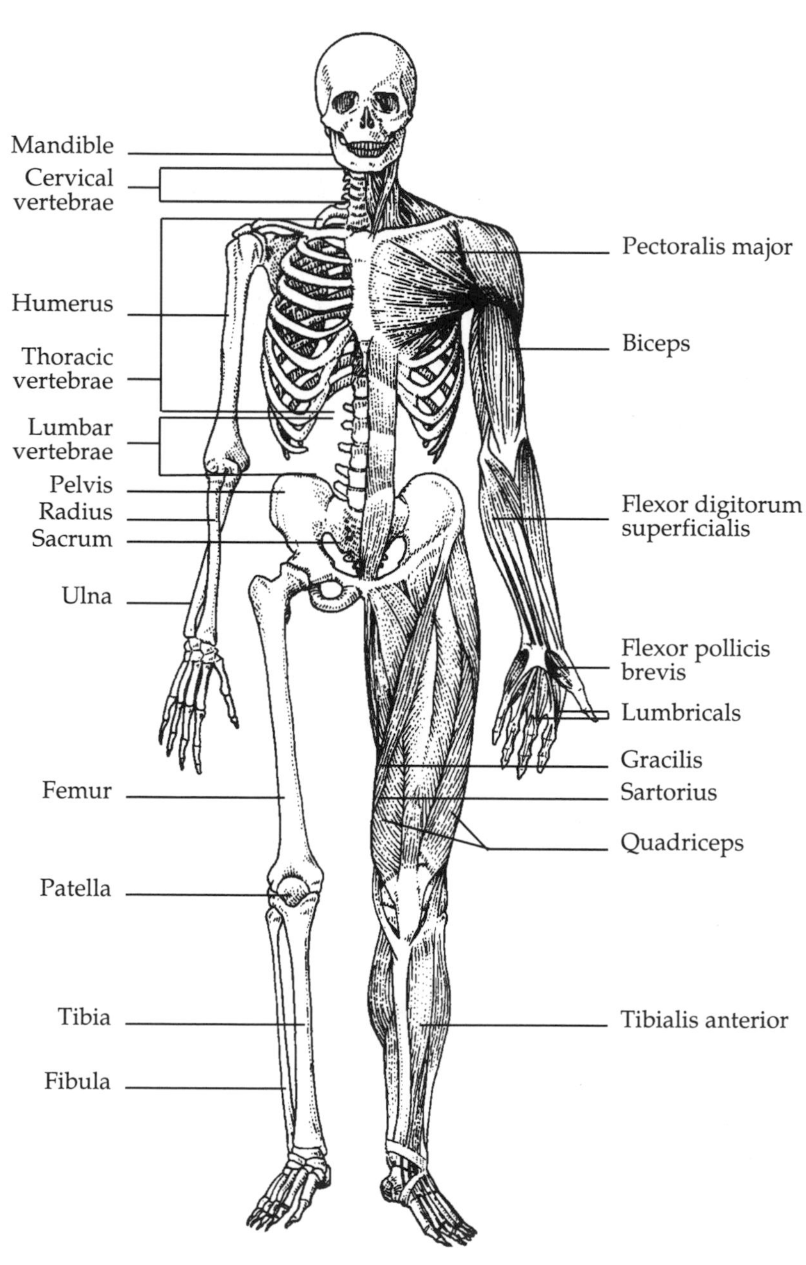

THE BONES, JOINTS AND MUSCLES - INTRODUCTION

This section covers the body's 'chassis': the frame on which the tissues hang. Connected to the bones are the muscles whose expansion and contraction, lengthening and shortening, provides movement. They have many common problems.

The symptoms of some diseases affecting bones, joints and muscles are unique to them alone. It is also true that few firm diagnoses are made in this area by family doctors, without additional information from X-rays, blood tests or other investigations. Further investigations may be needed after diagnosis and treatment in order to check progress.

In this section the usual order of symptoms has been varied in order to begin with some key general symptoms of muscles and bones occurring elsewhere in the body. We then move to specific bone, joint and muscle symptoms as experienced in different parts of the body, working from the shoulders downwards. Finally, under the heading FINGERS AND TOES, are grouped symptoms affecting the outer reaches, or extremities, of the body, which are vulnerable in certain special ways.

WASTING AND LOSS OF POWER IN THE MUSCLES

Muscular wasting, or atrophy, results from either damage to the nerve or blood supply to a muscle; lack of use because of illness or injury; or primary muscle disease.

PROBABLE

INJURY
GENERAL BODY WASTING

POSSIBLE

CARPAL TUNNEL SYNDROME
INJURY OF A NERVE OR NERVES
DIABETES
ALCOHOLIC NEUROPATHY
RHEUMATOID ARTHRITIS

RARE

MOTOR NEURONE DISEASE
DUCHENNE'S DYSTROPHY
TUBERCULOSIS
SUBACUTE COMBINED DEGENERATION OF THE SPINAL CORD

PROBABLE

■ INJURY

The body's normal protective response to immobilization of the

Muscles

affected part. One of the best examples of this is a damaged knee. The knee is held slightly flexed, and you try to prevent movement for a few days. By the end of a week, you may well see some wasting of the quadriceps muscle at the front of the thigh.

The weaker the muscle, the less safe the joint feels, and a vicious circle of disuse and further wasting then continues. This is why careful medical assessment and controlled exercises to maintain muscle bulk are important for all such injuries.

■ GENERAL BODY WASTING
Bed-bound patients can develop generalized disuse atrophy (wasting) of these muscles. This can be aggravated by the underlying condition.

POSSIBLE

■ CARPAL TUNNEL SYNDROME
See page 293.

■ INJURY OF A NERVE OR NERVES
See page 319.

■ DIABETES
See DIABETIC NEUROPATHY, page 317.

■ ALCOHOLIC NEUROPATHY
See page 318.

■ RHEUMATOID ARTHRITIS
See page 279.

RARE

■ MOTOR NEURONE DISEASE
A disease of the nervous system. There are several forms, but the main features are:
* Progressive onset of muscular weakness, accompanied by muscle wasting.
* Small muscles of the hand are affected first.
* 'Flickering' contractions of parts of muscles.

The disease progresses relentlessly, ultimately affecting speech, swallowing and breathing muscles.

■ DUCHENNE'S DYSTROPHY
This is a primary muscle disease, which starts during the first few years of life.
* Wasting and weakness of back and pelvic muscles; affects both sides of the body.
* Failure of function affecting both sides of the body leads to a 'waddling' gait while still mobile.
* Gradual degeneration leading to inability to walk and general immobility.
* Immobility leads to the muscles shortening, and deformity becomes inevitable.

The outlook is poor.

■ TUBERCULOSIS
See page 447.

■ SUBACUTE COMBINED DEGENERATION OF THE SPINAL CORD
See page 320.

CRAMPS, ACHES AND PAINS IN THE MUSCLES

Most are of little significance. If they die away within a few days they should not be taken seriously, unless they are recurrent.

PROBABLE
SIMPLE CRAMP
VIRAL OR BACTERIAL INFECTION
INJURY

POSSIBLE
INTERMITTENT CLAUDICATION
BIOCHEMICAL IMBALANCE

RARE
DRUGS
DERMATOMYOSITIS
POLYMYOSITIS
POLYMYALGIA RHEUMATICA
TETANUS

PROBABLE

■ SIMPLE CRAMP
* Sudden onset of muscle spasm, often while asleep.
* Muscle, often the calf, feels hard due to contraction.
* Relieved by massage.
* Often residual discomfort for a few hours.

■ VIRAL OR BACTERIAL INFECTION
Fleeting muscular pains are a common accompaniment of any infection. Most settle within a day or two. No specific treatment is required, apart from that for the underlying infection.

■ INJURY
A direct blow to a muscle can cause painful local swelling and bruising. Indirect injury, for instance straining to lift a heavy object, can make muscle fibres stretch and tear. Repetition of the movement reproduces the pain. Treatment for both is painkillers and resting the affected muscle.

POSSIBLE

■ INTERMITTENT CLAUDICATION
See PERIPHERAL VASCULAR DISEASE, page 318.

■ BIOCHEMICAL IMBALANCE
Loss of salt, typically after strenuous exercise, can precipitate painful cramps.

RARE

■ DRUGS
A number of drugs are known to cause muscle pains. These include lithium, alcohol, amphetamines and suxamethonium (used for general anaesthesia).

■ DERMATOMYOSITIS
A disease associated with disordered immunity. May be

associated with cancer. Develops from the age of 40 years onwards.
* Inflammation and pains in multiple muscle groups.
* Muscular weakness.
* Dermatitis.
* Oedema.

■ POLYMYOSITIS
Can be associated with many diseases, including collagen disorders and lung cancer. May remit and relapse.
* Progressive, painful inflammation of muscles — worse when used.
* Affects muscles in a variable manner, but those affected are weak.
* Fever.
* Malaise.
* Tachycardia.

■ POLYMYALGIA RHEUMATICA
A disease of the elderly.
* Painful, stiff upper limb muscles.
* Malaise.
* Fever.

■ TETANUS
Caused by the organism *Clostridia tetani* and acquired by contamination of open wounds. The damage is done by a very powerful toxin that attacks the nervous system. Symptoms may take two weeks to develop.
* Local muscular weakness near site of infection.
* Facial muscles go into spasm: the individual appears to be forcing a grin.
* Muscles of the body go into spasm at the slightest stimulus.
* Fever

Tetanus still claims victims, even when cared for in specialized units. Immunization is the essential precaution, and needs to be repeated every ten years. To help you remember your immunization, choose a convenient birthday (for example your twentieth) on or near which you can renew the cover.

POOR OR ABSENT MUSCLE CONTROL

See THE BRAIN AND NERVOUS SYSTEM, pages 377-409, especially CONVULSIONS, page 387 and PARALYSIS, pages 404-5.

INVOLUNTARY TWITCHING OR TREMBLING MUSCLES

See page 438.

UNUSUALLY WEAK MUSCLE

Muscle weakness without muscle wasting is rare. However, two conditions are worth considering. Both are very rare.

■ CUSHING'S SYNDROME
Caused by an excess of corticosteroids, and often the result of doctors giving steroids to treat other diseases such as rheumatoid arthritis.
* Weight gain, except for limbs.
* Moon face.

* Buffalo hump.
* Muscle weakness.
* Purple lines (striae) on abdomen, back and upper thighs.
* Osteoporosis.
* Diabetes.
* High blood pressure.
* Hair grows on body.
* Occasional psychiatric disorders.

■ PRIMARY ALDOSTERONISM
A very rare disease, also known as Conn's syndrome, caused by excess secretion of aldosterone by the adrenal gland.
* Muscle weakness.
* Excessive thirst.
* Excessive urine output.
* High blood pressure.

THE SKELETON

PAINFUL BONES

Pain in bones can be either localized — to part of one or more bones — or generalized.

PROBABLE
INJURY
OSTEOARTHRITIS
OSTEOPOROSIS

POSSIBLE
SECONDARY BONE CANCER

RARE
OSTEOMALACIA AND RICKETS
TUBERCULOSIS
INFLAMMATORY ARTHROPATHIES
PRIMARY BONE CANCER

PROBABLE

■ INJURY
Is it broken?

Signs of a break (fracture) are:
* Pain at the site of injury.
* Possibly deformity — the limb looks bent.
* Loss of function — typically inability to bear weight.

Depending on the site and force of the injury, skin, nerves and blood vessels may be involved.

Obviously, urgent medical attention is needed.

Persistent pain following an injury, particularly when accompanied by swelling, should raise the suspicion of a fracture. Seek medical help.

Lesser injury may not cause a break, but can still cause pain and loss of function.

See also SUBPERIOSTEAL HAEMATOMA, this page.

■ OSTEOARTHRITIS
See page 285.

■ OSTEOPOROSIS
See page 286.

POSSIBLE

■ SECONDARY CANCER
There is the possibility of localized bone pain being caused by a secondary (metastatic) deposit in someone with cancer. So if an individual has a *known* cancer elsewhere in the body, this possibility needs considering. In an otherwise fit person, it becomes a *rare* rather than *possible* diagnosis.

RARE

■ RICKETS AND OSTEOMALACIA
See page 287.

■ TUBERCULOSIS
See page 289.

■ INFLAMMATORY ARTHROPATHIES
A term for joint inflammation, e.g. rheumatoid arthritis or ankylosing spondylitis, *pages 279 and 287.*

■ PRIMARY BONE CANCER
See under CANCER OF BONE OR CARTILAGE, 276.

BONES, SWOLLEN OR MISSHAPEN

PROBABLE
CALLUS
SUBPERIOSTEAL HAEMATOMA

POSSIBLE
ACUTE OSTEOMYELITIS
CHRONIC OSTEOMYELITIS
RICKETS
MALUNION OF FRACTURE
ACROMEGALY
PAGET'S DISEASE OF BONE

RARE
BENIGN TUMOUR
CANCER OF BONE OR CARTILAGE
TUBERCULOSIS

PROBABLE

■ CALLUS
New bone formed after a fracture.
* Previous, definite bone fracture.
* Forms within a few weeks.
* The larger the bone, the greater the amount of callus.
* Pain-free when bone is fully healed.

■ SUBPERIOSTEAL HAEMATOMA
A direct injury to bone, typically the shin, but no fracture.
* Clear history of local injury.
* Swelling (bruising) noted almost

immediately.
* Painful for several weeks after the injury.
* A hard lump still apparent weeks or months afterwards.
* Common in those who play 'rough and tumble', or contact, sports.

POSSIBLE

■ ACUTE OSTEOMYELITIS
A bone infection which, if suspected, requires immediate treatment. A primary site of infection elsewhere in the body may be apparent, the bone being affected by bacteria carried in the bloodstream.
* High, persistent fever.
* Sudden onset of pain in bone with swelling, which may not be obvious.
* Overlying redness and swelling of the soft tissues, not the bone.
* Extreme pain on movement.
* Rigors.
* Malaise.

■ CHRONIC OSTEOMYELITIS
May occur after untreated or inadequately treated acute osteomyelitis; or after a compound fracture (where there is a fracture and a cut down to the bone).
* Thickening of bone.
* Wound (sinus) discharging pus.
* Local pain.
* Inflammation around wound.

■ RICKETS
See page 287.

■ MALUNION OF FRACTURE
Failure of adequate reduction — meaning a poorly joined break. Sometimes this occurs despite careful realignment or setting of the broken bone. It may give the appearance of deformity or swelling.

■ ACROMEGALY
General enlargement of the skeleton caused by excessive growth hormone from the pituitary gland. Jaws and hands appear especially large.

■ PAGET'S DISEASE OF BONE
See page 437.

RARE

■ BENIGN TUMOUR OF BONE AND CARTILAGE
Both bone and cartilage in any part of the body may give rise to benign tumours which present as:
* Pain-free hard lumps.
* Smooth surfaces.
* Slow-growing.

■ CANCER OF BONE OR CARTILAGE
Individuals with known cancer of other organs of the body (for example breast or lung) may develop secondary tumours (deposits) in the bones.
* Chronically and progressively painful.
* Pain may be very localized.
* A lump may *not* be present.

Other symptoms of advanced cancer may be present, but sometimes bone secondaries are the first indication of an as-yet undiagnosed cancer. This is why localized pain in a bone without a history of injury should be followed up with your doctor.

Primary malignant bone tumours are rarer than secondary tumours. They may form at any age, and there are several different types.

■ TUBERCULOSIS
See page 289.

BONES BREAKING EASILY

Meaning fractures occurring without an obvious history of injury. They divide into two types: those which are the result of disease (pathological) and those in apparently normal bones (spontaneous or stress fractures).

Spontaneous or stress fractures may occur because of repeated bending, as when athletes train; or after repeated compression, for instance jumping and running, that acts on the spine.
* Local pain.
* Local swelling.
* Relieved by rest over a few days.
* Pain recurs when activity is repeated.
* May not be seen initially on an X-ray.

Typical sites include the small bones of the foot (metatarsals); upper arm bone (humerus); upper thigh bone (neck of femur); knee cap (patella); and spine.

In pathological fractures, the bone is abnormally weak because of either local abnormality (for example, malignant tumours, tuberculosis, osteomyelitis) or general abnormality (for example, osteoporosis, osteomalacia). These abnormalities can be congenital (for example, brittle bone disease) or acquired (rheumatoid arthritis). Also, if a bone is unused, it becomes thinner and is prone to break.

PROBABLE
OSTEOPOROSIS

POSSIBLE
PAGET'S DISEASE OF BONE
OSTEOMALACIA
DISUSED BONE

RARE
OSTEOMYELITIS
BENIGN BONE TUMOURS
BONE CANCER
BRITTLE BONE DISEASE
MARBLE BONES

PROBABLE

■ OSTEOPOROSIS
The inclusion of osteoporotic fractures under pathological fractures is a little controversial, but the simple fact remains that osteoporotic bone is not normal bone. Gradual thinning of the bone, particularly in elderly females, may result in broken bones without significant injury. A fracture of the neck of the femur is very common. The symptoms are:
* Pain in the groin/hip (after or

causing a fall).
* Apparent shortening of the leg.
* Inability to bear weight on the affected side.
* The foot on the affected side may be turned outwards.

Most commonly treated with an operation to realign and fix the broken bone.

POSSIBLE

■ PAGET'S DISEASE OF BONE
See page 437.

■ OSTEOMALACIA
See RICKETS AND OSTEOMALACIA, page 287.

■ DISUSED BONE
Bone requires regular use to maintain its normal structure. If unused because of paralysis (for instance by a stroke, multiple sclerosis or spina bifida), the bones become weak and may even break when the individual is being carried, or turned in bed.
So, bone pain in any bedridden or partially paralysed individual may be caused by a fracture.

RARE

■ OSTEOMYELITIS
■ BENIGN BONE TUMOURS
■ BONE CANCER
See page 275.

■ BRITTLE BONE DISEASE
There are two main types of this disease, *osteogenesis imperfecta congenita*, where fractures develop in the womb and at birth; and

THE SKELETON

The skeleton

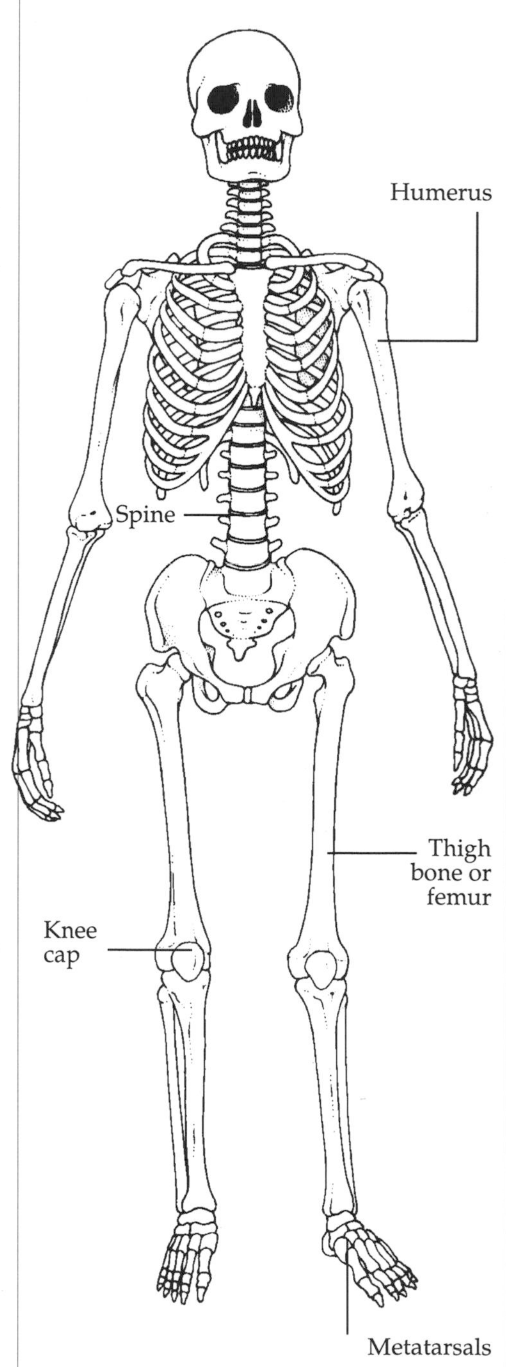

osteogenesis imperfecta tarda, a milder variant with fractures later in life. This a hereditary disorder of connective tissue, which prevents bones and other tissue forming properly. The symptoms are:
* Bones fracture with minimal injury.
* Whites of the eyes appear blue.
* Ligaments may be lax (allowing excess mobility of joints).
* Deafness may occur.
* Teeth may be deformed.
* General deformity because of repeated fractures.

■ MARBLE BONES
Also known as osteopetrosis. A very rare, inherited condition, in which bones become even more solid and hard than usual. As well as a increased likelihood of fractures, growth may be affected.

INFLAMED OR ACHING JOINTS

Virtually any generalized disease, such as influenza, gives symptoms of aching in joints and muscles. These are often fleeting, moving from one joint or muscle to another. Many diseases have major or primary involvement with joints, the most significant of which are:

PROBABLE
VIRAL INFECTION
OSTEOARTHRITIS

POSSIBLE
ANKYLOSING SPONDYLITIS
GOUT
RHEUMATOID ARTHRITIS
STILL'S DISEASE
SICKLE CELL ANAEMIA

RARE
REITER'S SYNDROME
PSORIATIC ARTHRITIS
GONOCOCCAL ARTHRITIS
SYSTEMIC LUPUS ERYTHEMATOSIS (SLE)
RHEUMATIC FEVER
HAEMOPHILIA
SYPHILIS

PROBABLE

■ VIRAL INFECTION

Any viral infection, such as the common cold or influenza, will give vague joint pains.
* General malaise.
* Fever.
* Cough, runny nose.
* Muscle pain.
* Joint pain.
* Normally cures itself in a few days.

■ OSTEOARTHRITIS
See page 285.

POSSIBLE

■ ANKYLOSING SPONDYLITIS
See page 287.

■ GOUT
Caused by excess uric acid in the blood.
* One joint affected to begin with (monarticular); most commonly, first affects the big toe joint.
* Sudden onset.
* Joint is hot, shiny, red and excruciatingly painful.
* There may be malaise and fever.
Attacks recur and involve other joints:
* Gouty tophi, lumpy collections of uric acid crystals, form in the skin, particularly on the ears and adjacent to joints.

The high levels of uric acid, if untreated, can cause kidney stones and kidney failure. Blood tests are needed to confirm the diagnosis, and drugs to control the symptoms.

■ RHEUMATOID ARTHRITIS
The commonest type of chronic, generalized inflammatory joint disease. It is actually a connective tissue disease and it may run in the family. Symptoms are caused by persistent inflammation of the synovial membrane, which lines joint capsules. Commonest in young women. This is a remitting and relapsing disease; treatment involves relief of pain and reduction of inflammation. At later stages, in severe cases, surgery may be necessary to improve function because of deformity.

An immunoglobulin called rheumatoid factor is commonly present in the blood of affected individuals. Features include:
* Painful swelling of joints (often symmetrical).
* Early morning stiffness.
* Progressive joint deformity. (See also sections on specific joints.)
* Progressive loss of function.
* Lumps may appear in skin and around joints.
* Osteoporosis may develop.
* Anaemia.
* Muscle wasting.

■ STILL'S DISEASE
This is the juvenile form of rheumatoid arthritis (above), occurring in childhood.

■ SICKLE CELL DISEASE
An inherited disease found in those of African origin. The red blood cells become sickle-shaped when low amounts of oxygen are available. These sickle cells are less pliable than normal cells and so block up capillaries (small blood vessels) causing damage to organs because of lack of oxygen and poor blood supply. Some individuals are less affected — they are described as having sickle cell trait. Those with full-blown disease have recurrent attacks of severe pains, in limbs and abdomen — sickle crises.

Features of the disease include:
* Anaemia.
* Increased predisposition to infection.
* Joint pains.
* Fever.
* Jaundice.
* Abdominal pains.

The Skeleton

Treatment is mainly aimed at relieving the symptoms. Blood transfusions, administering oxygen and strong painkillers are mainstays.

RARE

■ REITER'S SYNDROME
Virtually always in men after puberty. Its cause is unknown but there will be the following three symptoms:
* Urethritis — developing up to a month after sexual intercourse — not caused by bacteria.
* Conjunctivitis — up to three weeks after the urethritis.
* Arthritis — up to two weeks after the conjunctivitis. This is mild, and occurs in more than one small- to middle-sized joint.

■ PSORIATIC ARTHRITIS
Occasionally, arthritis can be a complication of psoriasis, a skin disease.
* Various joints, in different parts of the body, are affected.
* The distal interphalangeal joints may be the only ones involved.
* Possibly nail pitting.

■ GONOCOCCAL ARTHRITIS
One of many complications of the sexually transmitted disease gonorrhoea. In males the main symptom is:
* Urethral discharge.
In females up to 75per cent may have no symptoms. Those that do may have:
* Pain on passing urine.
* Vaginal discharge.

May develop in one joint with symptoms of infective arthritis (*see above*).

Distal interphalangeal joint

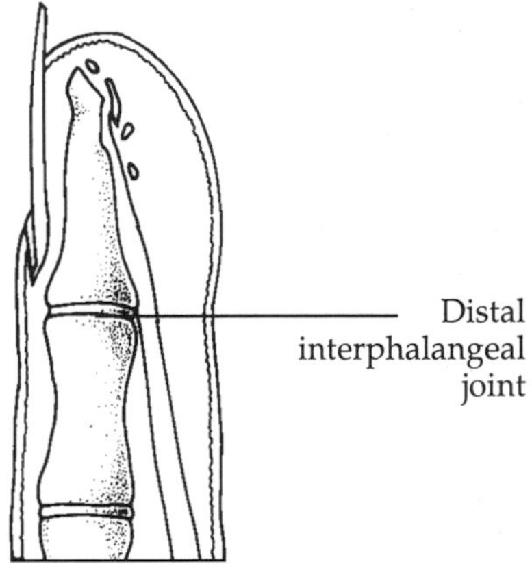

■ SYSTEMIC LUPUS ERYTHEMATOSIS (SLE)
See page 448.

■ RHEUMATIC FEVER
See page 448.

■ HAEMOPHILIA
See page 427.

■ SYPHILIS
See page 448.

SWOLLEN JOINT WITH NODULES

PROBABLE
BURSA
OSTEOARTHRITIS

POSSIBLE
RHEUMATOID ARTHRITIS
GOUT

RARE
CHARCOT'S JOINTS

PROBABLE

■ BURSA
Many joints have sacs, like empty balloons, overlying their surfaces. If damaged, these fill with fluid and enlarge. They feel like smooth, fluid-filled swellings and may be uncomfortable and irritating. In particular, the bursa in front of the knee may become swollen after kneeling: commonly known as housemaid's knee.

■ OSTEOARTHRITIS
See page 285.

POSSIBLE

■ RHEUMATOID ARTHRITIS
See page 279.

■ GOUT
See page 279.

RARE

■ CHARCOT'S JOINTS
Joints that have lost the sense of pain and position. If the joint is damaged, it can become progressively more deformed, as degeneration occurs rapidly. The joint looks as if it should be very painful, possibly with extreme swelling and deformity. Fluid, bony protuberances and loose pieces of bone may easily be felt in and around the joint. Dislocation is not uncommon. The commoner causes include syphilis, spina bifida, indeed anything that can damage the peripheral nerve system, including diabetes and alcohol.

PAINFUL JOINTS

See INFLAMED OR ACHING JOINTS, page 278.

STIFF JOINTS

See INFLAMED OR ACHING JOINTS, page 278.

PAINFUL SHOULDER

PROBABLE
FROZEN SHOULDER
OSTEOARTHRITIS

POSSIBLE
PAINFUL ARC SYNDROME
ROTATOR CUFF TEAR
DISLOCATION OF THE SHOULDER
RHEUMATOID ATHRITIS
FRACTURED COLLARBONE (CLAVICLE)
FRACTURED HUMERUS

RARE
RUPTURED BICEPS TENDON
POLYMYALGIA RHEUMATICA
TUBERCULOSIS
INTERNAL BLEEDING

PROBABLE

■ FROZEN SHOULDER
Commonest in later middle age.
* Slight injury to shoulder joint may or may not have occurred.
* Subsequently progressive pain and stiffness.
* Pain starts at shoulder tip and runs down outer arm to hand.
* Can be very disabling.
* Tends to cure itself.

Called 'frozen shoulder' because someone with this condition tends to hold their shoulder very still, due to the pain.

■ OSTEOARTHRITIS
See page 285.

POSSIBLE

■ PAINFUL ARC SYNDROME
Most common in a middle-aged or later middle-aged person.
* Pain at shoulder tip.
* Variable in intensity; worse at night.
* Limited shoulder movement.
* Local area of tenderness — can be identified with one fingertip.
* Pain worse over part of the 'arc' made by raising the arm from the side.

■ ROTATOR CUFF TEAR
Tendons lying at the upper part of the shoulder can tear or rupture without warning. Tends to occur with pre-existing wear and tear changes, and so typical of the elderly.
* May be associated with a fall or lifting.
* Sudden onset of pain.
* Arm cannot be moved outwards.

■ DISLOCATION OF THE SHOULDER
A common injury in 'contact' sports. The two components of the shoulder joint (scapula and humerus) articulate at the glenoid fossa and the humeral head . Forceful injury makes the humeral head slip down and forwards.
* Pain on movement.
* Loss of shoulder contour.
* Humeral head may be felt below the outer end of the clavicle.
* Arm is held out from the body at elbow.

■ RHEUMATOID ARTHRITIS
See page 279.

■ FRACTURED COLLARBONE (CLAVICLE)
The shoulder bone is know medically as the clavicle and may break as a result of direct or indirect injury.
* Pain at the point of the break.
* Pain on arm movement: often the individual holds the affected arm with the opposite hand to prevent movement.
* Deformity at fracture site.

■ FRACTURED HUMERUS
The upper end of the humerus can break in a number of ways, but the damage is almost always the result of a direct blow or a fall.
* Pain when attempting to move shoulder or arm.
* Often, substantial tracks of bruising down arm.
* Variable amount of deformity — dependent on the degree of displacement.

RARE

■ RUPTURED BICEPS TENDON
In the elderly. The top end of the biceps muscle runs over the top of the humeral head. Changes due to wear and tear can make it rupture.
* Sudden onset of pain at shoulder tip.
* Flexing arm against resistance allows upper end of biceps (now unattached) to bunch up and become visible in the upper arm.

■ POLYMYALGIA RHEUMATICA
See page 271.

■ TUBERCULOSIS
See page 289.

■ INTERNAL BLEEDING
Anyone who develops pain at a shoulder tip after abdominal injury, when lying flat, must be urgently investigated for internal abdominal bleeding. It is thought that blood from the bleeding point tracks up to the diaphragm, from where pain is referred to the

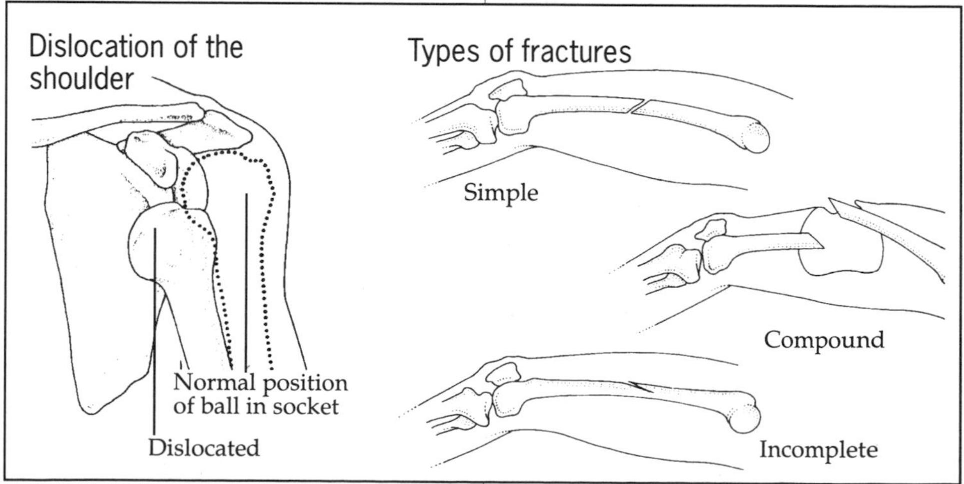

shoulder, which shares the same nerve supply.

CANNOT STRAIGHTEN BACK

See PAINFUL BACK, below.

ROUND OR HUNCHED SHOULDERS

See KYPHOSIS and SCOLIOSIS, covered under *A LUMP ON THE BACK, page 288.*

PAINFUL BACK

The back is taken here as the area from the neck down to the tail-bone (the coccyx). All of us will have at least one episode of back pain during our lives caused by either injury or disease.

Back pain lasting more than two to three weeks and which does not respond to simple painkillers must be reported to a doctor.

Pain may prevent you from straightening up, but may also be felt when in a 'normal' upright posture.

PROBABLE
MUSCULAR
ACUTE BACK STRAIN
CHRONIC BACK STRAIN
OSTEOARTHRITIS
SCIATICA
CERVICAL SPONDYLOSIS

POSSIBLE
PROLAPSED INTERVERTEBRAL DISC
SHINGLES
COCCYDYNIA
SCOLIOSIS
KYPHOSIS
OSTEOPOROSIS
ANKYLOSING SPONDYLITIS

RARE
CANCER OF THE SPINE
BENIGN TUMOUR
RICKETS AND OSTEOMALACIA
TUBERCULOSIS
GASTRO-INTESTINAL DISEASE

PROBABLE

■ MUSCULAR
Tearing or bruising of muscles or ligaments.
* Distinct history of injury — typically a blow, pulling or pushing.
* Dull ache initially, but the pain increases.
* Pain is local.
* Worse on movement, typically coughing or deep breathing.
* Resolves after a few days.
May need strong pain killers.

■ ACUTE BACK STRAIN
* May develop after a sudden twisting or bending movement, or lifting even a very small object.
* Often in the lower back.
* Often very painful at start, then less so.

* Worse on movement — may be impossible to move initially.
* Difficult to say exactly where the pain is.
* Lifting the leg straight while lying flat may aggravate the pain.
* Normally responds to bed rest and pain killers.

A physiotherapist, osteopath or chiropractor may be able to help.

■ CHRONIC BACK STRAIN

Low back pain that recurs. The individual has had similar episodes over a number of years and will be aware of the types of activity that cause it and relieve it. Symptoms can be made worse by obesity.
* Similar symptoms to acute back strain, but may be less intense.

■ OSTEOARTHRITIS

The wear and tear disease. Particularly vulnerable are weight-bearing joints such as hips and low lumbar spine, but any joint can be affected.
* Intermittent, non-specific low back pain.
* Worse after standing and at the end of the day.
* Relieved by rest.
* *However*, it is possible that discomfort remains even whilst lying in bed.
* Gradually, as the joint becomes stiffer, pain decreases, and some mobility is lost.

■ SCIATICA

Really a symptom itself, rather than a diagnosis, and a common one for many who suffer from bad backs. Caused by pressure on the sciatic nerve, which has its origins in the lower back. Can, rarely, be caused by actual damage to lumbo-sacral nerves, lumbar spine and the sciatic nerves. Persistent sciatica needs investigation as it can indicate serious underlying disease.
* Pain originates in low back or buttock.
* Pain radiates down the back of the thigh to the back and outer aspect of the calf and foot.
* Tingling or altered sensation may also be noted in the leg.
* Symptoms can be made worse by raising and straightening the leg.

■ CERVICAL SPONDYLOSIS

See page 135.

POSSIBLE

■ PROLAPSED INTERVERTEBRAL DISC

Often known as a 'slipped disc' (as are acute and chronic back strains and sciatica). The fibrous disc that acts as a buffer between the vertebrae has a gelatinous centre. Age or injury can cause this centre to bulge out, applying pressure on the nerves which emerge between the vertebrae and supply sensation to the body.
* Minor episodes of backache are an early warning.
* Sudden onset of severe back pain when bending or stooping: you may be unable to stand.
* Sciatica (above) may be present.
* Coughing and straining make the pain worse.
* Numbness or tingling may develop in a leg or foot.

THE SKELETON

Prolapsed intervertebral disc

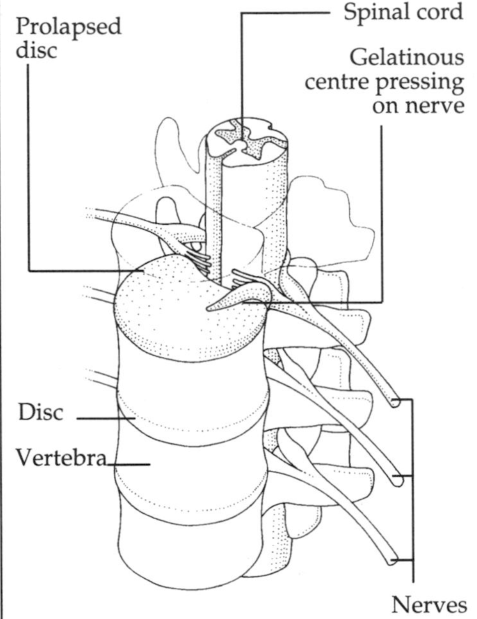

* Very occasionally, a slipped disc may cause urinary retention. This is a medical emergency.

The symptoms may subside in a few days or weeks; although a few may persist.

Numbness or tingling
If you have numbness or tingling in the feet or legs or in the genital region, and/or your ability to pass water seems to be affected, seek medical help urgently.

■ SHINGLES
* Initially, skin irritation.
* Red spots develop, often in a band a few inches wide on one side of the body.
* The spots develop into fluid-filled vesicles which burst and form crusts.
* Can become very painful.
* If suspected, can be treated with acyclovir, a strong anti-viral treatment, but best given before the spots develop.
* Tends to cure itself in 10 to 14 days.

Shingles is caused by the chicken pox virus. Those who have not had chicken pox can catch it from someone with shingles.

■ COCCYDYNIA
Pain associated with the coccyx or tail bone.
* Persistent pain after a fall.
* Pain aggravated by local pressure.
* Pain aggravated by sitting.

■ SCOLIOSIS
See page 288.

■ KYPHOSIS
See page 288.

■ OSTEOPOROSIS
Thinning of the bones caused by ageing. In women, this is especially a post-menopausal problem. Prevention of osteoporosis is one of the main reasons for hormone replacement therapy (HRT).
* There may be non-specific pain in the spine.
* Increased susceptibility to stress fractures, which may account for localized pain of sudden onset in vertebra after a fall.
* Occurs in otherwise fit individuals.
* Increasing deformity as age increases.
* Shortening of the vertebral column; height loss.

■ ANKYLOSING SPONDYLITIS
Essentially an inflammatory disorder, affecting the spine and sacroliliac joints — commonest in males during the late teenage years. It tends to occur in families.
* Intermittent backache at the early stage.
* Intermittent stiffness.
* Symptoms worst in the early morning.
* As the disease progresses, swelling and stiffness of other joints may develop.
* Occasionally, eyes, heart, lungs and ears may be affected.

RARE

■ CANCER OF THE SPINE (PRIMARY OR SECONDARY)
The spine is a well-recognized site of secondary cancer — meaning cancerous growth which has spread from another (primary) site. Anyone developing the following should see a doctor without delay:
* Localized, continuous pain in the back.
* Unremitting pain in the back which cannot be said to come from one particular place.
* Pain radiating from the back to the limbs.
* The development of pain, weakness or altered sensation in the limbs.

Other symptoms of cancer, including weight loss, malaise and loss of appetite may also be evident.

■ BENIGN TUMOUR OF THE BACK
Although benign tumours rarely give rise to pain, large ones, or ones adjacent to pressure areas, for example, at the level of a trouser waist band, may do so. Even if you think it is benign, report it to a doctor.

■ RICKETS AND OSTEOMALACIA
Both represent similar disease processes in children (rickets) and in adults (osteomalacia), and are caused by lack of Vitamin D.
The symptoms of rickets are:
* Skull deformity.
* Knee, ankle and wrist thickening.
* Enlargement of the bony cartilages of the chest ('rickety rosary').
* Lower limb deformities.
* Rarely, spinal curvature and pain.

The symptoms of osteomalacia are:
* General bone pain.
* Backache.
* Muscle pain.
* Loss of height due to vertebral collapse.
* Stress fractures.

■ GASTRO-INTESTINAL OR ABDOMINAL DISEASE
A number of small conditions may cause back symptoms, although very rarely in isolation.

Inflammation of the pancreas and peptic ulcer may cause pain (often centrally in the small of the back). Inflammatory bowel disease such as Crohn's disease or ulcerative colitis can cause back pain, either by referred pain from the diseased bowel or because of the joint inflammation that, rarely, may be associated with them.

■ TUBERCULOSIS
See page 289.

A LUMP ON THE BACK

PROBABLE
BENIGN TUMOUR OF SKIN STRUCTURES
INFECTION
NORMAL BODY PROMINENCE

POSSIBLE
KYPHOSIS
SCOLIOSIS

RARE
SPINA BIFIDA
CANCER
TUBERCULOSIS

PROBABLE

■ BENIGN TUMOUR OF SKIN STRUCTURES
Meaning a harmless lump, such as a lipoma or sebaceous cyst, which may occur in the skin anywhere in the body. Common features are:
* Pain-free.
* Slow increase in size.
* Otherwise sound health.

■ INFECTION
Commonest in those with acne, greasy skin or poor personal hygiene.
* Often sited on the upper back.
* Painful.
* Red.
* Localized swelling.
* Pus may ooze out.

Any infection may eventually become an abscess — a collection of pus. Often, it may discharge itself, but occasionally surgical drainage may be needed. Sometimes a cellulitis (*page 310)* develops, which requires antibiotics. If recurrent infections occur, then a doctor should ensure that diabetes is not to blame.

■ NORMAL BONY PROMINENCES
Occasionally, a previously unnoticed lump may become apparent. This often occurs after a loss of weight.The spine itself is a rather knobbly structure.

POSSIBLE

■ KYPHOSIS AND SCOLIOSIS
Deformities of the spine causing humps.

Kyphosis:
* Spine is unusually curved.
* Curve of the upper spine is exaggerated when viewed from side.
* Hump-back appearance.
* Some pain.

There are various causes: bad posture; disease; ankylosing spondylitis; rare congenital disease.

Scoliosis is a sideways deformity

of the spine:
* Usually a family history.
* Spine appears to curve more to one side when looked at from behind.
* Some pain.

May be associated with any disease that affects the spine.

RARE

■ SPINA BIFIDA
A congenital abnormality recognized at or soon after birth.

■ CANCER
People with known malignant disease may develop secondary growths in either the skin or skeletal structures of the back. Pain, irregular contour and rapid growth are ominous signs.

Usually, the cancer will have already made itself known.

■ TUBERCULOSIS
Unrecognized tuberculous infection of the spine or other bone(s) can cause sudden collapse of the affected part so that a bony lump can be felt. This may be known as a kyphus (and is a specific type of kyphosis — *see above*).
* Develops rapidly.
* Often associated with general malaise and occasional fever.
* Pain is often slight in the early stages, but can then become severe and constant.

BACK PAIN, WOMEN ONLY

PROBABLE
PERIOD PAIN
MITTELSCHMERZ

POSSIBLE
PELVIC INFLAMMATORY DISEASE

RARE
CANCER OF THE CERVIX, OVARIES AND WOMB

PROBABLE

■ PERIOD PAIN
Also called dysmenorrhoea.
* Low abdominal and back pain associated with periods.
* Occurs at each period and settles.
* Otherwise fit.

■ MITTELSCHMERZ
* Low back and abdominal pain developing in the middle of the menstrual cycle.
* Believed to be associated with ovulation.

POSSIBLE

■ PELVIC INFLAMMATORY DISEASE
Infection of the female genital tract. If suspected, requires

treatment to minimize the risk of infertility later.
* Fever.
* Low back and low abdominal pain, ranging from severe to very slight, or even non-existent.
* Vaginal discharge — yellow/green/brown.
* Discharge is often smelly.
* Possibly malaise and fever.

RARE

■ CANCER OF THE CERVIX, OVARIES AND WOMB
* There may be chronic, unremitting back or lower abdominal pain.
* Possibly offensive, bloody vaginal discharge (in cases of the uterus and cervix).
* Abdominal swelling: fluid collects in the abdominal cavity.
Other symptoms associated with malignant disease may be present:
* Weight loss.
* Anorexia.
* Anaemia.
* Malaise.

PAINFUL ELBOW

A number of structures around the elbow can give pain. The elbow joint is made up of three bones: the humerus, the radius and the ulna. A number of muscles and tendons attach near the joint, and nerves pass close by.

A direct blow can, of course, break or bruise the bone: the olecranon is the most prominent part and most often damaged. The lower end of the humerus may be broken, as may each epicondyle. The upper end of the radius may be broken indirectly if you fall on an outstretched hand: force is transmitted up the arm to its top end. The symptoms of a fracture are:
* Local pain.
* Local swelling.
* Loss of function– flexing/extending and twisting the forearm.
* Deformity may not be particularly noticeable.

Bruising can give similar symptoms, but the pain disappears relatively quickly and function returns.

One other elbow problem lies outside our conventional analysis of probable, possible and rare: knocking the 'funny bone'. The funny bone is not in fact a bone, but a nerve called the ulnar nerve, which runs round the back of the medial epicondyle. If you knock it:
* Exquisite pain on the medial epicondyle (and not knowing whether to laugh or cry).
* Pain and altered feeling (tingling) sensed down the fore-arm to the hand (mainly on the inner aspect), lasting a few seconds.

PROBABLE
TENNIS ELBOW
GOLFER'S ELBOW
JAVELIN THROWER'S ELBOW

The elbow bones

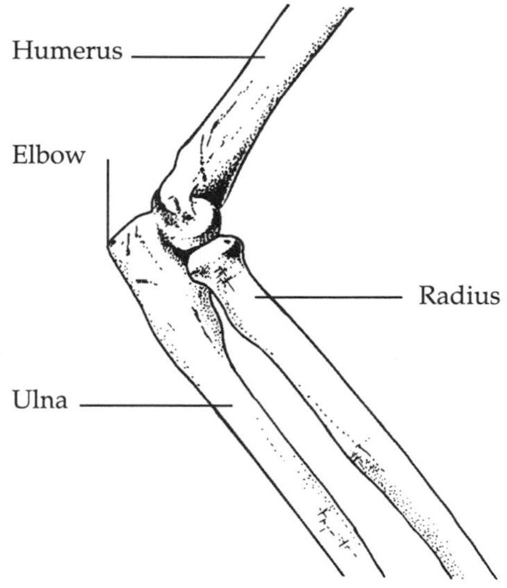

RARE
LOOSE BODIES
INFECTED BURSA

PROBABLE

■ TENNIS ELBOW
■ GOLFER'S ELBOW
■ JAVELIN THROWER'S ELBOW

These are 'repetitive strain injuries', typical of tennis players, golfers and javelin throwers, but not exclusive to them.
* Local pain: in tennis elbow, the lateral epicondyle is involved; in golfer's elbow, the medial epicondyle; in javelin thrower's, the olecranon.
* Pain worse on certain movements, for instance turning a door handle, shaking hands, lifting, serving at tennis; straightening the elbow with the palm face up; straightening the whole arm above the head when throwing.
* Patients are often middle-aged. May be treated with rest, or local injection of anaesthetic or steroid; occasionally surgery may help. Acupuncture may also be of benefit.

RARE

■ LOOSE BODIES

Pieces of bone may chip off and lie free in the joint as a result of injury, degeneration (perhaps from osteoarthritis), inflammation (perhaps from rheumatoid arthritis) or some unknown cause.
* Intermittent pain in joint.
* Joint locks.
* Cannot always fully extend or flex the elbow.
* Associated symptoms of other disease.

If symptoms persist or progress, surgical removal of the loose body may be necessary.

■ INFECTED BURSA

The bursa is a sac, like an empty balloon, that lies under the skin over the olecranon. Injury — a blow or friction — to the olecranon makes the bursa fill with fluid, which can then be seen as a lump on the point of the elbow. This is often pain-free. Occasionally, enlargement is associated with other disease such as gout or rheumatoid arthritis. If the overlying skin is damaged (cut or grazed), then the fluid may become infected.

PAINFUL WRIST

PROBABLE
SPRAIN
COLLES' FRACTURE
SCAPHOID FRACTURE

POSSIBLE
OSTEOARTHRITIS
RHEUMATOID ARTHRITIS
CARPAL TUNNEL SYNDROME

RARE
TUBERCULOSIS

PROBABLE

■ SPRAIN
Usually the result of a twisting or bending injury.
* Uncomfortable on movement, but no real limitation.
* No specific local tenderness.
Will settle within a few days.

■ COLLES' FRACTURE
Common in post-menopausal females who fall on to an outstretched hand. The ends of the radius and ulna are broken. A 'dinner fork deformity'.
* Pain in wrist.
* Deformity: lump on back of wrist.
* Pain on movement.
* Swelling can be extensive.
Requires realigning and immobilization in a plaster.

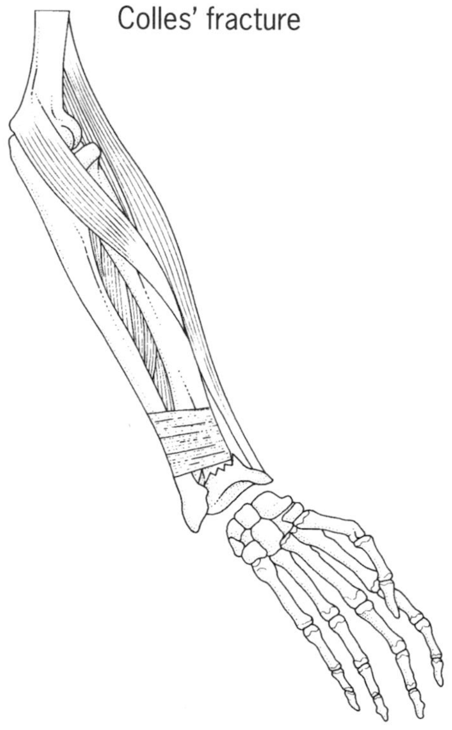

■ SCAPHOID FRACTURE
After falling on to an outstretched hand.
* Pain in wrist.
* Swelling.
* Pain on movement.
* Local pain at base of the back of the thumb.
If this fracture is untreated, the scaphoid, a small bone in the wrist, will degenerate, causing early osteoarthritis. Suspected scaphoid fractures must be immobilized initially, and X-rays reviewed after a week or so.

POSSIBLE

■ OSTEOARTHRITIS
See page 285.

■ RHEUMATOID ARTHRITIS
See page 279.

■ CARPAL TUNNEL SYNDROME
Although mainly causing symptoms in the hands and fingers, carpal tunnel syndrome may cause swollen, painful wrists.
* Pressure on nerves passing to the hand through the wrist gives rise to tingling and numbness.
* Common in pregnancy and pre-menstrually, or when fluid retention is a symptom. *See also SWOLLEN HANDS, page 294.*

RARE

■ TUBERCULOSIS
See page 289.

SWOLLEN WRIST

See PAINFUL WRIST, page 292.

A SWELLING AT THE WRIST

PROBABLE
GANGLION

POSSIBLE
OSTEOARTHRITIS
RHEUMATOID ARTHRITIS

RARE
TUBERCULOSIS

PROBABLE

■ GANGLION
A small, usually pea-sized, fluid-filled swelling adjacent to the wrist joint, capsule or tendon sheath.
* Localized smooth lump, normally on the back of the wrist.
* Cystic.
* Can shine a light through it.
* Mild discomfort; worse if knocked.

May need removal by surgery. Used to be treated by firm blow from the family Bible.

POSSIBLE

■ OSTEOARTHRITIS
See page 285.

■ RHEUMATOID ARTHRITIS
See page 279.

RARE

■ TUBERCULOSIS
See page 289.

UNUSUALLY LARGE HANDS

Will be a feature of *ACROMEGALY*, *page 275.*

SWOLLEN HANDS

PROBABLE
NORMAL VARIATION
PREGNANCY
INJURY

POSSIBLE
CARPAL TUNNEL SYNDROME
HYPOTHYROIDISM

RARE
AXILLARY VEIN THROMBOSIS
LYMPHOEDEMA

PROBABLE

■ NORMAL VARIATION
Intermittent swelling of one hand, or both, is a common, noticeable symptom. You may find it difficult to remove rings, or a wrist strap may make an indentation on the wrist. May be worse in hot weather or, for women, premenstrually.

Carpal tunnel syndrome

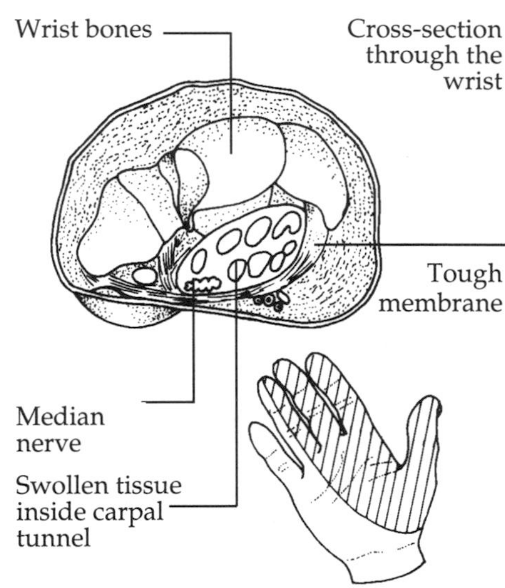

■ PREGNANCY
Particularly in the later stages, the body's normal response is to retain fluid and this tends to make the hands look puffy.

■ INJURY
Swelling would be a normal response to direct physical insult.

POSSIBLE

■ CARPAL TUNNEL SYNDROME
Certain conditions causing swelling of the tissues of the hand and wrist may also compress the median nerve which supplies sensation and power to part of the hand. Commonest in menopausal women, individuals with rheumatoid arthritis and, in pregnancy; it may also occur with myxoedema.
* Pain and tingling in the thumb, index, middle and half the ring finger.

* Waking at night with burning pain, tingling and numbness, as above.
* Weak opposition of thumb and little finger.
* Difficulty in fine movements, such as sewing or gripping a pen for writing.
* Possibly pain and heaviness in the arm.

Splints may give relief, but in some cases the nerve needs releasing by surgery.

■ HYPOTHYROIDISM

Carpal tunnel syndrome (*above*) can be feature of this condition, which is caused by an under-active thyroid gland. (Do not confuse this with *hyper*thyroidism, an over-active gland.) Other symptoms are:
* Skin becomes dry and rough.
* You 'feel the cold'.
* Voice becomes gruff, features coarsen.
* Weight gain, constipation, slow speech, slow thought.

The disorder is easily treated. For further details, *see HYPOTHYROIDISM, page 000.*

RARE

■ AXILLARY VEIN THROMBOSIS

Blockage of the main vein in the armpit or upper arm. May have no apparent cause, or occurs after vigorous exercise.
* Swelling of entire arm.
* No pain, but there may be a dull ache.
* Superficial veins of arm may appear more prominent because the deep veins are blocked.

■ LYMPHOEDEMA

Primary or secondary. *See page 311.*

TREMBLING HANDS

See TREMBLING OR SHAKING, page 438.

In addition to the diagnoses listed on *page 438*, a doctor might also consider two very rare diagnoses causing tremor of the hands which comes on when an individual wants to carry out a task. This is known as 'intention tremor', and is characteristic of Wilson's Disease and Friedrich's ataxia. The first is a metabolic disorder, causing excessive deposits of copper in the brain, eyes and liver. It affects those between 10 and 25 years, and besides intention tremor symptoms include rigidity, abnormal limb movements, eye pigmentation, mental deterioration and ultimately cirrhosis of the liver. Friedrich's ataxia, a hereditary degeneration of the brain and spinal cord, comes to light during the first ten or 20 years of life. Its symptoms include progressive unsteadiness of gait, clumsiness, speech difficulties, loss of sense of position and intention tremor.

Clubbed fingers

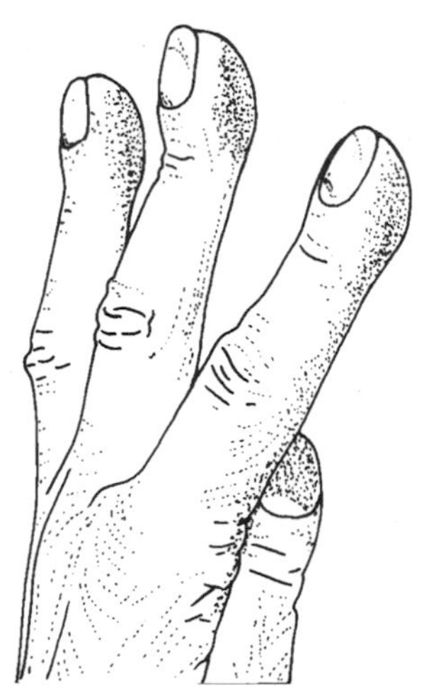

CLUBBED OR CURVED FINGERS OR NAILS

This means that:
* The end part of the finger becomes rounded.
* The nails appear larger and more curved lengthways and side to side.
* The angle between the nail bed and the skin on the back of the finger is lost; *see illustration above*.

If the fingers have been clubbed since birth, and there are similar finger-shapes in the family, then the symptom is not significant. But if clubbing develops during life, it may well be associated with other diseases, some of which are listed below. It is rare for clubbing alone to be the first indicator of these diseases. Medical science has not yet explained this phenomenon. Diseases of which clubbed fingers is a symptom:
* Lung diseases such as chronic bronchitis, emphysema, pleurisy, empyema, tuberculosis, cystic fibrosis, lung cancer.
* Heart disease: congenital heart disease, endocarditis.
* Gastro-intestinal disease: Crohns' disease, cystic fibrosis, liver cirrhosis, ulcerative colitis.
* Malignant disease.

See relevant sections for further details.

PROBLEMS WITH FINGERNAILS

It is said that over 60 diagnoses can be made from examining the nails alone. The appearance of the nail may be a clear sign of certain diseases, and the commonest variations are listed here along with the disease with which they are associated.
* Bitten fingernails: may, of course, be no more than a habit, or may point to an underlying tension, even anxiety or depression, particularly if of recent onset.
* Paronychia (sometimes known as 'a whitlow'): an abscess of the fingertip, which becomes red, tender, tense and throbbing; pus may accumulate. Often needs to be released by a surgical incision. Antibiotics may be required.
* Transverse fissures (lines): quite common after any illness and may be present for many months.
* Transverse ridges: often in association with eczema.
* Sub-ungual haematoma: discolouration after injury. The classic injury to a nail is a hammer blow, or an object dropped on the toes.

Paronychia
— 'a whitlow'

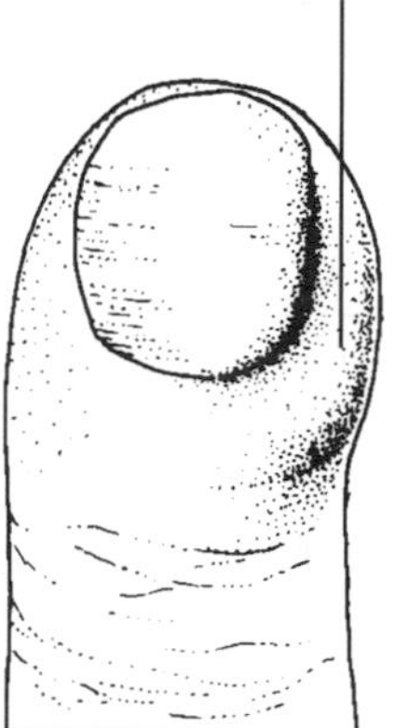

Within a few minutes, a blue, then a purplish, then dark brown or black area may appear. The toe feels painful and throbs, because blood, which causes the discolouration, builds up pressure under the nail.

The symptoms are easily relieved by piercing the nail over the haematoma with a heated paper clip or a needle, allowing the blood to escape. There are two reasons for heating the needle: easier penetration of the nail and sterilization.

* Pale nails or leuconychia: in association with pale mucosa and conjunctiva in the eye this symptom suggests anaemia.
* Bluish nails: suggests cyanosis. Often accompanies lung or heart disease. Examine also the lips and the ears — breathlessness may be a feature.
* Koilonychia or spoon-shaped nails: iron deficiency, anaemia.
* Glomus tumour: an exquisitely tender, red or violet coloured area a few millimetres across under the nail.
* Pitting of the nails: often occurs in association with psoriasis.
* Onycholysis: the nails separate from the nail bed — another feature of psoriasis, particularly at the end of the nail.
* Fungal infections of the nails give a markedly thickened, irregular and discoloured nail. The nail loses its usual colour, becoming uniformly cream-coloured and opaque. Other fungal infections may be present elsewhere.
* Onychogryphosis: enormous overgrowth and thickening of (mainly) the big toe nail, most commonly seen in the elderly. Advanced cases end up looking like a ram's horn.
* Brittle nails: may be due to excess manicuring and application of polish and polish remover.
* Splinter haemorrhages: longitudinal areas of redness that look like small splinters at the tips of the fingernails: may be associated with infection of the heart lining. Heart murmurs, malaise, shortness of breath, fever and anaemia are other signs.
* Coloured lunula or half moons: brown discolouration may be seen in chronic kidney failure, red discolouration in heart failure.
* White lines: short, white lines are frequently seen across nails. The exact cause is unclear. They may be a sign of a blow to the nail, or may appear after an illness. They are of little significance.

Other diseases associated with nail deformities are:
* Lichen planus: a rare, itchy skin disease that also affects the nails.

The whole skin may be affected. The nails (in about 10 per cent of cases) become flaky, striated (lined), spoon-shaped, or may be destroyed.
* Alopecia areata: hair loss from the scalp, in patches. The nails may be pitted.
* Nail-patella syndrome: a rare hereditary disease. Rudimentary or absent nails and small or absent patella (kneecap).
* Paronychia congenita: nails are thickened, as is the surrounding skin.
* Dystrophic epidermolysis bullosa: irregularity and thickening of the nails which makes the skin blister easily in response to injury.

EXTREMELY COLD OR FROZEN FINGERS

This symptom occurs with *CHILBLAINS and FROSTBITE: see under ITCHING OR NUMBNESS OF THE FINGERS AND TOES, page 320.*

SWOLLEN OR MISSHAPEN FINGERS

If a finger or thumb is severed, wrap it in clean material or clingfilm, surround it with ice, and rush to the nearest hospital. With new micro-surgical techiques, it is sometimes possible to save the digit.

PROBABLE
PULP SPACE INFECTION
FLEXOR SHEATH INFECTION
TRIGGER FINGER

POSSIBLE
MALLET FINGER AND THUMB
RHEUMATOID ARTHRITIS
HEBERDEN'S NODES
DUPUYTREN'S CONTRACTURE
GOUT

RARE
ISCHAEMIC CONTRACTURE
CONGENITAL DEFORMITIES
CONGENITAL CONTRACTURE
MALIGNANT TUMOURS
BENIGN TUMOURS

PROBABLE

■ PULP SPACE INFECTION
Infection, typically after a prick from plant or needle in the soft tissue at the finger tip.
* Swelling.
* Pain.
* Redness.
* Throbbing.
May require drainage or antibiotics.

■ FLEXOR SHEATH INFECTION
Infection in the sheath surrounding the tendons that bend the fingers (flexor tendons).
* Entire finger is red and swollen.

Swollen or misshapen fingers

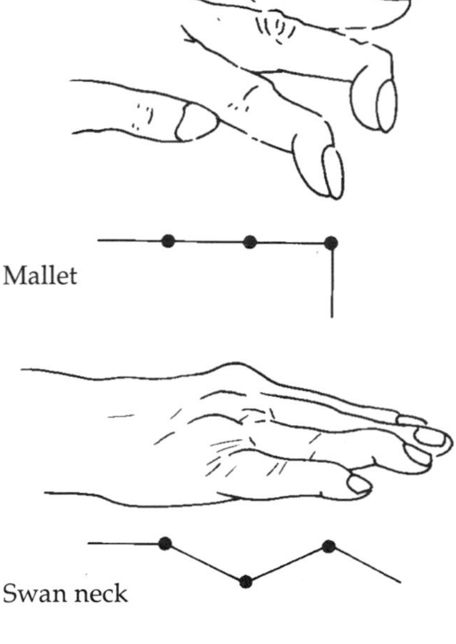

Mallet

Swan neck

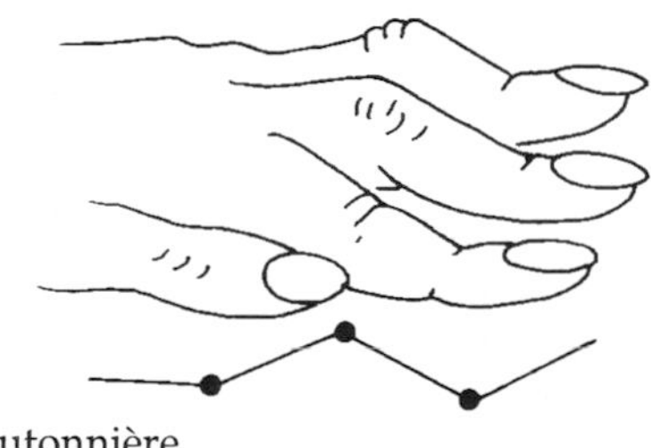

Boutonnière

* Pain.
* Loss of function.
* Pain worse on movement — finger is held crooked — the most comfortable position.
* Infection (untreated) may spread back into the palm of the hand.

This is an orthopaedic emergency, needing immediate treatment to prevent long-term loss of function and deformity.

■ TRIGGER FINGER

Thickening or inflammation of part of a flexor tendon in a finger or thumb causes:

* The digit to 'stick' when bending or straightening.
* May 'unstick' with a snap, spontaneously, or:
* May need to be forced to straighten.
* A small tender nodule may be felt at the base of the digit on the palm.
* This nodule can be felt clicking as the digit is flexed.

Recovery may be spontaneous, but persistent symptoms require surgery

POSSIBLE

■ MALLET FINGER AND THUMB

Damage to the tendon (extensor) which attaches to the dorsal surface of the terminal phalanx of each digit. The damage may be caused by injury to the end of the digit, or indirectly, after a wrist fracture. Occasionally, it happens in association with other disease — such as rheumatoid arthritis.

* Terminal phalanx of digit appears bent but cannot be straightened.

Splinting for six weeks may help cure cases caused by direct trauma.

In other situations, surgery may be needed.

■ RHEUMATOID ARTHRITIS

This disease affects the fingers and hands in a number of ways, including:

* Ulnar deviation of the fingers: the fingers appear to drift towards the side of the little finger, and the knuckle joints appear pronounced.

* Swan neck deformities; *see illustration.*
* Boutonnière's deformities; *see illustration.*
* Drop finger: the finger cannot be extended at the knuckle joint.
* Mallet thumb; *see above.*

■ HEBERDEN'S NODES
Caused by osteoarthritis.
* Distal interphalangeal joints *(see illustration page 280)* are painful.
* Bony overgrowth makes the joints appear enlarged and knobbly.

■ DUPUYTREN'S CONTRACTURE
* A fibrous contracture of (commonly) the little and ring fingers, which cannot be completely straightened.
* Sometimes the fingers are so bent that cleaning of the hand is a problem.
* Thickening can be felt on the palm side of affected fingers and on the palm.

Often of unknown cause, but has been linked with excessive drinking, and with certain drugs. It may also be hereditary.

■ GOUT
A generalized disease that may affect joints and skin. In the fingers and hands, the following may be seen:
* Tophi: lumps in the skin containing waxy, yellow material.
* Deformed joints of fingers and hand.

RARE

■ ISCHAEMIC CONTRACTURE
Also known as Volkmann's contracture. Direct or indirect injury to the blood supply of the forearm damages muscle, making it atrophy and shrink.
* Pale or bluish-looking skin on hand.
* Thin forearm.
* Hand is clawed — fingers flexed at both finger joints.
* Sensation diminished.
* Fingers can only be straightened when the hand is flexed at the wrist.
* Only able to grip when hand is flexed.

■ CONGENITAL DEFORMITIES
Present at birth.
* Failure of development — part or all of the fingers and hand may be deformed or absent.
* Syndactyly or webbing: fusion of adjacent fingers.
* 'Extra' digits: ranging from small lumps of flesh to entire digits (usually on the outer part of the limb).

■ CONGENITAL CONTRACTURE
* Present from birth.
* Fingers may be bent.
* Thickened tissue may be felt on the surface of the palm.
* May only affect one digit.

■ MALIGNANT TUMOURS
See LUMPS IN THE SKIN, page 250.

■ BENIGN TUMOURS
See LUMPS IN THE SKIN, page 250.

PAINFUL HIP

Likely to have different causes at different ages. Pain is often felt in the groin or the front of the hip, and may radiate down the thigh and to the knee. In children (who may not complain of pain) a limp may be the only evidence of pain. Accidental dislocation is excluded from this section because the cause – severe injury – is obvious.

PROBABLE
OSTEOARTHRITIS
FRACTURED NECK OF FEMUR

POSSIBLE
IRRITABLE HIP
PERTHES' DISEASE
SLIPPED EPIPHYSIS
RHEUMATOID ARTHRITIS

RARE
CONGENITAL DISLOCATION OF THE HIP
SUBLUXATION OF THE HIP
INFECTIVE DISLOCATION OF THE HIP

PROBABLE

■ OSTEOARTHRITIS
From about 50 years of age. Osteoarthritis is a problem of growing old — of degeneration. All of us are affected to some degree by this form of arthritis, sometimes described as 'wear and tear arthritis'. Some pre-existing conditions predispose to an early appearance of osteoarthritis, including congenital dislocation of the hip, infective arthritis, Perthes' disease, and slipped epiphysis — the risk is increased if the diagnosis is missed or treatment delayed.
* Pain radiating from groin to knee.
* Initially after exercise, progressing to pain at rest or disturbing sleep.
* Progressive stiffness of leg.
* Difficulty in putting on shoes and socks.
* Progressive limp.
* Apparent shortening of leg.

Treatment is first aimed at relieving the pain (painkillers); then at improving function (exercises and physiotherapy); eventually, severe cases may require joint replacement.

■ FRACTURED NECK OF FEMUR
See information on pathological fractures under BONES BREAKING EASILY, page 276.

POSSIBLE

■ IRRITABLE HIP
In children or adults.
* Pain in groin or front of thigh, often to the knee.
* Limp.
* All movement of hip limited by pain.

This diagnosis tends to be made if investigations for other causes lead to nothing. The hip settles

THE SKELETON

with bed rest and, occasionally, traction. It is important, particularly in the young, to seek a specialist opinion to exclude more serious disease.

■ PERTHES' DISEASE

The blood supply to the femoral head is compromised, and it dies. The course of the disease is up to four years. Surprisingly, the symptoms can be quite slight.

* Patient aged five to ten years, occasionally older or younger.
* Intermittent ache in hip.
* Intermittent limp.
* Painful movements.

It is important to distinguish between this serious disease and irritable hip.

The treatment of Perthes' disease varies, depending on the medical centre. In the past, treatments required many months of hospital attention and confinement to bed. Today this is often no longer the case, the disease being managed adequately by close supervision and surgical intervention if required. Seeking a second opinion is often helpful with this important condition.

■ SLIPPED EPIPHYSIS

A disease of adolescents, usually between 11 and 13; commonest in boys. The top part of the femoral head slips off the lower part at the epiphysis. Hip injury may play some part in its development, but not invariably. Individuals with this condition may be obese and may have delayed sexual and physical development. The

Slipped epiphysis

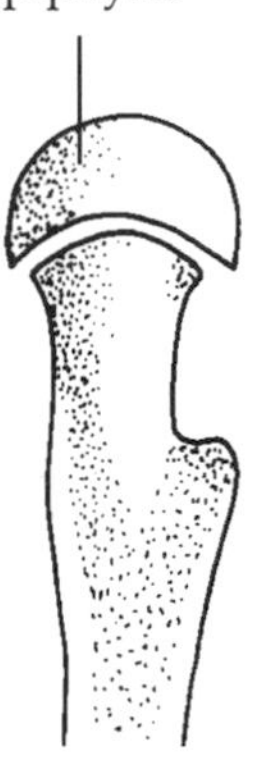

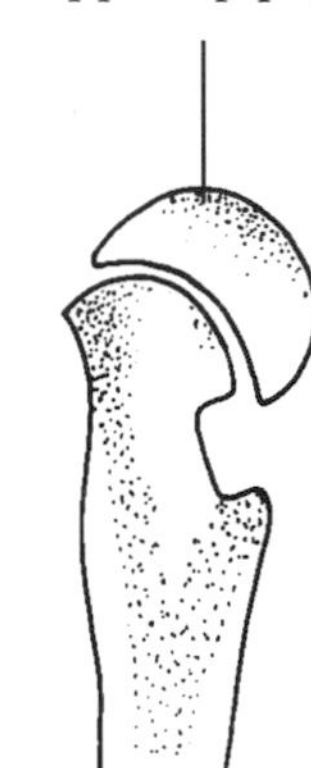

epiphysis may slip slowly, in which case the following symptoms develop:

* Slight irritability of hip with reduced range of movement.
* The limb appears shortened.
* The foot appears to be rotated outwards.
* Outward movement from and inward rotation towards the other leg are most often reduced.
* Limp may be apparent.
* There may be muscle wasting on the affected side.
* The upper part of the femur — the greater trochanter — may appear higher on the affected side when felt through the skin.

Sudden slipping of the epiphysis gives the same symptoms as a fractured neck of the femur. Probably some slipping has taken place, followed by a fall.

■ RHEUMATOID ARTHRITIS

Other generalized features of the disease will also be present. *See INFLAMMATORY ARTHRO–PATHIES, page 274.*

* Slow onset of groin pain.

* Limp which may be attributed to other joints.
* Muscle wasting can be severe.
* Both hips may be affected.
* Foot is turned outwards.
* Hip mobility is markedly reduced.

RARE

■ CONGENITAL DISLOCATION OF THE HIP
See DISLOCATED HIP, page 000.

■ SUBLUXATION OF THE HIP
Early degeneration of the hip due to abnormal shape of acetabulum. May well appear at about 20 years of age.
* Pain in groin.
* Worse on exercise.
* Progressive limp.

■ INFECTIVE DISLOCATION OF THE HIP
Most common in children and newborn babies. *See DISLOCATED HIP, below.*

DISLOCATED HIP

May be congenital (hereditary) or acquired, or caused by infection.

■ CONGENITAL DISLOCATION (CDH)
CDH tends to run in families and arises because of an abnormally-shaped hip socket, combined with lax joint ligaments. Breech birth (when the baby's feet, rather than the head, come out of the birth canal first) increases the likelihood. Symptoms before walking:
* Asymmetry of hip, seen at skin creases.
* Legs will not part fully.
* The baby may be late to start walking.
Symptoms after walking:
* Asymmetry of legs.
* Limp.

If both hips are dislocated, the waddling gait could pass as normal, in which case the dislocation will go undetected, causing damage. So the problem needs to be recognized at an early stage. Treatment is with different forms of splint.If untreated, the limp remains, and the hip joint is progressively distorted and damaged.

Ultimately, severe osteoarthritis develops and hip replacement may be needed as an adult.

CDH
This condition affects five times as many girls than boys. *Instability* of the hip — as opposed to outright dislocation — may be diagnosed in as many as 400 out of every 100,000 live births. However, this condition settles. True dislocation of the hip will not settle. Ultrasound can be used to check on the unborn baby, to avoid X-ray exposure.

■ ACQUIRED DISLOCATION
Acquired dislocation of the hip is caused either by injury or infection. Typically, a car or motorcycle accident, in which the individual is sitting with the knee bent, results in the femoral head being pushed backwards out of the

acetabulum. Extreme force is needed.
* Extreme pain.
* Deformity in extreme cases.
* Leg is shortened and twisted inwards.
* The knee is slightly bent.
* The leg cannot be moved.

The femoral head can be replaced in the acetabulum, but recovery can be a lengthy process, often because there are other injuries.

Much less commonly, the hip may also dislocate forwards; also centrally, when the femoral head pushes through the acetabulum into the pelvis.

■ INFECTIVE DISLOCATION OF THE HIP

Untreated infection (including tuberculosis) in any joint requires urgent orthopaedic attention to remove pus and clear the infection, as the joint surface and surrounding structures can be rapidly destroyed.

Features include:
* Pain (of variable intensity).
* A limp.
* Eventually, loss of function.
* Malaise.
* Fever.

Neglected, or mistreated, episodes of infective dislocation may mean surgery at a later date to correct deformity.

BOW-LEGGEDNESS

This is in most cases an innocent variation of the normal, occuring in childhood. Most children grow out of it.
* Feet together.
* Knees splayed.

May also, but much more rarely, be seen in rickets *(page 287)*, osteoarthritis *(page 285)*, and Paget's disease *(page 437)*.

LIMPING

Limping can be a symptom of many disorders and is caused by pain, or deformity or both. Look for a specific site of pain or deformity, and then refer to that section.

PAIN WHEN WALKING

Look at pages 316-21 first, then consider alternatives in the following pages covering leg and knee; also the preceding pages covering hip.

WALKING WITH A WADDLING GAIT

See CONGENITAL DISLOCATION OF THE HIP, page 303; and DUCHENNE'S DYSTROPHY, page 270.

PAINFUL LEG OR THIGH

See the general bone and muscles symptoms pages 269-81; also back symptoms, pages 284-90.

PARALYSED LEG

See pages 404-6.

VEIN OR VEINS STANDING OUT IN LEG

See VARICOSE VEINS, page 310.

SWOLLEN LEG

See SWOLLEN ANKLE, page 309.

WEAK LEG

See WASTING AND LOSS OF POWER IN THE MUSCLES, page 269; also page 272.

LEG UNUSUALLY WHITE

This may indicate sudden blockage of an artery — a medical emergency — as a result of *PERIPHERAL VASCULAR DISEASE, page 318.*

KNEE PAIN AFTER INJURY

The precise cause of the pain will be governed by the force of the injury, and its site — so 'probable', 'possible' and 'rare' are not relevant here.

The knee is made up from: bones — lower femur, upper tibia, patella; ligaments — medial and lateral collateral, anterior and posterior cruciate; the joint capsule; the menisci medial and lateral; and the surrounding soft tissues. All can be damaged.

The most significant injuries are listed below, plus their symptoms and an indication of the type of injury that may cause them. All require immediate treatment.

Delaying treatment, especially if the injury is severe, will increase the risk of complications. All injuries to a joint increase the risk of early onset of osteoarthritis.

■ DISLOCATION OF THE KNEE
Enormous force is needed to disrupt the knee joint, including its capsules and ligaments.
* Severe pain.
* Marked deformity.
* Marked bruising.

Nerves and arteries to the leg may be damaged.

■ DISLOCATION OF THE PATELLA
See LOCKED OR LOCKING KNEE, page 306.

■ FEMORAL CONDYLE FRACTURES
* May be sustained after a fall from a height.
* Severe pain in the knee, which cannot be moved.
* Immediate swelling and deformity.

■ LIGAMENTOUS TEAR
Can be complete or partial, and is often missed, the symptoms of swelling, pain and reduced

function being put down to 'sprain'. Often the worse the damage, for example, a complete rather than a partial tear, the less the pain. If someone has a severe injury to the knee which still allows some movement, the knee should be assessed for stability by an expert when symptoms have settled and before any sporting activities are started again.

■ FRACTURED PATELLA
Probably caused by a falling on to knee, or by a direct blow.
* Immediate swelling.
* The knee is bent.
* May be unable to straighten leg, either because of pain or disruption of the straightening mechanism.

■ SUPRACONDYLAR FRACTURE OF THE FEMUR
Caused by severe, direct injury.
* Severe pain — knee cannot be moved.
* Immediate swelling and deformity.

■ FRACTURED TIBIAL PLATEAU
Caused by a direct blow or a fall from a height.
* Severe pain - knee cannot be moved.
* Immediate swelling and deformity.

■ UPPER TIBIAL EPIPHYSIS AND APOPHYSIS
Injury to the upper lower leg, below the knee cap (the shin just below the knee), can damage the point of attachment of the quadriceps tendon to the tibia.
* Knee swollen, particularly below the kneecap.
* Local tenderness at the upper tibia.
* Raising the leg when it is straightened is painful or impossible.

A similar condition in young adults, which develops spontaneously, is known as Osgood Schlatter's Disease.

KNEE, SWOLLEN

See KNEE PAIN AFTER INJURY, page 305; KNEE, LOCKED OR LOCKING, below; INFLAMED OR ACHING JOINTS, page 278.

LOCKED OR LOCKING KNEE WHICH MAY COLLAPSE

The knee joint gets fixed at a particular angle. If it is completely locked it is not possible to straighten it. Some knees lock intermittently: they may appear to 'catch', and then to straighten.

These symptoms invariably suggest a problem within the knee itself, either a damaged cartilage (meniscus) or a loose body, which might be bone or cartilage. If injury to the knee predates the symptoms, it is important to remember exactly how it happened.

PROBABLE
LIGAMENT DAMAGE

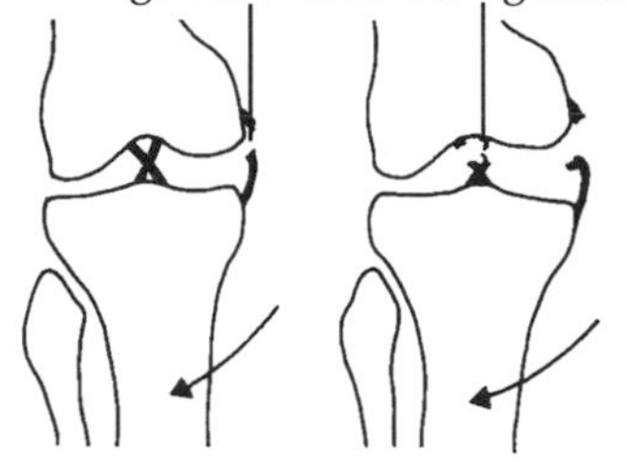

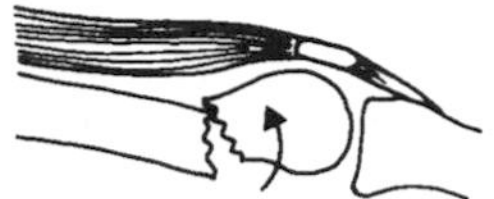

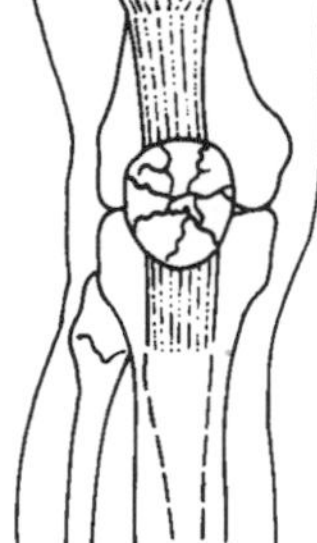

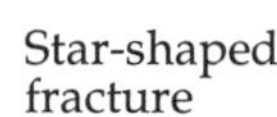

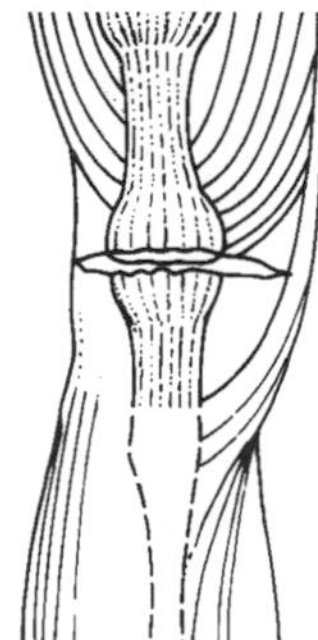

Knee injuries

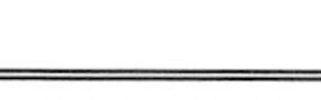

POSSIBLE
TORN MEDIAL MENISCUS
LOOSE BODY
OSTEOARTHRITIS

RARE
RECURRENT DISLOCATION OF THE PATELLA
TORN LATERAL MENISCUS
DISCOID LATERAL MENISCUS
CHONDROMALACIA PATELLA
OSTEOCHONDRITIS DISSECANS

PROBABLE

■ LIGAMENT DAMAGE
The most common reason for the knee to lock, collapse or give away is damage to one of the internal ligaments. Symptoms are often similar to those of damage to the cartilage; *see TORN MEDIAL MENISCUS, below.*

POSSIBLE

■ TORN MEDIAL MENISCUS
Typically, the meniscus is crushed and twisted between femur and tibia. Common in footballers and rugby players.
* Often immediate pain at the inner aspect of knee.
* Knee may lock — cannot be fully straightened.
* Swelling of the joint within a few hours.

After the first incident, symptoms may subside, only to recur with increasing frequency.

■ LOOSE BODY
Trapped between femur and tibia.

* Intermittent sudden pain on climbing or descending stairs.
* Inability to straighten leg.
* Swelling, due to fluid, may accompany each attack.
* Each attack resolves as the loose body moves from between the joints.
* The loose body may be felt in the joint, often above or at the side of the patella.

■ OSTEOARTHRITIS
Degenerative or osteoarthritic changes in the joint can cause formation of loose bodies; *see above*. Common in later middle age, and onwards.

RARE

■ RECURRENT DISLOCATION OF THE PATELLA
Anatomical peculiarities, which are often, in fact, normal variants of the ligaments, muscles, tendons or bones around the knee may allow the kneecap to slide sideways. Commonest in young females.
* Kneecap may appear very mobile from side to side.
* Knee gets stuck in a bent position (maybe only briefly), causing the individual to fall (collapsing knee).
* Kneecap can be felt to one side, and then moves.
* May occur in both knees.

■ TORN LATERAL MENISCUS
Less common than a torn medial meniscus; *see page 307*. Symptoms are the same, except pain is on the outer side of the knee.

Knee joint

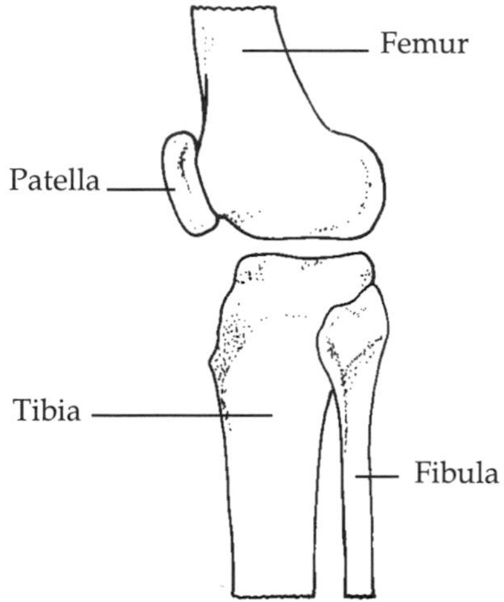

■ DISCOID LATERAL MENISCUS
An abnormally-shaped lateral meniscus slips between the femur and tibia and the knee gives way. A `clunking' sensation is experienced. Eventually, surgery will be needed.

■ CHONDROMALACIA PATELLA
Degeneration of the cartilage at the back of the kneecap. Young females are often affected
* May have had recurrent patella dislocation (*see above*) or a knee injury.
* Intermittent pain at the front of the knee, with swelling.
* Occasional locking of the knee.
* Knee occasionally gives away.

■ OSTEOCHONDRITIS DISSECANS
The lower part of the articular surface of the femur (the condyle) may be damaged after injury. Part of the articular cartilage flakes off,

creating a loose body. The individual is often in his or her late teens.
* Intermittent ache.
* Intermittent swelling.
* Intermittent locking.
* Knee feels unstable, as though it will collapse.

'KNOCK' KNEES AND BOW LEGS

In the great majority of cases, knock knees are a normal feature of childhood. As the child grows, the knees gradually begin to look normal, usually by the time the child is seven.
* Feet appear splayed.
* Knees press against each other.

Doctors often watch the leg shape over a period of six months to see how the appearance changes. At three to four years, the gap between a child's inner ankle bones, when standing comfortably, should be less than 4 in/10 cm.

May also, but rarely, be seen in rickets *(page 287)*, osteomalacia *(page 287)*, Paget's disease *(page 437)* and Charcot's joints *(page 281)*.

BOW LEGS
Bow legs are common in infants. If the child is lying flat, with feet together, and there is a gap of more than 2 in/5 cm between the bottom of the femurs at the knee, an X-ray may be a useful precaution to exclude rare causes, such as rickets and problems of bone development.

Bowing on one side only should always be investigated by a doctor.

PAINFUL KNEE

See INFLAMED OR ACHING JOINTS, page 278; LOCKED OR LOCKING KNEE; page 306; PAINFUL HIP, page 301.

SWOLLEN ANKLE

Can be on one or both sides.

PROBABLE
ACUTE OR CHRONIC INJURY

POSSIBLE
VARICOSE VEINS
DEEP VENOUS THROMBOSIS
POST-PHLEBITIC LIMB
CELLULITIS
HEART FAILURE

RARE
ANAEMIA
LYMPHOEDEMA
MISSED FRACTURE
NEPHRITIS

PROBABLE

■ ACUTE OR CHRONIC INJURY
See WEAK AND PAINFUL ANKLE, pages 311-12.

POSSIBLE

■ VARICOSE VEINS
Enlarged leg veins caused by damage to valves in the veins. Blood fails to return to the heart at the proper rate and stays in the leg. This in turn can cause a swollen ankle and lower leg, often only on one side.
* Varicose veins visible.
* Increases during day or after exercise.
* Discomfort rather than pain.
* Disappears when leg is elevated, and at night.
* May be associated with ulcers, particularly inner-ankle swelling.
* Long-standing varicose veins cause brownish discoloration of the lower legs and feet. Sometimes described as varicose eczema.

■ DEEP VENOUS THROMBOSIS
Blockage of the veins by a thrombosis or blood clot deep inside the leg. May occur for no reason; or after an operation or prolonged bed rest. More likely in the elderly, the obese, smokers, and those on the contraceptive pill or with known malignant disease. If suspected, requires urgent medical attention.
* Sudden onset.
* Initially no pain, then mild discomfort.
* Calf and sometimes the thigh also swell.
* Pain may be aroused by pressure on the back of the calf.
* Swelling is persistent and does not decrease.

If a piece of the clot moves from the legs to the chest, there will be chest pain and shortness of breath. (*See also PULMONARY EMBOLUS, page 218.*) If the clot is large enough, death can follow in rare cases.

■ POST-PHLEBITIC LIMB
For months or years after a deep venous thrombosis (*above*) the limb may remain swollen and tender. Ulcers may develop at the ankle, plus discoloration of the skin. It is best treated with support bandages.

■ CELLULITIS
A bacterial infection of the soft tissues. It may be localized in part of the foot, ankle or leg, or it may spread. Caused by a simple puncture wound, or by bacteria gaining access through broken skin on the foot or ankle (for example, via an ulcer or Athlete's foot).
* Redness; swelling.
* Can be very painful.
* Skin may be shiny, due to stretching.
* Malaise.
* Fever.

Rest and antibiotics will be needed to treat this condition.

■ HEART FAILURE
If the heart fails to pump as well as it should, the body retains fluid. At worst this can cause congestion of the lungs, which makes breath-

ing difficult. A mild case may cause ankle swelling.
* Swelling on both sides.
* Legs feel cool.
* May be intermittent.
* May be associated with shortness of breath.
* In bad (and untreated) heart failure, swelling may progress all the way up the leg.
* Associated symptoms can include distended neck veins and cyanosis.

The symptoms can be cured by diuretic tablets.

RARE

■ ANAEMIA
Ankle swelling may be the first symptoms noted by an anaemic individual. This is because anaemia may precipitate mild heart failure *(see above)*.

■ LYMPHOEDEMA
Obstruction to drainage of fluid via the lymphatic system. It may be primary (no underlying cause); the result of congenital abnormality; or it can arise from absence of the lymphatic system in that limb. A congenital form, known as Milroy's Disease, also exists. Secondary lymphoedema can be caused by operation on the lymph glands in the groin (for example to control malignant disease), or by parasite infection — filariasis.
* Firm swelling.
* Does not vary in size.
* Infection or inflammation may develop; *see CELLULITIS, page 310.*
* Skin becomes thickened.
* In severe cases the skin may acquire the texture of elephant hide — elephantiasis.

■ MISSED FRACTURE
Occasionally a small fracture of an ankle bone may go unrecognized at the time of injury, resulting in long-term swelling, pain and instability.

■ NEPHRITIS
Damage, acute or chronic, to the kidneys caused by disease, not injury, may also cause swelling of the ankles.

Other symptoms may include:
* Puffy face (particularly around the eyes).
* Protein and/or blood in urine.
* Malaise.
* Shortness of breath.
* Nausea and vomiting.

WEAK AND PAINFUL ANKLE

Almost always the result of injury, such as a twist (often caused by slipping on a step) or jumping from a height. The ankle joint is made up of three main bones: the tibia, fibula and calcaneum. Each may be damaged. The injury also damages the soft tissues (ligaments, tendons and muscles) surrounding the ankle. Pain originates from these structures. The ankle feels 'weak' and likely to 'give away'. The symptoms only relate to the affected ankle.

Ankle injuries should be regarded seriously, since even untreated sprains can cause long-term disability. Pain killers, rest

THE SKELETON

and physiotherapy are often appropriate treatments if there is no fracture.

PROBABLE
ACUTE INJURY (SPRAIN)

POSSIBLE
CHRONIC INJURY CELLULITIS

RARE
FRACTURE

PROBABLE

■ ACUTE TRAUMA (SPRAIN).
* Clear story of injury.
* Painful to stand or bear weight.
* Swelling, local or general.
* Swelling appears after a few hours or the following day.
* Ankle feels as though it will 'give away'.

POSSIBLE

■ CHRONIC INJURY
* Injury some time in past — weeks, months or even years.
* Symptoms have persisted for some time.
* Feeling of 'weakness' or 'about to give away' predominates.
* Pain not so intense as with acute trauma.
* Swelling after exercise.

Bones of the foot and ankle

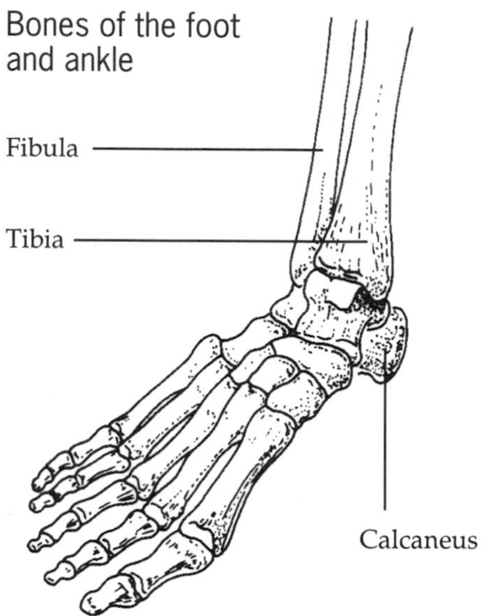

■ CELLULITIS
See page 310.

RARE

■ FRACTURE
In general, the symptoms are very obvious and confined to the affected bone.
* Pain severe.
* Unable to bear weight.
* Immediate swelling.
* Bruising within a few hours.

A break to the lower end of the tibia will cause symptoms on the inner aspect of the ankle; to the lower fibula on the outer aspect; to the calcaneus (heel bone) on both sides and at the back over the heel.

UNUSUALLY LARGE FEET

PROBABLE
NORMAL VARIANT

RARE
ACROMEGALY

PROBABLE

■ NORMAL VARIANT
Most individuals worried about their foot size have no physical abnormality or underlying disease. The size of their feet merely reflects the variation in size that would be expected in any population. And many people worry that their feet are too small.

RARE

■ ACROMEGALY
See page 275.

FLAT FEET

The term really means flattening of the arches. It can be a postural problem, in association with knock knees and a short Achilles' tendon. It may occasionally be congenital, in association with spina bifida, but this is rare. It may also develop as a result of general lack of fitness, say after being bed-ridden. The muscles and tendons that support the arches become wasted and flat feet develop.
* Feet look flat — no arch on instep.
* Shoe soles wear badly.
* Pain is rare, but may develop later in the foot and leg muscles.
Treatment is rarely needed, although instep supports may be of some help.

Most commonly, no cause for flat feet is found, and unfortunately specialists can offer little in the way of help.

The French believe in encouraging very young children to walk in barefoot on different surfaces (sand on a beach is a favoured one), to help develop the arches. Flat feet often run in families.

PAINFUL ARCHES OF FEET

See FLAT FEET, this page.

PAINFUL FEET

PROBABLE
VERRUCA

POSSIBLE
PLANTAR FASCIITIS
HALLUX VALGUS
HALLUX RIGIDUS

The Skeleton

RARE
CLAW TOES
MORTON'S METATARSALGIA
PES CAVUS

PROBABLE

■ VERRUCA
Also called a plantar wart; caused by a viral infection, hence outbreaks in schools and swimming pools.
* Local tenderness on sole of foot, where the verruca is pushed into the surface.
* The plantar wart is visible and there may be several — normally on the weight-bearing areas.
* May vanish spontaneously.

Most schools no longer undertake verruca checks. There is no need to prevent a child swimming because he or she has a verruca. As this is a viral infection, the body will eventually overcome it, and the verruca will go.

Only painful or unusually troublesome verrucas should be treated. Unnecessary treatment often merely enlarges the area affected. An old, hard verruca is not very infectious.

POSSIBLE

■ PLANTAR FASCIITIS
An inflammation of the layers of membrane, called fascia, which lie in the sole of the foot.
* Common after the age of 40.

Hallux valgus

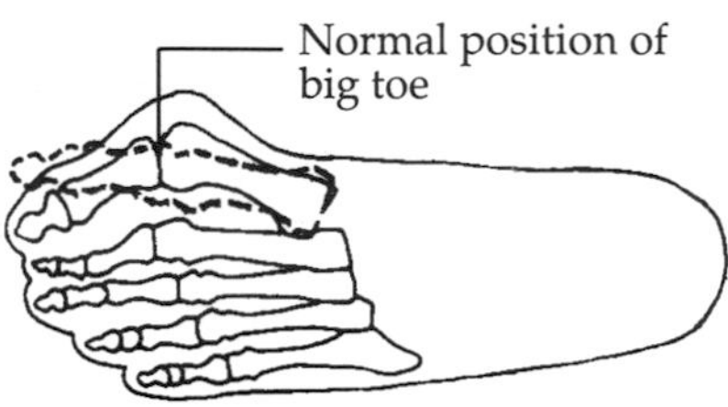

Morton's metatarsalgia

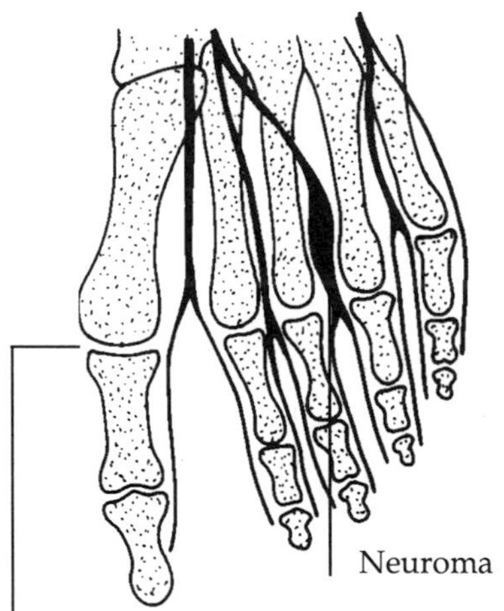

* Local tenderness underneath the heel.
* Worse on walking/running.
* Commonest in occupations requiring individuals to be on their feet for long periods — a penalty of being a traffic warden.

■ HALLUX VALGUS
The big toe becomes deformed. commonest in women beyond middle age.
* Big toe tip points to outer side of foot.
* Base of big toe is prominent.
* The end of the metatarsal bone points to the inner side of the foot.
* A lump of bone is therefore felt

under the skin.
* The overlying skin becomes thickened and painful (bunion) as does the bone on the sole of the foot. May eventually need surgery .

■ HALLUX RIGIDUS
Caused by osteoarthritis of the first metatarsophalangeal joint.
* Pain on movement.
* Bony outgrowths may develop, appearing as lumps around the joint.
* Thickened skin may develop on the upper surface of the joint.
* Range of movement of the joint is eventually limited by stiffness and pain.

RARE

■ CLAW TOES
See PES CAVUS, below.

■ MORTON'S METATARSALGIA
Affects the middle-aged.
* Enlargement of the nerve (neuroma) between the heads of metatarsal bones.
* Local pain, worse if foot is squeezed from side to side.
* Pain radiates to toes.
May require surgery.

■ PES CAVUS
The opposite of a flat foot: the arch of the foot is raised. Often associated with curling of the toes (claw toes). Thought to be caused by imbalance of the muscles that support the arches, and most likely to be seen in those with neurological disease of the lower limb, for instance poliomyelitis, spina bifida, cerebral palsy.
* Curled or clawed toes.
* High arch on instep.
* Callosities eventually develop on pressure points.
* Metatarsalgia (pain on the metatarsal heads) may develop.

SWOLLEN FEET

See SWOLLEN ANKLE, page 309.

ULCERATED OR INFECTED FEET

PROBABLE
INGROWN TOENAIL
ATHLETE'S FOOT
VERRUCA

POSSIBLE
DERMATITIS
DIABETIC COMPLICATION
VARICOSE VEINS
DEEP VENOUS THROMBOSIS
POST-PHLEBITIC LIMB
CELLULITIS
ATHEROSCLEROSIS

RARE
ALCOHOLIC NEUROPATHY
MULTIPLE SCLEROSIS
RAYNAUD'S DISEASE
BUERGER'S DISEASE
FROSTBITE
SYPHILIS

THE SKELETON

PROBABLE

■ INGROWN TOENAIL
The big toe is the one almost always affected. The side of the nail cuts into the toe tissue causing local infection (paronychia). Caused by ill-fitting shoes and cutting the nail too short.
* Outer side of nail most commonly affected.
* Often on both feet.
* Recurrent pain.
* Recurrent infection — with redness, swelling and pus.

May ultimately need surgery to the nail bed.

■ ATHLETE'S FOOT
See ITCHING OR NUMBNESS OF THE FINGERS AND TOES, page 320.

■ VERRUCA
See page 314.

POSSIBLE

These diagnoses are discussed in detail on pages *321; under DIABETIC NEUROPATHY, page 317; on page 310; and under PERIPHERAL VASCULAR DISEASE on page 318.*

RARE

These diagnoses are discussed in detail on pages *318, 317, 488, 321, 448 and 318.* respectively. Buerger's disease is painful ulceration caused by obliteration of blood vessels in the limbs; particularly in young male smokers of eastern European origin.

CORNS ON THE FEET

See page 255.

FINGERS AND TOES

Collected here is a group of symptoms which can particularly affect the fingers and toes (but also the arms and legs): parts of the body at the outer reaches of the blood's circulation. The nose and ears are similarly placed, and certain symptoms such as numbness, itching or discolouration (for example chilblains) can affect them just as they do the fingers and toes.

NUMB FINGERS AND TOES

The onset of numbness in any part of the body should be taken seriously. It is not a common symptom in isolation and may be an accompaniment to underlying disease. Its main danger is that the 'warning sign' of pain is not present: therefore skin damage, skin breakdown and ulcers may develop because the individual cannot feel the discomfort. This is particularly common over pressure points (eg heel, medial and lateral malleolus, sole of the foot).

THE SKELETON

Pressure points of the feet

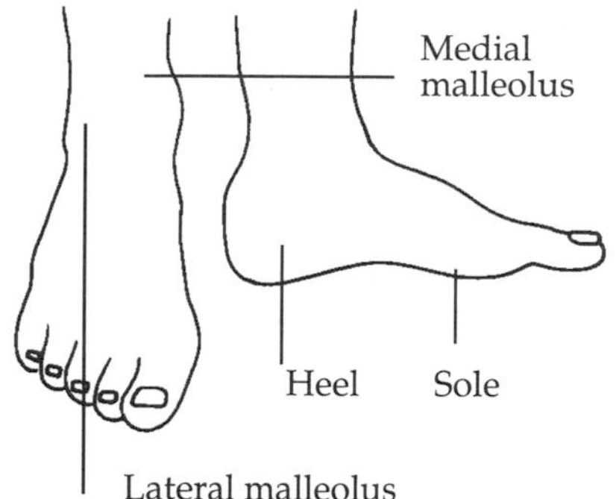

Numbness of fingers and toes accompanied by back or neck pain is a serious symptom, and should be reported to your doctor immediately. It can be a sign of direct pressure applied to a nerve by a disc or from a bone injury.

POSSIBLE

CERVICAL SPONDYLOSIS
DIABETIC NEUROPATHY
MULTIPLE SCLEROSIS
PERIPHERAL VASCULAR DISEASE
ALCOHOLIC NEUROPATHY

RARE

GUILLAIN-BARRE SYNDROME
FROSTBITE
LEPROSY

POSSIBLE

■ CERVICAL SPONDYLOSIS

See page 135.

■ DIABETIC NEUROPATHY

A long-standing complication of diabetes. Neuropathy means disease of the nerves. If you have diabetes, you may notice:

* Some tingling and pain (lower limbs).
* Stocking anaesthesia (numbness over a leg to the upper thigh — the area covered by a stocking).
* Some muscle wasting and weakness.
* Painless ulceration over pressure points on feet.
* Cellulitis (*see above*) associated with ulcers.

Occasionally, only one nerve may be affected, causing numbness, muscle wasting and weakness in one limb.

Other neurological symptoms of diabetes may be:

* Radiculitis — localized scalding and painful sensory changes.
* Irregular shape to pupils.
* Impotence.
* Failure of orgasm.
* Nocturnal diarrhoea.
* Feeling of dizziness on standing or changing position (postural hypotension).
* Loss of sweating in lower limbs.

■ MULTIPLE SCLEROSIS

Used to be known as disseminated sclerosis. Nervous tissue in the central nervous system is affected. Features may include:

* Numbness and tingling in hand(s) or feet (allowing ulcers to develop if pressure points are not treated carefully).
* Visual disturbance (poor vision, double vision).
* Weakness in limbs.
* Muscle wasting.

THE SKELETON

* Loss of postural sense.
* Vertigo.
* Bladder disturbance.
* Tremor.
* Speech disturbance.
* Swallowing difficulties.

May take several years to be diagnosed as it remits and relapses. The outlook is mixed: some unfortunate cases suffer, eventually, from paralysis and disability; in many, symptoms remain mild and can be helped with medication. But, as yet, no specific treatment exists.

■ PERIPHERAL VASCULAR DISEASE

As individuals age, the arteries begin to 'fur up' with fatty and calcified deposits: a normal part of the ageing process, known as atherosclerosis. In certain individuals, particularly smokers and those with a genetic disposition, the arteries fur up more extensively and at a younger age. Progressive atherosclerosis will result particularly in reduction of blood supply to the legs, with:
* Cold limbs (predominantly the legs).
* Legs may appear pale if lifted in the air.
* Cramp-like pain, particularly in the calf muscles, on walking any distance (intermittent claudication).
* Pain settles when walking stops.
* Occasionally sensory changes, including numbness.
* Pulses may not be felt in the usual places.

■ ALCOHOLIC NEUROPATHY

Most chronic alcoholics have damaged nerves, giving:
* Numbness in the lower limbs. Ulcers may develop.
* Tingling in the lower limbs.
* Burning in the lower limbs (especially in the feet).
* Weakness of the lower limbs.
* Wasting of the muscles of the lower limbs.

Walking will be affected. The problems can be reversed by giving up alcohol; proper diet; taking B vitamin supplements.

RARE

■ GUILLAIN-BARRE SYNDROME

Also known as acute inflammatory polyneuropathy.

An illness affecting the peripheral nervous system. It can occur at any age, often one to three weeks after an acute viral infection.
* Initially, tingling in the hands and feet.
* Weakness develops in the arms and legs and ultimately, in severe cases, the muscles controlling the lungs. Sometimes the individual needs artificial ventilation.
* Loss of sensation may be severe or minimal.
* Facial weakness is a possibility.

Gradual improvement takes place over weeks or months: complete recovery is normal.

■ FROSTBITE

See page 321.

■ LEPROSY

Essentially a disease of under–developed countries acquired by close contact with an infected individual over a prolonged period. Under these circumstances, the diagnosis will probably be obvious. One of the early signs is numbness and tingling in the ends of the arms and legs. There are many other symptoms

COLD FINGERS AND TOES

See FEELING THE COLD, page 488.

ALTERED SENSATION IN THE FINGERS AND TOES

Any disease or injury of a nerve can cause altered sensation in the area of the skin supplied by that nerve. It can take many forms, from tingling, through pins and needles and burning, to complete absence of sensation if the nerve is destroyed.

PROBABLE
DISEASE OR INJURY OF A NERVE OR NERVES

POSSIBLE
DIABETIC NEUROPATHY
MULTIPLE SCLEROSIS
PERIPHERAL VASCULAR DISEASE
ALCOHOLIC NEUROPATHY
SUBACUTE COMBINED DEGENERATION OF THE (SPINAL) CORD

RARE
GUILLAIN-BARRÉ SYNDROME
FROSTBITE
LEPROSY

PROBABLE

■ DISEASE OR INJURY OF A NERVE OR NERVES
Perhaps the commonest form is pressure neuropathy — or nerve palsy. This can occur if you fall asleep in an awkward position. Nerves usually affected are the ulnar (at the elbow); the radial (at the upper arm); and the peroneal nerve by the knee.

Common to all these palsies are:
* Initial numbness on waking in the area served by the nerve.
* Initial loss of function of the affected part.
* Within a few minutes, sensation returns.
* At first this is a mild tingling, but it progresses to painful pins and needles.
* After several more minutes, or longer, the sensations settle and full function returns.

Occasionally, if the local pressure on the nerve has been unduly prolonged, full function may take weeks to return.

POSSIBLE

■ DIABETIC NEUROPATHY
■ MULTIPLE SCLEROSIS
■ PERIPHERAL VASCULAR DISEASE, *page 318.*

■ ALCOHOLIC NEUROPATHY
See pages 317 and 318.

■ SUBACUTE COMBINED DEGENERATION OF THE SPINAL CORD
SACD for short. This is a result of vitamin B12 deficiency, caused by a number of of factors, the most significant being pernicious anaemia. Other causes include poor diet, extreme vegetarianism, malabsorption, certain drugs, and excessive drinking. Damage is done to parts of the white matter in the spinal cord, giving:
* Pins and needles (paraesthesia) in the feet (hands and arms rarely affected).
* Inability to feel vibration and to sense position — affecting legs and body.
* Weakness in the legs; muscle wasting.
* Unsteady gait.

Obviously other symptoms of the disorder causing SACD may also be present.

RARE

■ GUILLAIN-BARRE SYNDROME
■ FROSTBITE
■ LEPROSY
See pages 318, 321 and 318 respectively.

TINGLING FINGERS AND TOES

See ALTERED SENSATION IN THE FINGERS AND TOES, page 319.

ITCHING OR NUMBNESS OF THE FINGERS AND TOES

In an otherwise normal individual.

PROBABLE
ATHLETE'S FOOT
CHILBLAINS

POSSIBLE
DERMATITIS

RARE
FROST BITE

PROBABLE

■ ATHLETE'S FOOT
A fungal infection of the feet.
* Irritation between the toes.
* Burning and itching between the toes.
* Some redness, as a result of inflammation.
* Crusting and further infection can take place.
* Smelly feet.
* Cracking of skin, particularly between the toes.

■ CHILBLAINS
Damage to blood vessels in the skin caused by exposure to cold. Treated best by slow rewarming.
* Local pain in fingers or toes.

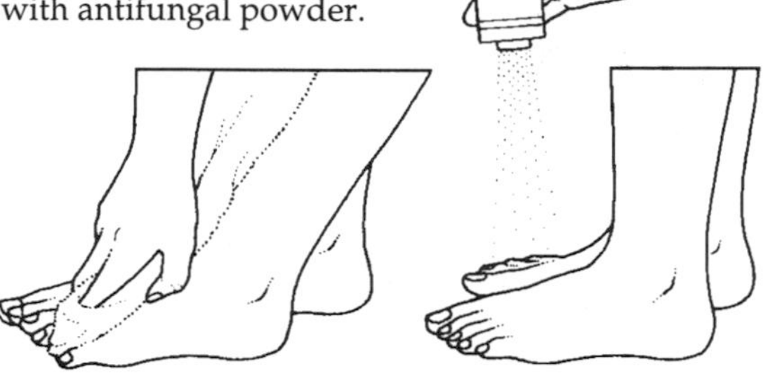
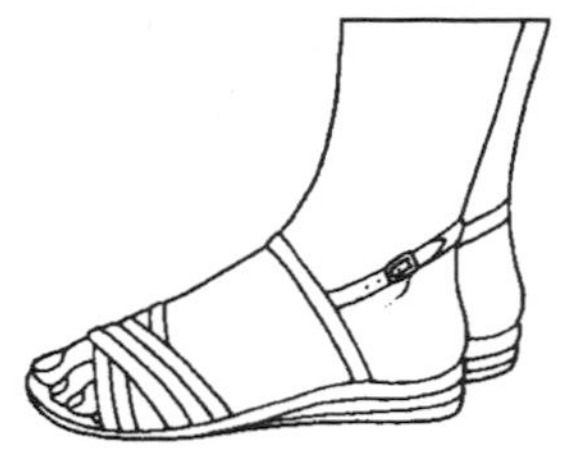

Athlete's foot
To prevent fungal infection spreading keep the skin between the toes dry and treat with antifungal powder.

Keep the feet dry and well ventilated by wearing open toed sandals.

* Itching and burning at first, followed by:
* Swelling .
* Local discolouration (reddish/ purple) at the site of pain.
* Blister formation.

POSSIBLE

■ DERMATITIS
Acute dermatitis — inflammation of the skin — may be caused by an allergy to chemicals (for instance, deodorants or washing powders). So dermatits can be caused by socks washed in a detergent to which an individual is allergic.
* Irritation.
* Burning.
* Inflammation, including weeping and crusting skin.
* Symptoms confined to areas which come in contact with the source of the allergy.

RARE

■ FROST BITE
In prolonged below-freezing temperatures, all extremities are at risk, including ears, nose, toes and fingers. People with poor circulation, typically the elderly, or those who lose heat fastest (for instance children) are most at risk.
* Initial pain and tingling in affected part.
* May become numb (pain-free) — a bad sign.
* Discolouration: may at first be reddish purple, but when the affected part becomes white, then the frostbite is serious.
* If untreated, the frostbitten areas will develop gangrene — death of tissue — because blood is no longer supplied. Ulcers develop and rapidly become infected.

Urgent medical help is needed to supervise the rewarming of the affected part, and to minimize the final damage

The Reproductive and Sexual Organs

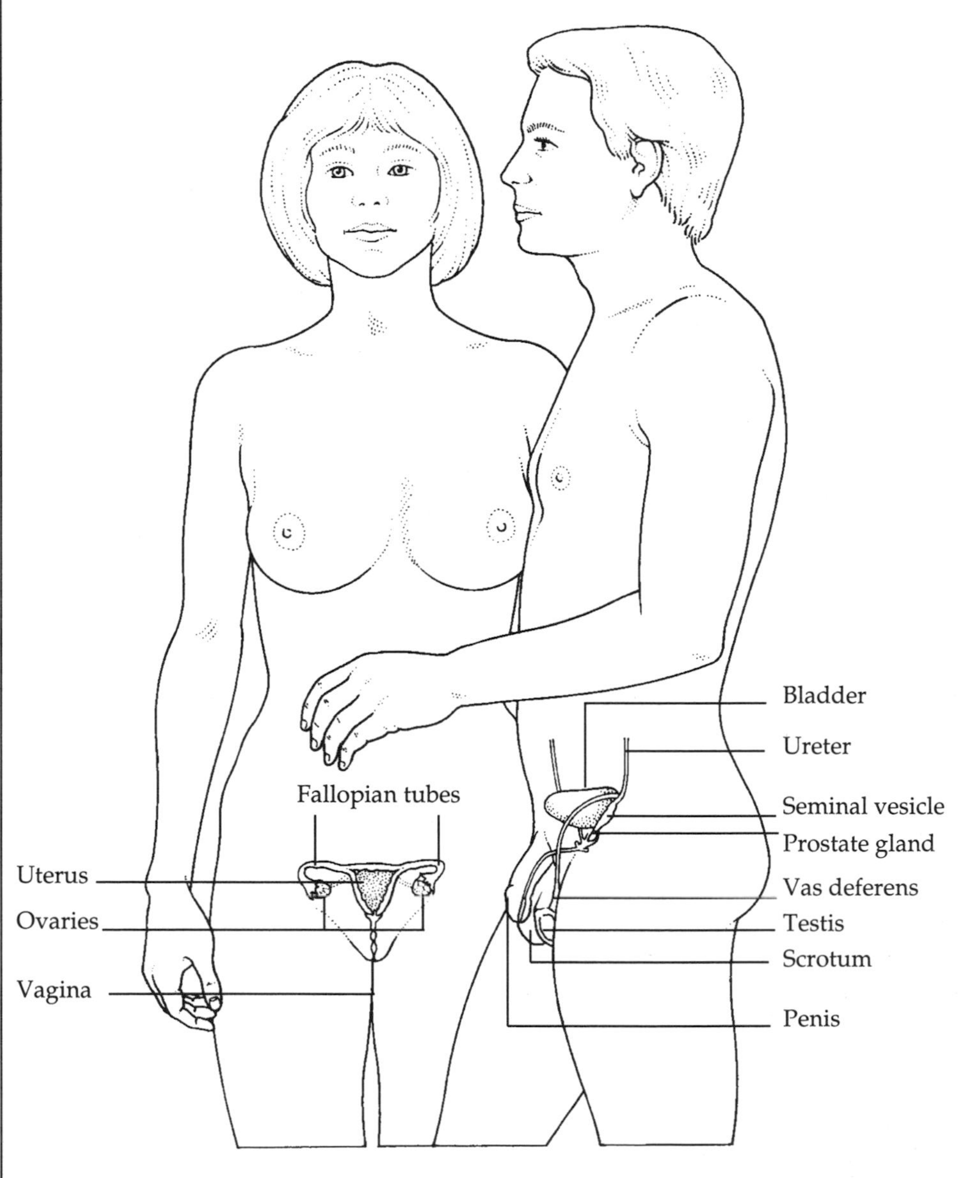

BLISTERS ON OR AROUND THE GENITALIA

PROBABLE
HERPES

POSSIBLE
MOLLUSCUM CONTAGIOSUM

PROBABLE

■ HERPES
The same virus that causes cold sores can cause these blisters on and around the genitalia. Commonest in women.
* A few blisters crop up from time to time.
* Intensely painful when they appear.

Anti-viral drugs may be helpful. It is especially important, if you are pregnant, to report any previous or current attacks of herpes to your doctor or midwife. This enables measures to be taken to diminish the risk of infecting the baby at birth.

POSSIBLE

■ MOLLUSCUM CONTAGIOSUM
Harmless, blister-like lumps, that occur in many parts of the body. Caused by a virus.
* Painless, unless they become infected.
* Dimple in the centre.

These usually disappear on their own; simple treatment can speed the process.

GENITAL LUMPS, ULCERS AND SORES

Minor infections of the genitals are very common, and are frequently obvious to an untrained eye. It is important to be alert to early symptoms of venereal disease, being especially careful if you have many sexual partners. You owe this not just to yourself but to your sexual partners, too.

PROBABLE
FURUNCLES
SCABIES OR CRAB LICE
WARTS

POSSIBLE
CYSTS
SYPHILIS

RARE
BEHCET'S DISEASE
TROPICAL VENEREAL DISEASES
CANCER

THE REPRODUCTIVE AND SEXUAL ORGANS

PROBABLE

■ FURUNCLES
Tiny pimples on the skin, or at the base of pubic hairs.
* Tender, rapidly-appearing lumps.
* Come to a yellow head.
* Discharge pus and blood, then disappear.
Simple antiseptic creams help these go. Severe cases may require a course of antibiotics.

■ SCABIES OR CRAB LICE
Mites which bite the skin, causing:
* Itch, worse at night.
* Several small lumps appearing rapidly around the genitals.
* Scabies commonly bite between the fingers, and on the wrist.
Treatment is with shampoos and skin applications, plus careful decontamination of bedding and clothing.

■ WARTS
Fleshy growths a few millimetres in length are fairly common, and as harmless on the genitals as elsewhere. Quite different are masses of spreading warts:
* Appear like tiny, branching corals.
* Often also found around the back passage.
As these may be associated with syphilis, go to a specialist in sexually transmitted diseases.

POSSIBLE

■ CYSTS
Women commonly develop a Bartholin's cyst.
* Painless swelling in one lip of the vagina.
* May cause no other problem.
* If infected, becomes very swollen and tender; fever.
Surgical drainage is needed.

■ SYPHILIS
The symptoms of infection with syphilis appear two to four weeks after contact. Either partner may be infected.
* Painless ulcer on the genitals, turning into a firm lump. The ulcer, known as a chancre, may appear around or in the vagina, in the mouth, or around the back passage, depending on the nature of the sexual activity.
* Local lymph nodes enlarge.
* Heals over several weeks.
* After a few months, secondary features appear, such as rashes on the palms and soles, joint pains, swollen lymph nodes, genital warts. Years later, syphilis can rampage through the body, affecting just about every organ and causing dementia. Early disease is cured by penicillin.

RARE

■ BEHCET'S DISEASE
A combination of:
* Painful, single ulcers on genitals and in the mouth.
* Red eyes, either conjunctivitis or iritis.
* Symptoms tend to recur.

■ TROPICAL VENEREAL DISEASES
By rare, we mean rare in Europe

and the U.S.A; sexually promiscuous travellers to the tropics are at risk. These diseases are chancroid, *lymphogranuloma venerium* and *granuloma inguinale*. They all produce:
* Genital ulcer, within a few days of infection.
* May remain small, or become very large.
* Usually painful.
* Swollen local lymph glands.

The diagnosis is made on appearance, and results of swabs; treatment with antibiotics usually leads to a cure.

■ CANCER
Skin cancer may be the reason for a persistent, ulcerated area on the penis or vagina: see a doctor.

Delay reduces the chance of a complete cure.

LUMPS IN THE GROIN

The groin is the region at the top of the thighs, by the side of the genitals in front of the hip joints. Lumps on the genitals themselves are considered under specific headings. Lumps in the groin are very common and are noticed early, being such a visible part of the body. They are not usually serious.

There are several different structures in the groin. Lumps in that region may have many causes. In practice, it is usually possible to make a confident diagnosis based only on the appearance of the lump and an examination.

PROBABLE
INGUINAL HERNIA
ENLARGED LYMPH NODES

POSSIBLE
VEINS
FEMORAL HERNIA
LIPOMA
UNDESCENDED TESTICLE

RARE
ANEURYSM OF BLOOD VESSEL
TUMOURS AND ABSCESSES

PROBABLE

■ INGUINAL HERNIA
An extremely common type of hernia, caused by weakness in the muscle wall of the abdomen, which bulges forward as a soft lump. Although typically a problem of adulthood, and made worse by lifting and straining, it may also be seen in very young babies.
* Bulges noticeably on straining.
* Often completely disappears when relaxed, lying flat.
* Slight aching is common.
* If it becomes painful and firm, bowel may be trapped within it. Seek medical help immediately.
Hernias in children should always be treated. Inguinal hernias in adults who are engaged in physical activity or lifting of weights

(for example, labourers) can be extremely troublesome. In an elderly person who is not particularly active, repair may not be necessary.

■ ENLARGED LYMPH NODES
Just like the neck, the groin has groups of lymph glands, whose job is to protect against infection. It is normal to feel a few small glands in the groin; they are about half a centimetre in size, painless and mobile under your finger. Minor scratches on the legs, or pimples around the groin, will cause these glands to enlarge for a few days, and it is best to keep an eye on these until they shrink again. Glands which remain swollen for longer, which are painful or unusually large, need to be thoroughly checked. There are so many possibilities that enlarged glands are treated as a separate topic in *SWOLLEN LYMPH NODES, page 489.*

Enlarged glands accompanied by any of the following symptoms should be taken seriously.
* Enlarged glands elsewhere, such as neck, armpits.
* Sores on the genitals.
* Bleeding from the back passage.
* Fever, malaise.
* Anaemia.
* Bruising.

POSSIBLE

■ VARICOSE VEINS
Enlarged veins are often seen and felt in the groin.
* Swelling is very soft, easily squeezed by finger pressure.
* A bluish tinge may be noticeable.
* Usually varicose veins further down the leg.
* Slight aching after standing.

■ FEMORAL HERNIA
A femoral hernia arises from a weakness at the very top of the thigh, and is different from an inguinal hernia. It carries a higher chance of blockage, and also requires surgical treatment.
* Commonest in older women.
* Often appears rapidly as a small tender lump..
* Blockage causes a painful, hard lump, vomiting, intestinal obstruction.

■ LIPOMA
A soft mass, present for many weeks and growing slowly, if at all, is probably a lipoma — a fat lump.
* Painless.
* Often others elsewhere.

There is no need to the remove the lump unless there is any doubt about the diagnosis.

■ UNDESCENDED TESTICLE
In males, the testicle may lodge just above the groin.
* Noticeable in babies and children, when it may be seen soon after birth. The scrotum is checked during the first year to make sure both testicles are present.
* No testicle felt in that side of the scrotum.

The testicle should be surgically brought down into the scrotum, ideally as early as possible and preferably before the third birthday. Failure to do so increases the risk of impaired fertility and the appearance of cancer in the affected testicle.

RARE

■ ANEURYSM OF BLOOD VESSEL
The large femoral artery, which carries blood to the leg, passes near to the surface in the groin. Its wall can weaken and it expands like a balloon, producing:
* A lump, pulsating in time with your heart beat, but delayed by a fraction of a second.
* Often tender.
Can be repaired surgically.

■ TUMOURS AND ABSCESSES
As with lumps anywhere on the body, the possibility of a tumour or an abscess has to kept in mind. In such cases the lump may:
* Be tender.
* Feel as if it is attached to surrounding tissues.
* You may be generally unwell.
These are very unusual.

LOSS OF PUBIC HAIR

Although this is not a common problem, it is alarming to the individual when it happens. Thinning of the hair is a normal feature of ageing, and it occurs as an expected side effect of chemo–therapy for cancer. Otherwise, it is probably caused by hormone disturbances.

PROBABLE
ALOPECIA

POSSIBLE
ADDISON'S DISEASE
CIRRHOSIS OF LIVER

RARE
UNDERACTIVE PITUITARY GLAND

PROBABLE

■ ALOPECIA
A general term for hair loss of unknown cause. In the most common form, it causes thinning of hair, perhaps with some actual hairless patches. Only in severe cases is there complete, generalized hair loss.
* Baldness in men or women.
* Loss of eyebrows, armpit hair.
Usually cures itself. *See also LOSS OF HAIR OR BALDNESS, page 263.*

POSSIBLE

■ ADDISON'S DISEASE
A consequence of underactive adrenal glands, causing:
* Profound weakness.
* Dark patches in the mouth, on the gums or on old scars.
* Weight loss.
* Nausea, stomach cramps.
Treatment is by hormone replacement, once the underlying cause has been established.

■ CIRRHOSIS OF THE LIVER
Usually due to alcoholism.
* Hair thins rather than

disappears.
* Small, dilated veins appear on face, chest.
* Red palms.
* Impotence.
* Swollen ankles.
* Nausea, indigestion.
* Easy bruising.
* Possibly blood in vomit, or in motions.
* Variable degree of confusion.

Treatment, of course, requires complete abstention from alcohol.

RARE

■ PITUITARY GLAND DISEASE
Failure of this gland in the brain, which is involved in so many functions of the body, causes:
* Striking pallor.
* Hairlessness.
* Great tiredness, weakness.
* In women, cessation of periods.

Lifelong hormone replacement allows a return to health.

HOT FLUSHES

Sudden waves of heat passing over the whole body, occurring at any time. Often worse at night, and in social gatherings.

PROBABLE
MENOPAUSE

POSSIBLE
OVERACTIVE THYROID GLAND

RARE
CAUSES OF FEVERS OR SWEATS

PROBABLE

■ MENOPAUSE
Known also as 'the Change', or 'the change of life', and linked to the drop in the level of female hormones present in the blood.

Conventionally, menopause is said to have begun if a woman has not had a period for one year. However, hot flushes can begin before periods stop — blood tests are a useful check. On average, the menopause begins at about 50 years. But, it is entirely normal to enter menopause in the early 30s or late 50s. The best guide is the age at which your mother began her menopause. Other symptoms are:

* Periods become erratic and lighter.
* Skin becomes coarser.
* The skin of the vagina becomes drier.
* Aches and pains are common.

Some features are more controversial, perhaps more a reflection of personal adjustment to this major event in a women's life:
* Loss of sexual desire.
* Headaches.
* Depression.
* Irritability.

Hot flushes usually continue for two to three years; a few unlucky individuals continue to have them for ten years or more. This is not a symptom of disease.

For some women, it is a relief for periods to end; for others, it is a matter of deep emotion: the beginning of old age. The reaction of the majority of women lies somewhere between the two, and is intimately connected with support from their partners and families, and their own self-esteem.

Hormone replacement therapy (HRT) is a useful treatment for the irksome symptoms of the menopause, relieving hot flushes, vaginal dryness and reducing the aches and pains. Whether it relieves the psychological symptoms is more controversial. A decision about HRT needs detailed discussion with your doctor about the many pros and cons. The treatment is particulary advisable if you go into a very early menopause, when it is clear that hormone replacement therapy protects again thinning of the bones in old age. Often, a short course of HRT, perhaps taken for just a few years, helps a woman who is otherwise reluctant to take hormones for years on end.

POSSIBLE

■ <u>OVERACTIVE THYROID GLAND</u>
* Occurs at any age.
* Sweating, increased appetite, weight loss.
* Intolerance to heat.
* Tremor of hands.
* Consistently rapid pulse, possibly palpitations.
* Protruding eyes (in some cases).

Treatment aims to reduce the output of thyroid hormone from the thyroid gland.

RARE

■ <u>PERSISTENT FEVER OR SWEATS</u>
It is worth considering whether any of the many causes of fevers or sweats might be responsible. The subject is covered in detail on *pages 440-51 and 456-460,* but your suspicions might be aroused by:
* Menopausal symptoms beginning abruptly.
* Periods still regular.
* Drenching sweats at night.
* Malaise, weight loss.
* Exposure to unusual infections through travel, occupation.
* Enlarged glands.

MASCULINE CHANGES

Male features in a woman may reflect upsets in the balance between male and female hormones, unless this is clearly a feature of your family or race. If periods are normal, there is probably not a serious underlying hormonal problem. Typical masculine changes are:
* Growth of hair on the face, chest, abdomen.
* Balding.
* Deepening voice.
* Disruption of periods.

PROBABLE
HEREDITARY

POSSIBLE
HYPOTHYROIDISM
POLYCYSTIC OVARIES
DRUGS

RARE
OVARIAN TUMOUR
CUSHING'S SYNDROME

PROBABLE

■ HEREDITARY
Racial and family differences in hairiness are well known; for example, both men and women from Mediterranean races tend to be hairier than Nordic peoples, for example. There is no effect on fertility.

POSSIBLE

■ HYPOTHYROIDISM
An underactive gland may often be the reason for masculinization, as it causes:
* Gruff voice, coarse skin.
* Periods to stop, or be heavy.

Additional features of an underactive thyroid gland are:
* Weight gain.
* Slow thought.
* Slow pulse.
* Weakness.

The diagnosis is made on the basis of blood tests.

■ POLYCYSTIC OVARIES
A disease in which the ovaries have many cysts, and produce male hormones. It is *not* a form of cancer. It affects women in their teens or early 20s, and its symptoms are:
* Hairiness.
* Absent periods.
* Severe acne.
* Overweight.

However, the severity varies. In practice, polycystic ovaries would be a possibility if a woman had complained of two or more of the symptoms listed. Ultrasound examination of the ovaries, together with measurement of hormones, has made this disease easy to diagnose. Treatment can improve fertility, as well as dealing with the other features.

■ DRUGS
Hairiness is a side effect of several widely used drugs. The most common is phenytoin, used to control epilepsy; steroids, used to treat a range of arthritic diseases, may also be to blame.

RARE

■ OVARIAN TUMOUR
Suspected in a previously healthy woman who develops signs of masculinization. There are no other symptoms of an early tumour, which must be detected by examination and ultrasound investigation.

■ CUSHING'S SYNDROME
There are many causes of this syndrome, which involves the production of excessive amounts of natural male hormones and steroids by the body's glands. Among its symptoms are:
* Obese body, but thin limbs.
* Masculine features.
* Easy bruising.
* Excessive production of urine.
* Purple stripes across the hip, and other fat-bearing areas.

PAIN IN THE PELVIS

Pains in the lower abdomen are common in women, and are frequently difficult to diagnose. Apart from gynaecological causes (problems in the womb and ovaries), there are plenty of other pelvic organs to consider: the intestines, the bladder and kidneys; pain from irritation of nerves in the back; diseases of the major arteries which run through the lower abdomen. The abdomen is also a sensitive index of emotional turmoil, at all ages and in both sexes. The abdomens of women criss-crossed by the scars of fruitless surgical investigations are a warning: take time early on for an honest review of emotional factors which may be contributing to the problem.

Pains associated with the following symptoms suggest a gynaecological cause:
* Painful periods.
* Unusual vaginal discharge.
* Abnormal vaginal bleeding.
* Pain on intercourse.
* Infertility.

For further details *see pages 343-61, 335 and 332.*

Symptoms pointing to a non-gynaecological cause are:
* Diarrhoea.
* Frequent desire to urinate; stinging or burning when you do.
* Pain varies depending on your posture.
* Pulsation in your abdomen, pain in legs on walking.
* Depression, marital problems.

Your overall condition may point to one of the many non-gynaecological diseases which can cause recurrent abdominal pains. Your doctors will rely on the pattern of symptoms, and the results of tests, before making a diagnosis.

INFERTILITY

Fifteen per cent of couples who have regular sexual intercourse will not have conceived after one year and may be termed sterile. About 10 per cent of all couples remain sterile. Before anything else, it is essential to establish that normal intercourse is taking place, as history teaches that pregnancy cannot follow an ejaculation into the belly button. Also, a sperm count should be taken early on, to avoid fruitless and unpleasant investigations for the woman. About 30 per cent of cases are due to problems in the woman's reproductive system.

PROBABLE
FAILURE OF EGG PRODUCTION
BLOCKED FALLOPIAN TUBES
CAUSE UNKNOWN

POSSIBLE
ENDOMETRIOSIS
GENERAL DISEASE

RARE
WOMB ABNORMALITIES

PROBABLE

■ FAILURE OF EGG PRODUCTION
This involves hormone imbalance, and would be suspected if there are:
* Irregular periods.
* Absent periods, or delay in beginning periods.

See specific headings on pages 343-353.

■ BLOCKED FALLOPIAN TUBES
These are the tubes through which eggs travel to the womb. Blocked tubes usually follow repeated pelvic infections, suspected from:
* Recurrent pelvic pain.
* Recurrent, infected vaginal discharges.
* Deep pain on intercourse.

See also PAINFUL PERIODS, page 351 and PAIN IN THE PELVIS, page 331.

■ CAUSE UNKNOWN
Despite thorough investigation, many cases remain unexplained.

POSSIBLE

■ ENDOMETRIOSIS
See page 349.
* Deep pain on intercourse.

■ GENERAL DISEASE
Any serious, general disease can reduce fertility, but should already be obvious.

RARE

■ WOMB ABNORMALITIES
Investigations sometimes show a range of unsuspected abnormalities, such as a malformed womb, which prevents implantation of the egg.

LACK OF INTEREST IN SEX (FRIGIDITY)

Most enduring relationships eventually balance the partners' sexual desires so that neither partner is left feeling frustrated or guilty. The road to that adjustment can be a difficult one. Blame does not enter into this, nor is it ever the fault of one party alone: recognizing that there is a problem is the first step to resolving it.

Natural variations in a woman's sexual desire occur during the monthly cycle, reaching a peak in mid-cycle (before ovulation) for some women. Major illness and childbirth will usually decrease sexual desire.

PROBABLE
PSYCHOLOGICAL FACTORS

POSSIBLE
ADVERSE SEXUAL EXPERIENCES

RARE
DEPRESSION

PROBABLE

■ PSYCHOLOGICAL FACTORS
Psychological factors are most likely if you feel:
* Sex is dirty.
* An aversion to being touched sexually by your partner.
* That things should be better than they are.
* Guilty about your lack of enjoyment of sex.

Sex counsellors can help this problem. Other counsellors, including individual and marriage guidance counsellors, can also contribute.

POSSIBLE

■ ADVERSE SEXUAL EXPERIENCES
Meaning traumatic events such as painful intercourse, misunderstanding about sexual anatomy and sexual response, fear of falling pregnant. Most important is the memory of early sexual experiences, particularly if either partner was abused. The techniques for dealing with such problems involve explanation, honesty and patience. Gradually exploring your anatomy and sexual response, without initially indulging in sexual intercourse, may be helpful.

RARE

■ DEPRESSION
A decreasing interest in sex in either a man or a woman may signal depression. Some other features of depression are:
* Feelings of sadness.
* Loss of self-worth.
* Disturbed sleep.
* Easy crying.
* Thoughts of suicide.
* Slowing of thought.

ORGASMIC FAILURE

A popular view places orgasm during intercourse right up there alongside other major goals of Western society, such as ensuring your children's white shirts dazzle the teacher, cooking meals that make your family swoon and having floors clean enough to eat off. There may be an element of unreality about all these.

Men may be unable to achieve orgasm for much the same reasons as women.

Some facts about female orgasm:

* It is a real physical and psychological event.
* Stimulation of the clitoris is usually important.
* It is not necessary for enjoyable sex each time.
* It may take longer to achieve for a woman than for a man.
* Women are capable of multiple orgasms; they do not need a resting period like most men.

It will be clear that failure to achieve orgasm may well not be a failure at all on the woman's part, but may possibly be due to difficulty within the partnership, or because of the techniques used during intercourse. Some women are unable to experience orgasm until they start to masturbate. It is helpful to share and explore with your partner what forms of stimulation lead to orgasm so that they can be enjoyed together.

PROBABLE
PSYCHOLOGICAL
POOR TECHNIQUE

POSSIBLE
PARTNER'S PROBLEM

PROBABLE

■ PSYCHOLOGICAL

This refers to the array of experiences that make a relationship: affection, trust, previous positive experiences. It is common knowledge that uncertainty in these, and other, aspects will lead to problems with sex and orgasm.

■ POOR TECHNIQUE

It is necessary to take the female anatomy into account. Female orgasm requires:

* Adequate foreplay.
* Clitoral stimulation.
* Avoidance of pain.
* Proper lubrication.

This is a matter of trial and error.

POSSIBLE

■ PARTNER'S PROBLEM

Failure to achieve orgasm can be a result of a partner's:

* Premature ejaculation;
* Impotence.

See pages 365, 366 and 363.

PAINFUL SEXUAL INTERCOURSE

PROBABLE
VAGINAL INFECTION
VAGINAL SPASM (VAGINISMUS)

POSSIBLE
VAGINAL DRYNESS
ENDOMETRIOSIS
CHRONIC PELVIC INFECTION

RARE
PHYSICAL BARRIER TO INTERCOURSE

PROBABLE

■ VAGINAL INFECTION
Perhaps a raw area in or near the vagina.
* Pain is superficial, not deep inside.
* Probably discharge.
* Probably an itch.
Possible causes are thrush and herpes. *See page 357.*

■ VAGINAL SPASM
Vaginismus. A term for a contraction of the muscles around the vagina which will prevent intercourse. This important symptom is nearly always the result of a psychological fear of penetration. Occasionally, it follows an unpleasant injury to the vagina, such as a painful tear or cut (episiotomy) after childbirth.
* Other aspects of sexual behaviour may be normal.
* Gynaecological examination may be impossible; this frequently gives the first clue to the problem.
Treatment encourages familiarity with one's own genitalia, building up gradually to sexual intercourse.

POSSIBLE

■ VAGINAL DRYNESS
See also BLEEDING AFTER THE MENOPAUSE, page 352. Mainly a post-menopausal problem:
* Vagina feels generally sore.
* Watery discharge, possibly bloodstained.
This can be greatly helped by the use of locally applied oestrogen creams or hormone replacement therapy (HRT). *See page 329.*

■ ENDOMETRIOSIS
* Intercourse causes pain deep inside.
* Heavy periods.
* Infertility.
See page 349.

■ CHRONIC PELVIC INFECTION
Also causes:
* Deep pain on intercourse.
* Heavy periods.
See PELVIC INFLAMMATORY DISEASE, page 349.

RARE

■ PHYSICAL BARRIER TO INTERCOURSE

The hymen, the membrane across the entrance to the vagina that is normally broken at first sexual intercourse, can be too thick to break. Rarely the entrance to the vagina is unusually narrow. Surgical help is needed here.
* You may see or feel an obstruction.
* Pain on attempting intercourse.
* Pain around entrance to vagina.

BREAST DISORDERS INTRODUCTION

It is wise for women to check their breasts from time to time, aiming to familiarize themselves with how they feel normally so that changes can be spotted early. Remember that the tissues of the breast extend into the armpit, so checks should include that area. Some countries now offer screening programmes, using X-rays (mammography) to detect changes in the breasts before *you* notice a problem. Such screening is not 100 per cent reliable, and it may turn up many apparent abnormalities which, on further investigation, prove harmless. However, these false alarms are a price worth paying in order to detect more serious disease earlier.

Many women believe that the only breast disease is breast cancer, and that any change whatsoever in their breast must be a symptom of this disease. Certainly, breast cancer is a possibility with many of the symptoms in this section. But it is not usually the most likely cause.

Fear of a breast cancer diagnosis puts some women off reporting symptoms. This is a great pity, since more often than not, skilled examination alone will produce a reassuring diagnosis, while investigations will show that all is well. Also, when cancer is confirmed, any delay in reporting symptoms will delay treatment. Every doctor would rather see a hundred women with false alarms than one woman with an obvious growth.

LUMP IN THE BREAST

At some time in their lives, most women will feel a lump in one of their breasts. Breasts are frequently lumpy, and some of these lumps are easily felt. In nine out of ten cases it will be entirely harmless. It will frequently turn out to be not a single lump at all. That leaves a one in ten chance of a lump being cancerous. That diagnosis must not be taken as a death sentence because, like all cancers, breast cancer is not one disease but a group of diseases, whose growth depends on the exact nature of the cancer, the age of the woman, and how early it is detected.

Breast cancer is one of the most closely studied forms of cancer, but doctors will admit that there is still an enormous amount they do not know about it. Fundamental questions remain unanswered, such as why the cancer starts, how quickly it grows and how best to treat it. Expert opinion about therapy is constantly changing, following the results of treatment trials which are being carried out worldwide.

In this situation, some women are tempted to search for miracle cures and get-well-quick treatments. Be very careful. There is a big difference between unconventional approaches that give support, hope, and self-reliance, and those which are just a means of peddling treatment which does not, and will not, stand up to the simplest scientific assessment.

There is a notion that doctors wash their hands of women who do not wish to follow conventional treatment. This is a myth. Whatever your views may be, begin by seeing your doctor as soon as you feel an abnormality in your breast. Your doctor will often be able to reassure you on the basis of examination alone.

PROBABLE
FIBROADENOMA
FIBROCYSTIC DISEASE
DUCT PAPILLOMA

POSSIBLE
BREAST CANCER
FAT NECROSIS

RARE
OTHER TUMOURS

PROBABLE

■ FIBROADENOMA

Commonest in women between 20 and 40 years old.
* Firm, painless lump.
* Freely mobile: which is why this lump has been described as a 'breast mouse'.

Some women have several of these over many years, but each one should be surgically removed. They are not thought to lead to cancer.

■ FIBROCYSTIC DISEASE

This is a misleading technical term for something that is not really a disease at all. The breasts are generally lumpy, and within that lumpiness there may be more definite, large lumps which are usually fluid-filled cysts.
* Commonest in women 30 to 50 years of age.
* Lumpiness varies during the menstrual cycle.
* Often pain before a period.
* Often areas of the breast are tender.

Mammography (X-rays of the breast) are useful in differentiating these lumps from cancer. Many surgeons will drain obvious cysts, using a needle and syringe, and send the contents for detailed analysis. No other treatment is necessarily needed.

THE REPRODUCTIVE AND SEXUAL ORGANS

■ DUCT PAPILLOMA
A lump felt just behind the nipple, and associated with a bloody discharge from the nipple. This should always be reported to your doctor.
See page 341.

POSSIBLE

■ BREAST CANCER
You feel a lump; it may be tiny but you are sure it has appeared recently. Some of the features that would suggest that a lump is likely to be cancerous are:
* A firm, irregular lump.
* Not freely mobile, seems stuck in one place.
* Skin over it is dimpled and puckered.
* A newly indrawn nipple, or any nipple changes occurring at the same time.
* Swollen glands felt in armpit.
* Pain in the region of the lump.
* Bleeding from the nipple.

It may be possible to take a biopsy from the lump, allowing a definite diagnosis before any surgery is planned. Mammography also helps with diagnosis. In other cases, the diagnosis may not be made until the lump has been removed and analysed.

Treatment for pre-menopausal women is a combination of surgery, radiotherapy and chemotherapy in varying proportions. In post-menopausal women, surgery is commonly combined with radiotherapy and anti-oestrogen drugs, such as tamoxifen.

■ FAT NECROSIS
A hard knock to the breast can damage fat cells, leading to a lump that feels indistinguishable from a cancer.
* A firm lump.
* Does not move freely.
* Skin over it may be dimpled.

The only safe way to deal with this is a biopsy.

RARE

■ OTHER TUMOURS
It is possible for cancers elsewhere to spread into the breast. The diagnosis will probably only be made on biopsy.

PAIN IN THE BREASTS

If pain is felt over the whole breast, it is usually caused by a variation in hormone levels. It may be confined to one area, when you should feel for a localized abnormality, such as a lump or dimpled skin. Breast pain may be no more than a nuisance, but for some women it is a great problem, which has only attracted recent attention. Mammography makes it possible to be confident that there is no underlying disease. Treatments currently under trial include hormones, Vitamin B6, and evening primrose oil.

PROBABLE
BREAST ABSCESS
FIBROCYSTIC DISEASE

POSSIBLE
BREAST CANCER
PAIN FROM THE RIBS
PREGNANCY

PROBABLE

■ BREAST ABSCESS
See DISCHARGE FROM NIPPLE, page 341.
* Pain.
* Redness of one breast.
* Fever.

■ FIBROCYSTIC DISEASE
See page 337.
A frequent cause for a general ache in one or both breasts, with localized areas being especially tender.

POSSIBLE

■ BREAST CANCER
See page 338. Pain is unusual as an early symptom of breast cancer; though it can be present at an advanced stage.

■ PAIN FROM THE RIBS
Inflammation of the muscles between ribs, or where the rib and the breast bone meet.
* One breast affected.
* Pain is sharp, and highly localized.
* Pain reproduced by pressing between the ribs, or by pressing on the breast bone.

A harmless symptom that settles over a few weeks.

POSSIBLE

■ PREGNANCY
Aching in the breasts due to pregnancy often occurs even before a period has been missed. Other early symptoms of pregnancy are:
* Increased urge to pass urine frequently.
* A vague tiredness.

BREAST SIZE

The popular Western attitude to breast size equates large size with femininity. This attitude is largely shaped by male opinion, but many women are dissatisfied with the size of their breasts, considering them either too small or too large. Breast size does not affect the ability to breast feed a child. It is normal for the two breasts to be slightly different in size and shape.

PROBABLE
HEREDITARY

POSSIBLE
HORMONAL

RARE
LYMPHATIC OBSTRUCTION

PROBABLE

■ HEREDITARY
Breast size is mainly determined by in-built factors, with influence from grandparents on both the mother's and the father's side. Race also plays a part, with Asiatic women generally having smaller breasts. Reasons for breast surgery might include:
* Psychological distress.
* Neck and back pains from very heavy breasts.

POSSIBLE

■ HORMONAL
The contraceptive pill and hormone replacement therapy often cause a slight increase in breast size. Pregnancy, of course, makes the breasts enlarge, also under the influence of hormones. Many women notice a slight variation in size during their menstrual cycle. Breast size bears no relationship to a woman's ability to have children.

RARE

■ LYMPHATIC OBSTRUCTION
Interference with normal drainage of tissue fluid from the breast via the armpit will lead to one swollen breast.
* Often after radiotherapy to the chest wall, when the arm on that side is also very swollen.
* You may feel glands in the armpit; if so, report immediately.
* Breast becomes generally firm. Unfortunately, little can usually be done to cure this problem.

DISCHARGE FROM THE NIPPLE

During pregnancy it is normal for a milky fluid to ooze from the breasts. Mothers who breast feed will find not only that suckling causes a discharge of milk, but that even the sound of the baby crying will trigger this response, and again this is entirely normal. Abnormal discharges may be of milk in the absence of pregnancy, clear fluid, of blood or of yellow/green pus. Discharges are commonly due to disease of the duct system, that is, one of the 20 or so channels through which milk flows to the nipple from the milk-producing glands deeper within the breast.

PROBABLE
BREAST ABSCESS
HORMONE DISTURBANCE

POSSIBLE
DUCT PAPILLOMA
CANCER OF DUCTS
DUCT ECTASIA

RARE
BREAST CANCER
PAGET'S DISEASE OF THE NIPPLE

PROBABLE

■ BREAST ABSCESS

A frequent problem in the first few weeks of breast feeding, and thought to be caused simply by infection entering the breast via the constantly damp and sometimes cracked nipple.

* Symptoms build up over a few hours.
* Aching in one part of the breast.
* Often you see a firm red area of the breast.
* Bloody discharge, mixed with milk, may be present.
* Frequently rigors, high temperatures, sweats.
* Pain can be severe.

Antibiotics nearly always settle this disorder. Occasionally there is a chronic abscess, caused by persistent infection deep within the breast.

■ HORMONE DISTURBANCE

Milk production is controlled by a hormone, prolactin, secreted by the pituitary gland within the brain. An excess of prolactin causes:

* Discharge of milk from both breasts for months on end.
* Periods become scanty or stop altogether.

Blood tests will show abnormal levels of prolactin. The usual reason is a tiny growth in the pituitary gland; this can be controlled with appropriate drugs. A few medically prescribed drugs can cause this problem, particularly powerful sedatives and methyldopa, widely used to treat high blood pressure.

The breast

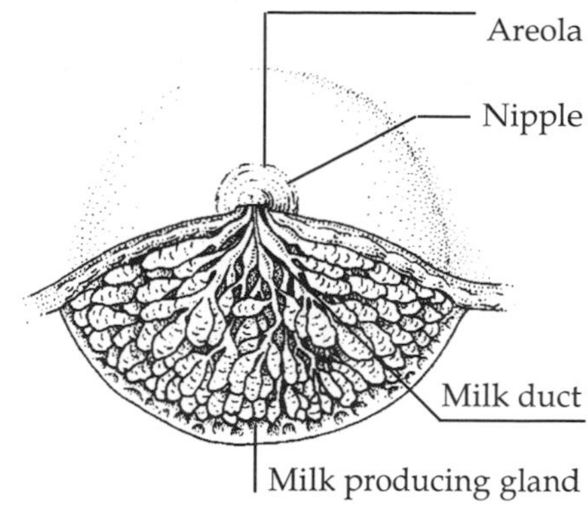

POSSIBLE

The three following possibilities give similar symptoms, and in all cases will require further investigation, since examination alone is not enough to decide definitely between them.

■ DUCT PAPILLOMA

A wart-like, benign growth within one of the ducts leading to the nipple.

* A bloody discharge, perhaps just a spot of blood on the bra.
* Sometimes just a clear, yellowish discharge.
* A lump may be felt near the nipple.

■ CANCER OF DUCTS

* Bloody discharge.
* Possibly a prickling sensation behind the nipple.

■ DUCT ECTASIA

In this condition, enlarged ducts allow the build-up of normal secretions, which then appear as:

* A brown or green discharge.
* Discharge is firm, cheese-like.

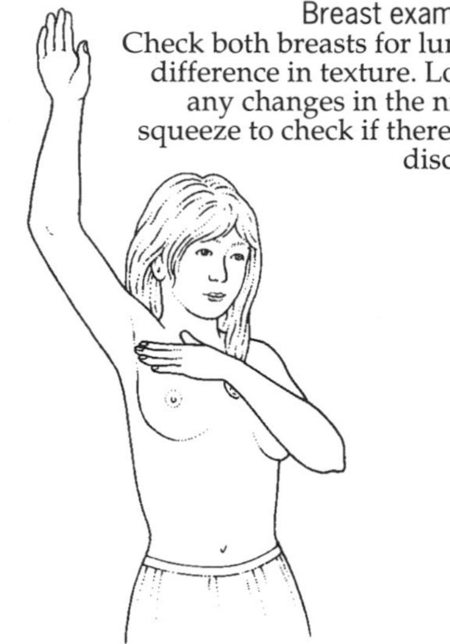

Breast examination
Check both breasts for lumps or difference in texture. Look for any changes in the nipples, squeeze to check if there is any discharge.

RARE

■ BREAST CANCER
See page 338. Occasionally a breast cancer some distance from the nipple causes bleeding.
* A breast lump is likely.
* Some discomfort is likely.

■ PAGET'S DISEASE OF THE NIPPLE
A distinctive condition, most common in older women:
* Cracked dry, red skin around one nipple.
* Oozes blood.
* The nipple becomes distorted.

This disease is nearly always due to breast cancer.

RETRACTION OF THE NIPPLE

Both nipples normally project a little, becoming flatter when warm or relaxed, and more protuberant if cold, or sometimes if sexually aroused. Retracted nipples appear sunken into the breast.

PROBABLE
CONGENITAL

POSSIBLE
BREAST CANCER

PROBABLE

■ CONGENITAL
Commonly seen in baby girls who grow up with one or both nipples retracted. It is not a sign of disease, but might affect the ability to breast feed.

There are many 'cures' for retracted nipples, but there is little evidence that they work.

POSSIBLE

■ BREAST CANCER
The retraction of a previously normal nipple must be taken as a symptom of breast cancer until proven otherwise. You should search for:
* Lump in the breast.
* Discharge from the nipple.

Always inform your doctor of any changes to your nipples. Don't delay.

MENSTRUATION INTRODUCTION

During the monthly cycle, the lining of the womb thickens and prepares to accept a fertilized egg. If conception does not take place, the lining breaks down and is shed — this is the menstrual discharge. This complex process involves hormones from the brain, the ovaries and the egg, all directed towards a common goal: a successful pregnancy. It is aptly said that menstruation is the womb crying for want of a pregnancy. Problem-free menstruation depends on a healthy balance between mind and body: it is more likely to be upset by psychological factors than most other bodily functions.

The length, frequency and heaviness of menstruation vary enormously, from person to person and from month to month, and this is not necessarily a symptom of any abnormality. Sudden changes are a different matter and should be heeded.

ABSENT OR INFREQUENT PERIODS

This section concerns women who have previously had normal periods. In the case of periods which have never started, *see DELAY IN BEGINNING MENSTRUATION, page 347.* In young women, stress is so often the reason for irregular periods that further investigation is usually unnecessary, except for reassurance, or to exclude pregnancy. Irregularities in women in their late 30s or early 40s are likely to have a physical or hormonal cause. In particular, women with infrequent periods should be examined to make quite sure that normal but infrequent periods are just that, and are not in fact occasional, abnormal episodes of bleeding from the womb or cervix. Bleeding out of the blue, without your usual pre-menstrual symptoms, should definitely be investigated.

PROBABLE

PREGNANCY
STRESS
BREAST FEEDING

POSSIBLE

MENOPAUSE
RAISED PROLACTIN
MAJOR WEIGHT CHANGE
POLYCYSTIC OVARIES
POST-PILL ABSENT PERIODS
SERIOUS GENERAL DISEASE

THE REPRODUCTIVE AND SEXUAL ORGANS

RARE

THYROID DISEASE
ADRENAL DISEASE

PROBABLE

■ PREGNANCY

It is a useful and proven medical rule of thumb that, if in doubt, any woman of child-bearing age with absent periods should have a pregnancy test if intercourse has taken place. After any missed period, you should be on the look-out for other symptoms of pregnancy, such as:

* Morning sickness.
* Tender breasts.
* Lethargy, weight gain.
* Passing urine more frequently than usual.
* Appetite changes.

Have a pregnancy test if you are uncertain.

■ STRESS

An extremely common reason, especially in young women. Stress is caused not just by obvious emotional turmoil but major changes in lifestyle, such as changes of job, travel, illness. Even what appears to be 'everyday' stress, such as preparing for exams, can be sufficient to stop periods.

* In conditions of obvious tension, the absence of periods for two or three months should not be a worry, as long as pregnancy is excluded.

Investigations are rarely needed, unless symptoms persist for more than six months.

■ BREAST FEEDING

Periods stop or are scanty during breast feeding, since hormones delay the normal return of the menstrual cycle. It is, however, possible to become pregnant while breast feeding, for ovulation may still occur.

POSSIBLE

■ MENOPAUSE

To be considered in women from 30 years of age onwards, especially given a family history of early menopause. Any woman whose ovaries have been removed, for example, in the treatment of breast cancer or at a hysterectomy, will experience rapid onset of menopausal symptoms.

■ RAISED PROLACTIN

See HORMONE DISTURBANCE, page 341. Absent periods, plus a milky discharge from the breasts, suggest an excess of prolactin, one of the hormones that normally contribute to the production of breast milk.

Rarely, the condition can be caused by a tumour in the brain. Blood tests and simple X-rays can sometimes detect this.

■ MAJOR WEIGHT CHANGE

Both excessive weight gain and dieting will disrupt periods, because they affect some brain centres. The most extreme form is *anorexia nervosa*:

* Skeletal thinness.
* Obsession with weight.
* Fine hair grows on body.

■ POLYCYSTIC OVARIES.
In a young woman, a diagnosis suggested by:
* Absent periods.
* Hairiness.
* Acne.
* Above-average weight.
See page 330.

■ POST-PILL ABSENT PERIODS
Commonest in women whose periods were irregular before they began to take oral contraception.
* Otherwise sound health.
* Periods return after three to six months.

If you have not had a period for more than six months after you stop taking the pill, seek professional advice.

■ SERIOUS GENERAL DISEASE
Remember that tension can stop your menstrual cycle (*see above*). The strain of another illness on your body may well cause this tension. Other symptoms might be:
* Weight loss.
* Tiredness.
* Chronic cough.
* Fever, diarrhoea.

Periods should return after recovery.

RARE

■ THYROID DISEASE
Over-excitability or lethargy, combined with disturbed periods, may suggest an over or under-active thyroid gland. *See page 350.*

■ ADRENAL DISEASE
A possibility if absent periods are accompanied by:
* Hairiness.
* Weight gain.
* Weakness.
See also MASCULINE CHANGES, pages 330-1.

BLEEDING BETWEEN PERIODS OR AFTER INTERCOURSE

The older the woman, the greater the significance of this symptom. Causes are frequently obvious to the trained eye: you should always obtain your doctor's advice. Check that the cause is not blood in your partner's semen.

PROBABLE
BREAKTHROUGH BLEEDING ON THE PILL
EROSION OF THE CERVIX
HORMONE IMBALANCE

POSSIBLE
POLYP OF THE CERVIX
CANCER OF CERVIX
CANCER OF THE WOMB
INFLAMMATION OF THE VAGINA

RARE
URETHRAL CARUNCLE

THE REPRODUCTIVE AND SEXUAL ORGANS

PROBABLE

■ BREAKTHROUGH BLEEDING ON THE PILL
In a young woman:
* Otherwise normal cycle.
* Scanty show of blood for a day or two.
* Occurs at about the same time each month.

If this occurs for more than a few months, a change of pill may be advised. This bleeding does not, however, mean that the pill is not working. Don't stop taking the pill because you see bleeding. Finish the packet as you would normally.

■ EROSION OF THE CERVIX
A harmless raw area on the cervix, which may cause:
* Heavy, clear vaginal discharge.
* Bleeding after intercourse.
* Brief, irregular blood-spotting between periods. Blood appears on underclothing and lavatory paper unexpectedly.

Treatment involves cauterizing that part of the cervix, a painless procedure.

■ HORMONE IMBALANCE
Caused by changes in natural oestrogen levels during the cycle.
* A possibility in young women.
* Regular, scanty, intermenstrual bleeding.
* Periods are otherwise normal.

The diagnosis is made only after the other possibilities have been ruled out.

POSSIBLE

■ POLYP OF THE CERVIX
A small fleshy outgrowth, which causes no other symptoms, and which may be visible on examination. Polyps should always be removed and biopsied, though it is rare for one to be malignant.

■ CANCER OF THE CERVIX
It is hoped that widespread cervical smear screening will reduce the frequency of this disease. Publicity may give the impression that it is a disease of young women; in fact, it is most common in women in their 40s and 50s. It is suspected that early sexual activity and having many partners increase the risks significantly. Though early cancer of the cervix has no symptoms, the disease later causes:
* Irregular bleeding.
* Unusual vaginal discharge.
* Pain, though this is unusual unless the cancer has spread inside the pelvis.

Treatment, at an early stage, is a minor operation. The diseased part of the cervix is removed, and this usually cures the problem. Advanced disease requires extensive surgery and radiotherapy. All sexually active women should have regular smears — at least every three years. Annual smears are recommended for those people who have either had a previously abnormal smear, or who have the wart virus (human papilloma virus — HPV), or herpes virus, present on the cervix.

■ CANCER OF THE WOMB
Many older women with irregular bleeding are offered a 'D&C', meaning dilatation and curettage. This simple operation, sometimes called a scrape, involves removal of part of the womb's lining: the object is to relieve symptoms and to provide material for analysis. The analysis may detect cancer cells as a cause of the bleeding. For further details, *see page 353.*

■ INFLAMMATION OF THE VAGINA
Through infection or, in post-menopausal women, when vaginal skin becomes thin and raw.
* Dry vagina.
* Itch.
* Thin, watery, blood-tinged discharge.

Treatment aims to eradicate the infection, and put female hormones back into the walls of the vagina, with oestrogen cream or hormone replacement therapy (HRT).

RARE

■ URETHRAL CARUNCLE
An outgrowth at the outlet from the bladder, causing pain and bleeding. *See page 353.*

DELAY IN BEGINNING MENSTRUATION

By the age of 16, most Western girls are menstruating, and it is reasonable to be concerned about those who are not.

PROBABLE
NORMAL BUT DELAYED

POSSIBLE
HORMONE DISORDERS
ANOREXIA NERVOSA

RARE
OBSTRUCTION TO MENSTRUAL FLOW
GENETIC DISORDERS OR CONGENITAL MALFORMATION

PROBABLE

■ NORMAL BUT DELAYED
This is likely if there is:
* Normal development of breasts and pubic hair (including armpits).
* Normal growth.
* Family history of menstruation starting late.

In addition, hormone tests would be normal. In these circumstances, it is a matter of 'wait and see', sometimes using hormones to kick start the system.

POSSIBLE

■ HORMONE DISORDERS
Suggested if the girl has the following symptoms:
* Short stature.
* Poor development of breasts.
* Either an absence or an excess of body hair.
* Obesity.
* Very severe acne.

Investigation of the girl's hormones, and treatment with hormones, may be needed.

■ ANOEREXIA NERVOSA
See page 424.

RARE

■ OBSTRUCTION TO MENSTRUAL FLOW
A membrane across the vagina can block the discharge of normal menstrual blood.
* Normal sexual development.
* Recurrent, lower abdominal pain.
* A bulge may protrude from the vagina, containing menstrual blood.

Treatment is simply the removal of the membrane.

■ GENETIC DISORDERS OR CONGENITAL MALFORMATION
There is a wide range of disorders which can lead to malformation of the womb, ovaries and vagina, or even a complete absence of these organs. There are no characteristic symptoms; it is a matter of specialist assessment, after all other causes have been excluded.

HEAVY PERIODS

Just what constitutes a heavy period is a highly individual matter, but a reasonable definition would be periods which:
* Involve flooding.
* Last for more than seven days each month.
* Produce clots of blood.
* Cause anaemia, with weakness, tiredness, pallor.

Blood loss which is significantly heavier than you would expect is worth discussing with your doctor.

PROBABLE
DYSFUNCTIONAL BLEEDING

POSSIBLE
ENDOMETRIOSIS
FIBROIDS
PELVIC INFECTION
MISCARRIAGE

RARE
THYROID DISEASE
ABNORMAL BLOOD CLOTTING
TUMOURS OF THE CERVIX AND WOMB

PROBABLE

■ DYSFUNCTIONAL BLEEDING
A medical way of saying ‘we don’t think there is anything very

wrong; this is a time when, for one reason or another, your bleeding pattern is disturbed.' This diagnosis should only be made when serious causes and other possibilities have been investigated and discounted. It is the commonest diagnosis in young women, less so in older women, where other causes are more likely. Treatment is with various combinations of hormones, and it can be expected to settle with time. Emotional upset may play a part.

POSSIBLE

■ ENDOMETRIOSIS
A puzzling disease, in which tissue that is an entirely normal part of the womb grows outside the womb, rather like garden seedlings. Frequently-affected sites are the ovaries and the lining of the abdomen. The reason is unknown, though there are many theories. Whatever the cause, it is a disease that brings much misery and heartache.
* Commonest in women who are in their 20s to 40s.
* Periods may be heavy, painful, or irregular.
* Difficulty in conceiving.
* Deep pain on intercourse.

Treatment involves hormones, destruction of localized deposits of endometriosis, or — as a last resort — hysterectomy.

■ FIBROIDS
The womb has walls of powerful muscle; fibroids are overgrowths of muscle fibres, which form swellings in the wall of the womb. They can be tiny or enormous; they are not cancerous.
* Commonest between 30 to 55 years of age, especially in women who have not borne children.
* Heavy, sometimes irregular, periods.
* Swelling of lower abdomen, if the fibroids are very large.
* Occasionally, sudden pain (if a fibroid becomes inflamed).

Fibroids are easy to diagnose and can then be safely ignored unless causing problems. Single fibroids can sometimes be cut out, but usually the only effective treatment if fibroids are very troublesome is a hysterectomy.

■ PELVIC INFECTION
A wide range of infections can smoulder within the womb and Fallopian tubes. Risk factors are:
* Having intercourse with many partners.
* Previous, acute pelvic infections, with pain, fever and vaginal discharge.
* Deep pain on intercourse.
* Irregular periods.
* Infertility.
* Presence of an intra-uterine contraceptive device (IUCD) — the coil.

A surgical inspection of the tubes is often needed to confirm the diagnosis, followed by prolonged, intensive antibiotic therapy.

■ MISCARRIAGE
It is thought that as many as one in eight pregnancies miscarries. Heavy bleeding or a 'late period' may be a miscarriage.

Sudden, severe bleeding in any

woman of childbearing years raises the possibility of pregnancy and its complications — regardless of contraception, moral rectitude or denial, as every doctor knows to their dismay. A negative pregnancy test does not exclude the diagnosis.
* A period may or may not have been missed.
* Other symptoms of pregnancy, such as nausea, tender breasts.
* Lower abdominal pain.
* Heavy bleeding.
* Passage of jelly-like material.

A reliable diagnosis can sometimes be obtained by having an ultrasound scan of the womb and Fallopian tubes.

RARE

■ THYROID DISEASE
Both overactive and underactive glands are associated with heavy periods. *See also HOT FLUSHES, page 328, and MASCULINE CHANGES, page 330.*

■ ABNORMAL BLOOD CLOTTING
Heavy menstrual flow may result from any condition which makes the blood clot less well than it should. Also look for:
* Easy bruising.
* Gums which bleed easily.
* Pallor.
* Enlarged lymph glands.
* Blood in urine, vomit or from bowels.

■ TUMOURS OF THE CERVIX AND WOMB
Though heavy periods are a possible symptom, these diseases are more likely to cause:
* Irregular bleeding.
* Unusual discharges.
* Post-menopausal bleeding, especially cancer of the womb.

Routine investigations of heavy periods will discover these tumours. *See also page 353.*

IRREGULAR PERIODS

Common at the beginning and end of a woman's reproductive life. The caution about distinguishing this from intermenstrual bleeding applies; *see ABSENT OR INFREQUENT PERIODS, page 343.*

PROBABLE
DYSFUNCTIONAL BLEEDING

POSSIBLE
PRE-MENOPAUSE
POST-MENOPAUSE

PROBABLE

■ DYSFUNCTIONAL BLEEDING
See page 348.

Irregularity in the mechanism of menstrual control is particularly common in teenage girls. Most women experience at least one episode of dysfunctional bleeding at some time in their life. It needs investigation if symptoms are at all troublesome or severe. Again, it is very important to distinguish

between irregular periods and either heavy periods *(see page 348)* or bleeding between periods or after intercourse *(see page 345)*.
See also DELAY IN BEGINNING MENSTRUATION, page 347.

POSSIBLE

■ PRE-MENOPAUSE
While irregular periods are common, caution is needed if you notice:
* Bleeding between periods.
* Bleeding after intercourse.
* Heavy, painful periods.

As there is often doubt about the health of the womb, further investigations are commonly carried out as a precaution.

■ POST-MENOPAUSE
All bleeding after the menopause, or after one year without menstruation, must be investigated. Never ignore bleeding after the menopause. Always check with your doctor since this can be due to serious, but treatable, disease. Early treatment is important. Don't delay.

See also BLEEDING AFTER THE MENOPAUSE, page 352.

PAINFUL PERIODS

Lucky is the woman who has no pain with her periods. Otherwise, levels of pain vary widely, as does the amount which different women find they are able to tolerate. Pain can certainly be regarded as abnormal when time is regularly lost from work, or when periods are accompanied by debilitating cramps, faintness and vomiting. In older women, these symptoms should be investigated, particularly if previously acceptable periods become intolerable, and are acompanied by pain on intercourse or heavy bleeding.

However, it is often the case that no disease is positively identified.

PROBABLE
UNKNOWN ORIGIN

POSSIBLE
ENDOMETRIOSIS
FIBROIDS
PELVIC INFLAMMATORY DISEASE

RARE
ABNORMAL SHEDDING OF THE WOMB LINING

PROBABLE

■ UNKNOWN ORIGIN
Painful periods are common in young women for the first few years of menstruation. They are thought to be caused by painful contractions of the womb during menstruation.
* Pain begins 12-24 hours before period.
* Continues for first one to two days of period.
* Pain frequently felt in tops of legs and back.

Drugs related to aspirin have a specific effect on this pain and are extremely helpful in relieving symptoms. One particular drug called mefenamic acid is increasingly used and can be very effective. The contraceptive pill can be useful for cases resistant to these drugs. The problem is sometimes relieved after a first pregnancy.

POSSIBLE

■ ENDOMETRIOSIS
Suggested by a combination of:
* Pain for several days before the period.
* Heavy periods.
* Deep pain on intercourse.
* Infertility.

This is a fairly common condition. *See also page 349.*

■ FIBROIDS
Benign muscular growths in the wall of the womb, also responsible for many heavy periods. *See page 349.*

■ PELVIC INFLAMMATORY DISEASE
Painful periods are one part of a picture which may include:
* Recurrent lower abdominal pain.
* Heavy periods.
* Deep pain on intercourse.
* Symptoms of infection.

It is especially important to catch this condition early, and treat it quickly. Otherwise, it may lead to infertility. *See the section on PELVIC INFECTION, page 349.*

RARE

■ ABNORMAL SHEDDING OF THE WOMB LINING
During a period, the lining of the womb is shed, but in many small pieces. With this condition, technically called membranous dysmenorrhea, the whole lining is lost in a few large pieces.
* Very severe abdominal pain.
* Passage of fleshy material.

This can happen once, or on a regular basis, in which case hormonal treatment is given.

BLEEDING AFTER THE MENOPAUSE

Bleeding more than a year after periods have apparently finished. This is a very important symptom, which should not be ignored, even if it happens only once, or if the blood looks pink rather than the usual full red.

There can easily be confusion with bleeding in urine, or from the back passage, so be prepared for your doctor to examine those regions, too.

PROBABLE
THIN VAGINAL SKIN
POLYP

POSSIBLE
CANCER OF THE WOMB
CANCER OF THE CERVIX

RARE
URETHRAL CARUNCLE

PROBABLE

■ THIN VAGINAL SKIN
An effect of low oestrogen levels.
* Vagina feels dry.
* A pink discharge is more common than outright blood.
* Skin feels sore.

Treatment is with oestrogen creams.

■ POLYP
A fleshy outgrowth from the cervix, which oozes blood.
* Intermittent, fresh blood.
* Possibly a heavy or offensive discharge.

A polyp can be seen on examination, but always needs to be biopsied to ensure that it is benign.

POSSIBLE

■ CANCER OF THE WOMB
There is no escaping the fact that this disease is a possibility. Unless the tumour is advanced, when pain arises, there will be no symptoms other than bleeding.

Diagnosis is made by scraping the lining of the womb, and treatment is hysterectomy plus radiotherapy of the pelvis. If it is caught early, the outlook is positive, but advanced cancer has a poor outlook, underlining the need to report post-menopausal bleeding as soon as possible.

■ CANCER OF THE CERVIX
* Possibly bleeding after intercourse, as well as at other times.
* Possibly an offensive discharge.

Diagnosed by examination plus cervical smear. Treatment depends on the size of the tumour, varying from a local removal, to removal of the womb and all surrounding tissues.

RARE

■ URETHRAL CARUNCLE
An oddity in which the outlet from the bladder, the urethra lying just in front of the vagina, becomes swollen and inflamed.
* Painful to touch.
* Pain on intercourse.
* Pain when passing urine.

The inflamed area is easily removed.

PRE-MENSTRUAL TENSION

Feelings of tension and stress are are just two from an array of physical and mental changes, which appear up to two weeks before menstruation and which go soon after bleeding begins. Among the many possible symptoms, the commonest are:
* Feeling bloated.
* Irritability.
* Tiredness.
* Headache.
* Tender breasts.
* Depression.

No one reason satisfactorily explains the symptoms, nor is

there any agreed treatment. However, women report benefit from many different remedies. The most promising are:

Vitamin B6: taken premenstrually, this undoubtedly helps some women.

Diuretics ('water pills'): increase the output of urine and so relieve bloating.

Evening primrose oil: taken as six capsules daily, this has been shown to benefit some women.

Herbal and alternative remedies: many different substances are for sale. Price is no indication of their likely efficacy. Doctors are sceptical of their benefits. It is usually worth trying conventional treatments first.

Hormonal preparations: doctors may advise a trial, either of progesterone (a female hormone), to be taken premenstrually, or the contraceptive pill. Both may possibly decrease premenstrual symptoms.

Beta-blockers: these drugs, originally introduced for control of blood pressure, can sometimes help to decrease physical symptoms of tension and irritability.

Some women find that simply knowing that they have a real condition, albeit one which medicine is relatively ignorant about, enables them and their families to adjust to their swings of mood.

FEMALE REPRODUCTIVE SYSTEM: THE VAGINA

BLEEDING FROM THE VAGINA

This topic refers to bleeding which is unexpected. Menstrual problems are dealt with under specific headings.

PROBABLE

MISCARRIAGE
ECTOPIC PREGNANCY

POSSIBLE

COMPLICATIONS LATE IN PREGNANCY
DISEASE OF THE CERVIX
DISEASE OF THE WOMB
ATROPHIC VAGINITIS

RARE

DISORDERS OF BLOOD CLOTTING

PROBABLE

■ MISCARRIAGE

It cannot be repeated too often that pregnancy is a possibility for any woman of childbearing years who

experiences unusual vaginal bleeding. The chances are increased in the presence of:
* A missed period.
* Tender breasts, morning sickness.
* Lower abdominal pain.

There is often great difficulty in deciding between a miscarriage and an ectopic pregnancy (*see below*). Miscarriages up to the twelfth week after conception happen in as many as one in eight pregnancies, and possibly more often. They are emotionally traumatic.

■ ECTOPIC PREGNANCY
Occurs if a fertilized egg implants not within the womb, but somewhere else, usually inside a Fallopian tube. The egg can only grow a little before its size starts to distend the tube, causing:
* Severe, one-sided lower abdominal pain.
* Bleeding.
* Faintness, if internal bleeding is severe.
* These may occur in women using a contraceptive coil.

This is a life-threatening emergency. Urgent removal of the egg and tube is needed. Later fertility can be affected.

POSSIBLE

■ COMPLICATIONS LATE IN PREGNANCY
In an established pregnancy, bleeding suggests a possible abnormality of the placenta. Painless bleeding happens if the placenta is lying too low in the womb (termed *placenta praevia*). Painful bleeding, especially after 26 weeks, may mean that part of the placenta has detached from the womb (abruption). In either case, a full and urgent obstetric assessment is essential.

■ DISEASE OF THE CERVIX
A possibility if the symptoms include any of the following, each of which is dealt with under specific headings:
* Heavy vaginal discharge.
* Irregular bleeding.
* Bleeding after intercourse.

See page 346.

■ DISEASE OF THE WOMB
This is the likeliest cause of vaginal bleeding after menopause, an extremely important symptom. *See page 353.*

■ ATROPHIC VAGINITIS
A thin, watery, bloody discharge. *See THIN VAGINAL SKIN, page 353.*

RARE

■ DISORDERS OF BLOOD CLOTTING
As well as bleeding from the vagina, there will probably be:
* Easy bruising.
* Blood from bowels, in urine.

See also pages 426-8.

DISCHARGE FROM THE VAGINA

Normal discharge from the vagina is clear, or slightly yellow. It varies in volume and consistency during the monthly cycle, reaching a peak at the time of ovulation, which is roughly mid-cycle. If you have a coil fitted, the amount of discharge may increase. Any change in the amount, consistency or smell of the discharge from what you would normally expect can be considered abnormal.

PROBABLE
THRUSH
CERVICAL EROSION

POSSIBLE
ATROPHIC VAGINITIS
CERVICAL POLYP
VAGINAL INFECTION
PELVIC INFECTION
FOREIGN BODY

RARE
GONORRHEA
TUMOUR
SEXUAL ABUSE

PROBABLE

■ THRUSH
This, the commonest cause, is a yeast infection. It is not something you 'catch' from your partner: it occurs as the normal balance of the various vaginal constituents is disturbed, allowing the yeast to grow until it gives rise to symptoms. It is possible for your partner to develop some symptoms on his penis as a result of contact with the yeast. Both partners should be treated at the same time.
* Itchy, white discharge.
* Curd-like deposits, visible on the walls of the vagina.

The risk increases after a course of antibiotics. There is a wide range of treaments, including creams, pessaries and tablets. For some women, thrush can be a recurring problem. Any woman with frequent attacks should have a urine test for diabetes.

■ CERVICAL EROSION
A cause of persistent, heavy, usually clear discharge. *See page 346.*

POSSIBLE

■ ATROPHIC VAGINITIS
Mainly a post-menopausal condition.
* Watery, possibly blood-tinged discharge.

See THIN VAGINAL SKIN, page 353.

■ CERVICAL POLYP
These fleshy outgrowths may also cause a persistent, heavy sometimes bloody discharge. *See*

POLYP, page 353.

■ VAGINAL INFECTION

Apart from thrush, three other infections are commonly caused by these organisms:

Trichomonas: a greenish, frothy discharge.

Gardenerella: a grey discharge, with a fishy smell.

Chlamydia: a recurrent discharge. Your partner may have had a penile discharge, termed non-specific urethritis.

There are specific antibiotic treatments for each of these.

Chlamydia, in particular, can lead to pelvic infection and infertility, making it especially important to diagnose. It requires special tests to make a diagnosis for chlamydia.

■ PELVIC INFECTION

See page 349.

An acute pelvic infection causes:

* Heavy, yellow or green vaginal discharge.
* Severe pelvic pain.
* Fever, malaise.

Vigorous treatment aims to reduce any internal damage which might lead to infertility.

■ FOREIGN BODY

Probably the commonest is a tampon lodged deep inside the vagina. Young children sometimes push small toys inside themselves.

* Yellow or green discharge, increasingly heavy.
* Very smelly.
* Possibly fever.

Tampons and the like are easily removed; children may need a specialist's help.

RARE

■ GONORRHEA

Unfortunately, this venereal disease causes only slight symptoms in women, so that cases are usually detected by tracing the contacts of men who have had this diagnosis confirmed.

* A slight increase in discharge.
* Possibly persistent burning on passing urine.
* Possibly a yellow discharge.

Gonorrhea can progress to pelvic infection with pain, profuse discharge and fever. It can cause infertility.

■ TUMOUR

Growths in and around the vagina may be a rare cause of a persistent discharge, but should be visible on gynaecological inspection.

■ SEXUAL ABUSE

This upsetting possibility needs to be considered for girls who have recurrent or unusual vaginal discharges. Signs of sexual interference might include:

* Tears, bruising around vagina or back passage.
* Disturbed behaviour.

This highly-charged topic needs the utmost care, both to avoid false conclusions and yet to uncover hidden misery. If suspected, the case should be placed in professional hands.

VAGINAL PROTRUSION

Nearly always a prolapse of the womb, caused by weakening of the muscles around the vagina. Part of the womb `drops' down into the vagina.

PROBABLE
PROLAPSE OF THE WOMB

POSSIBLE
PROLAPSE OF THE BLADDER OR RECTUM

RARE
TUMOUR

PROBABLE

■ PROLAPSE OF THE WOMB
* A firm lump, felt to be central in the vagina.
* Worse on coughing, straining.
* Lessens on lying flat or relaxing.
Surgical repair is possible.

POSSIBLE

■ PROLAPSE OF THE BLADDER OR RECTUM
* Bladder prolapse is felt in the front of the vagina.
* Usually causes leakage of urine on coughing, laughing.
* Rectal prolapse is felt at the back of the vagina.
Surgical repair is possible.

RARE

■ TUMOUR
The growth could arise from the womb, or the walls of the vagina; gynaecological examination will pinpoint this.

VAGINAL ODOUR

PROBABLE
NORMAL

POSSIBLE
INFECTION
RETAINED FOREIGN BODY
PSYCHOLOGICAL

RARE
CANCER

PROBABLE

■ NORMAL
* Some vaginal odour is unavoidable, and is probably a sexual cue.

POSSIBLE

■ INFECTION
See page 357. Suggested by odours

which are:
* Very smelly, or fishy.
* Accompanied by itch and discharge.

■ RETAINED FOREIGN BODY
It is not unusual for a forgotten tampon to cause a foul-smelling discharge.
* Brown discharge.
* Unpleasant odour.
* No pain or symptoms of illness.

Other possible causes are contraceptive sponges or condoms which have been left in the vagina in error. Doctors or nurses can remove these easily if you have difficulty.

■ PSYCHOLOGICAL
* An odour, but your partner or doctor smell nothing unusual.
* A worry that the odour is obvious to others.

A sympathetic ear may allow worries to be expressed, typically about cancer of the womb.

RARE

■ CANCER
Cancer of the cervix, womb, or even of the bowel, may cause:
* A persistent, foul-smelling vaginal discharge.
* Bleeding.
* Pain.

Things should not reach this stage unless warning symptoms have been neglected, such as unusual vaginal bleeding, discharges and changes of bowel habit.

VAGINAL PAIN

The causes overlap with those symptoms described under *PAINFUL SEXUAL INTERCOURSE , page 335.*

PROBABLE
INFECTIONS
ATROPHY OF VAGINAL SKIN

POSSIBLE
VAGINISMUS

RARE
CANCER

PROBABLE

■ INFECTIONS
Any vaginal infection will cause tenderness, plus:
* Itch.
* Discharge.
* Vaginal odour.

See page 357.

■ ATROPHY
In post-menopausal women, discomfort is due to thinning of the skin of the vagina, which becomes tender. This is easily remedied by oestrogen creams or hormone replacement therapy (HRT).

See THIN VAGINAL SKIN, page 353.

THE REPRODUCTIVE AND SEXUAL ORGANS

POSSIBLE

■ VAGINISMUS
Spasm of the muscles around the vagina. The effect is pain, which prevents intercourse. It has a psychological cause: *see VAGINAL SPASM, page 335.*

RARE

■ CANCER
Cancer growing within the vagina can cause pain, but it is highly unlikely to be an early or only symptom. Previously there is likely to have been:
* Bleeding after intercourse.
* Discharge.

See also pages 345 and under CANCER OF THE CERVIX, page 353.

VULVAL ITCH

PROBABLE
INFECTION

POSSIBLE
ALLERGY
THREADWORMS/CRAB LICE
ECZEMA OR PSORIASIS

RARE
LEUKOPLAKIA
CANCER
GENERAL DISEASE

PROBABLE

■ INFECTION
* Rapid onset of intense itch.
* White or coloured discharge.

The appearance of the associated discharge is usually diagnostic, for example, thrush, trichomonas (*see VAGINAL DISCHARGE, page 357*). If thrush is recurrent, diabetes may be a possibility and should be tested for..

POSSIBLE

■ ALLERGY
The sensitive skin in and around the vagina may itch because of allergy to over-vigorous washing, bubble baths, vaginal deodorants or condoms. Diagnosis is arrived at by cutting out all possible irritants, and then testing each one individually. Special low-allergy condoms are available.

■ THREADWORMS/CRAB LICE
Threadworms are extremely common, particularly in childhood.
* Intense itch.
* Especially at night.
* Itching around the back passage.

Worms or lice will be visible on careful inspection. Treatment is easy.

■ ECZEMA/PSORIASIS
Common skin disorders, causing:
* Dry flaking areas.
* Psoriasis spreads around back passage.
* Usually skin elsewhere is affected.

RARE

■ LEUKOPLAKIA
* Whitish, cracked skin.
* Spreads around back passage.
* Commonest in the elderly.

As this may progress to skin cancer, biopsy and follow-up is usual.

■ CANCER
Skin cancer may present the following symptoms:
* An itchy sore.
* Slowly grows.
* Bleeds.

Treatment is usually curative, but the earlier the diagnosis the better.

■ GENERAL DISEASE
Several disorders may cause generalized itch. Specific features might include:
* Swollen lymph nodes.
* Jaundice.
* Changes in volume of urine produced.
* Widespread skin involvement.
* Joint pains.

See also ITCHING — WITHOUT A RASH, page 259.

FEMINIZATION

Adult men who start to develop female features need a full hormonal assessment. Female features include loss of body hair, development of breasts, loss of sexual drive, and shrinking testicles.

PROBABLE
DRUG EFFECTS

POSSIBLE
GENETIC PROBLEMS
ALCOHOLISM

RARE
TUMOURS

PROBABLE

■ DRUG EFFECTS
Common culprits are cimetidine, used for treating peptic ulcers; oestrogens for treating cancer of the prostate; spironolactone and digoxin in heart disease.

POSSIBLE

■ GENETIC PROBLEMS
* Unusually tall individuals.
* Infertile.

■ ALCOHOLISM
* Impotence.
* Breast development.
* Decreased fertility due to diminished sperm count.

RARE

■ TUMOURS
If the above causes are excluded, it is essential to search for cancers in the testicles, lungs or elsewhere, which may be secreting female hormones. Possible symptoms include:
* Lump in or on a testicle.
* Coughing blood, chest pains, weight loss.

PAIN BETWEEN THE LEGS

PROBABLE
INJURY

POSSIBLE
PROSTATITIS

RARE
CANCER OF PROSTATE

PROBABLE

■ INJURY
Injury between the legs may irritate the prostate gland, giving rise to:
* A dull ache between the legs.
* Slight discomfort on passing urine.
* Blood in urine, if there has been a severe injury, such as falling astride something.

POSSIBLE

■ PROSTATITIS
Infection of the prostate gland causes:
* Pain.
* Fever, even rigors.
* Burning sensation when passing urine.
* Urine may appear cloudy.

This can be an awkward problem to eradicate, often needing extended courses of antibiotics.

RARE

■ CANCER OF PROSTATE
An advanced cancer may produce the following:
* Ache or pain between legs.
* Pain in back or pelvis because of spread to bones..

More usually, cancer of the prostate is painless, and is found on investigation after:
* Difficulty passing urine, caused by enlargement of the prostate, which obstructs the passage of urine.

Other symptoms of an enlarging prostate, not normally cancerous, include:
* Difficulty in starting to pass urine.
* Dribbling at the end of passing urine.
* Frequency of passing urine inceases: typically, you start having to get up in the night.

BLOOD IN SEMEN

A fairly common symptom, which looks alarming but one which hardly ever has an underlying cause. In fact, the reason remains unknown for the vast majority of cases.
* Commonest in elderly men.
* Blood may obviously be in the semen.
* May be mistaken for bleeding from the vagina after intercourse.

It is sensible to have your genitalia examined, plus a urine check, to ensure that the blood does come from the bladder. Otherwise, nothing else needs to be done unless the symptom recurs, when an internal check of the bladder and prostate gland may be advisable.

IMPOTENCE

Impotence means difficulty in achieving, or maintaining, a firm erection. It is a common disorder, admitted to far less often than it is experienced. Brief episodes of impotence accompany tiredness, and any serious, general ill-health. After ejaculation, there is loss of erection which takes longer and longer to recover with age, perhaps several hours by old age. This may cause confusion if the true disorder is premature ejaculation. Psychological factors are still the most likely reasons for impotence, but it is increasingly clear that physical disorders are more common than once thought, especially problems with blood flow to the penis. This probably reflects an openness to discuss and investigate sexual activity in the elderly. There is, accordingly, a great range of physical treatments now available at specialized centres, such as drugs injected into the penis, and pump devices.

See also PREMATURE EJACULATION, page 366.

PROBABLE
PSYCHOLOGICAL

POSSIBLE
DIABETES MELLITUS
BLOOD FLOW PROBLEMS
DRUGS
ALCOHOL
POST-OPERATIVE

RARE
NEUROLOGICAL DISEASE
HORMONE DISORDERS

The Reproductive and Sexual Organs

PROBABLE

■ PSYCHOLOGICAL
Factors here include depression, problems between partners and, most especially, the vicious circle of past impotence causing impotence again. Symptoms strongly suggestive of a psychological cause are:
* Normal erections during sleep or on awakening.
* Ejaculation during sleep.
* Impotence with one particular partner.
* Sudden onset of impotence.

Therapy will include explanation, exploration of psychological problems, and gradual return to sexual intercourse.

POSSIBLE

■ DIABETES MELLITUS
Diabetes affects the nerves and blood supply involved in erection. Undiagnosed diabetes may cause:
* Excessive passage of urine at night and during the day.
* Thirst.

■ BLOOD FLOW PROBLEMS
An erection is caused by engorgement of the penis's spongy tissues with blood. If the veins carrying this blood supply are leaking, inadequate erection may follow. Arterial disease can also affect the blood supply, both to the penis and to the nerves controlling erection.

Sophisticated tests of blood flow are available.

■ DRUGS
Many drugs used to treat high blood pressure may cause impotence, as do tranquillizers and heroin. Numerous other drugs may be implicated and are always worth checking for.

■ ALCOHOL
Shakespeare sums it up in *Macbeth:*
* 'It provokes the desire, but it takes away the performance'.

Chronic alcoholism actually leads to hormonal and neurological changes that make permanent impotence a risk.

■ POST-OPERATIVE
Surgery to the bowel, and to the prostate gland, runs the risk of damaging the nerves involved in an erection.

RARE

■ NEUROLOGICAL DISEASE
Of these, the commonest is multiple sclerosis, giving rise to:
* Numbness in various parts of the body.
* Unsteady gait.
* Visual disturbances, transient blindness in one eye.
* Difficulty in controlling passage of urine.

Anything else damaging the lower spine may cause impotence.

■ HORMONE DISORDERS
A wide range of possibilities. A possible cause if the individual has:
* Absent or small testicles.
* Lack of body hair.

* Breasts.
* Unusually short or tall stature.
* Extreme obesity.

Hormone treatment may help such cases.

See also HORMONAL, page 480.

MALE INFERTILITY

Male disorders account for about 30 per cent of infertility cases where couples have been trying to conceive for a year or more without success (the conventional definition of infertility). An early sperm count is always advisable, looking for low numbers of sperm, or increased numbers of abnormal sperm. Obviously, normal sexual intercourse should be taking place at regular intervals. Temporary infertility can follow a severe illness, after which it takes a few months for sperm production to recover. Research is showing that there are subtle disorders of sperm, accounting for hitherto unexplained cases of infertility.

See also INFERTILITY (female), page 332.

PROBABLE
DAMAGE TO TESTICLES

POSSIBLE
DRUGS
VARICOCELE
ALCOHOLISM
HORMONE DISORDERS

RARE
CHROMOSOME DISORDERS

PROBABLE

■ DAMAGE TO TESTICLES

The testicles may:
* Feel small.
* Be soft.

A number of different testicular problems may account for damage or impaired function. One example is undescended testicles, when the testicles may not be in the scrotum at birth and surgery is required to draw them down from the groin into the scrotal sac. Failure to do this at an early age, ideally before three years of age, can lead to impaired fertility later in life.

Torsion of the testicles, mumps, radiation and chemotherapy for cancer may all lead to a diminished sperm count.

Cigarette smoking, drinking, and high temperatures in the area of the scrotum can also decrease sperm production.

See also PAIN IN TESTICLES, page 372.

POSSIBLE

■ DRUGS

Several drugs reduce sperm production. The drugs used to treat cancer in children may damage the testicles.

■ VARICOCELE

See page 373.

These soft masses in the scrotum, which are enlarged veins, may cause reduced sperm production.

■ ALCOHOLISM
See also IMPOTENCE, page 363.
Chronic drinking reduces sperm production.

■ HORMONE DISORDERS
See page 364.
A possibility if there is:
* Absent body hair.
* Development of breasts.

RARE

■ CHROMOSOME DISORDERS
* Unusual height.
* Enlarged breasts.
* Small or absent testicles.
* Absent body hair.
* Abnormally-formed penis.

PRECOCIOUS PUBERTY

Sexual development before the age of nine years is abnormal; that includes the appearance of body hair, enlarged penis, deepening voice. All cases are rare; all require urgent investigation.

POSSIBLE
HYPOTHALAMIC DISEASE

RARE
TESTICULAR TUMOURS
ADRENAL DISEASE

POSSIBLE

■ HYPOTHALAMIC DISEASE
This gland in the brain controls many hormones. A disorder is likeliest if:
* The boy was normal at birth, and during early childhood.
* Later, shows abnormal growth, either too short or too tall.

RARE

■ TESTICULAR TUMOURS
* A lump may be felt.
* There may be a change or swelling in one testicle.

Blood tests may detect abnormally high levels of hormones in the blood.

■ ADRENAL DISEASE
Disease of the adrenal glands, which lie over the kidneys, usually makes a baby very ill within days of birth. Hormone treatment prevents masculine changes appearing during very early childhood.

PREMATURE EJACULATION

This means ejaculation before the penis enters the vagina, or very soon after entry. While this is not a disease, it can be very troublesome for many men. Considerable time and patience, as well as courage to explore the problem, will be required.

PROBABLE

■ PSYCHOLOGICAL FACTORS
With experience, sexual relationships expand to include more than intercourse alone, perhaps explaining why premature ejaculation is commonest in young men. Psychological approaches encourage concentration on aspects of sexual behaviour other than intercourse, for example stroking and massaging.

An aid to this is the 'squeeze technique', when the partner, told that ejaculation is near, squeezes around the base of the penis for some seconds. This usually delays progress to orgasm without destroying the erection. Further information should be sought from psychosexual therapists.

CURVED PENIS

Known medically as chordee. Extreme curvature may prevent sexual intercourse.

PROBABLE
CONGENITAL

POSSIBLE
PEYRONIE'S DISEASE

RARE
INJURY

PROBABLE

■ CONGENITAL
* Noticed at birth.
* The opening for urine (external meatus) is underneath the penis, not at the end — medical term, hypospadias.

Delicate surgery to correct these abnormalities makes use of the foreskin, which should therefore not be circumcised.

POSSIBLE

■ PEYRONIE'S DISEASE
A band of firm tissue forms on part of the shaft of the penis. In the middle-aged, or older.
* Pain and curvature on erection.
* A firm area felt on the shaft.

Treatment is difficult. Sometimes disappears spontaneously.

RARE

■ INJURY
Vigorous sexual intercourse or other injury may fracture the erect penis. Needs early treatment.
* Sudden pain; bruising.

DISCHARGE FROM PENIS

Whether clear or coloured, is highly suggestive of venereal disease, with non-specific urethritis and GONORRHEA, *both page 357*, the likeliest. *Must* be seen at a specialist clinic; partner also likely to be infected.

DISEASED FORESKIN

The foreskin is subject to infection, resulting in cracking and scar tissue formation. It may cause pain, interfere with passing urine and make sexual intercourse difficult.

PROBABLE
BALANITIS
PHIMOSIS

POSSIBLE
PARAPHIMOSIS

RARE
CANCER OF THE PENIS

PROBABLE

■ BALANITIS
An infection of the foreskin and adjacent penis.
* Mild pain.
* Discharge around the foreskin, not from the opening of the penis itself.
* Itch.

Antibiotics, plus salt baths, are the treatment. Diabetes may underlie recurrent balanitis.

■ PHIMOSIS
Inability to retract the foreskin over the tip of the penis. In boys it is normal to be unable to retract the foreskin until the child is five years old and it is wrong to attempt to do so. It may be abnormal if there is:
* Recurrent balanitis.
* Ballooning of the foreskin on passing urine.

Circumcision or stretching of the foreskin is then advisable.

POSSIBLE

■ PARAPHIMOSIS
* The foreskin becomes stuck, rolled behind the tip of the penis.
* Pain.
* Swelling of tip of penis prevents unrolling of foreskin back over the tip of the penis.

This calls for rapid treatment to reduce swelling; sometimes the only remedy is surgical, by making an incision or performing surgery.

RARE

■ CANCER OF THE PENIS
A rarity in the West, but common in some Far Eastern countries. It is unusual among circumcised men, the exact reason being unclear.
* Begins as a red area on tip of penis, or hidden within the foreskin.
* Grows, ulcerates.
* Discharge, pain, bleeding.

Treatment is radiotherapy and surgery.

PAINFUL PENIS

PROBABLE
INFECTION
DISEASE OF FORESKIN

POSSIBLE
STONE

RARE
PEYRONIE'S DISEASE

PROBABLE

■ <u>INFECTION</u>
* Pain, burning on passing urine.
* Need to urinate frequently.
* Possibly blood in urine.
* Urine cloudy.
* A discharge suggests venereal disease.

Infection, whether in a boy or adult, should always be investigated, since underlying causes are common.

■ <u>DISEASE OF FORESKIN</u>
* Tender, swollen foreskin.

See page 368.

POSSIBLE

■ <u>STONE</u>
See KIDNEY STONES, page 184.
* Pain radiating to tip of penis from groin, or from kidney region.
* Blood in urine.
* Nausea, sweating.

Stones can lodge anywhere in the urinary tract, from the kidney to the tip of the penis. Strong painkillers make it possible to tolerate the severe pain, and some may even aid the passage of the stone.

RARE

■ <u>PEYRONIE'S DISEASE</u>
See page 367.
* Pain and curvature of penis when erect.

PROLONGED ERECTION

Also known as priapism.
A very painful, prolonged erection in the absence of sexual desire. The tip of the penis remains soft. Whatever the cause, it needs urgent treatment to avoid long-term damage to the penis.

PROBABLE
UNKNOWN CAUSE

POSSIBLE
BLOOD DISORDERS

RARE
ALL OTHER CAUSES

PROBABLE

■ CAUSE UNKNOWN
Accounting for about three out of five cases: it may follow prolonged sexual activity.
* Otherwise sound health.

POSSIBLE

■ BLOOD DISORDERS
Blood tests will seek leukaemia or sickle cell disease.
* Easy bruising, malaise, enlarged glands suggest leukaemia.
* Recurrent joint or abdominal pains suggest sickle cell disease.
See pages 419 and 487.

RARE

■ ALL OTHER CAUSES
A routine search is always made for growths in the pelvis, drugs affecting erection, or damage to the spinal cord.

SMALL PENIS

An objective assessment of size is difficult because of variations at different temperatures, and degrees of erection. Worry about a small penis may be justified in the presence of some of the following features:
* Absent or small testicles.
* Absence of body hair.
* Excessive height.
* Breast development.
* Obesity.
* Previous injury, torsion of testicles.

In boys, a normal penis may appear very small if it is sunk in fat in the groin.

Investigations such as chromosome analysis, hormone profiles and brain scans may be needed. As treatment is possible for boys, cases of true micro-penis are worth reporting to a doctor, sooner rather than later.

ABSENT TESTICLE

Absence should be discovered at routine child health checks.
* A testicle which is not brought down into the scrotum is at risk of decreased fertility and also at greater risk of a malignant change in later life.

PROBABLE
UNDESCENDED TESTICLE

POSSIBLE
RETRACTILE TESTICLE

RARE
ECTOPIC

PROBABLE

■ UNDESCENDED TESTICLE
* Normal general development.
* Testicle often felt as a lump in the groin.

Three to four per cent of male babies have undescended testicles at birth. By the age of one, only 0.8 per cent will still have the condition: the testicles tend to descend into the scrotum of their own accord.

Undescended testicles should be surgically brought down into the scrotum, ideally around the age of two and, if possible, before three years old. This helps to reduce the risk of future subfertility.

POSSIBLE

■ RETRACTILE TESTICLE
An exaggeration of a normal reflex, which pulls the testicles up into the groin.
* Testicle is present at certain times.
* Cold, and emotion, can cause retraction.

Usually no treatment is needed for this condition.

RARE

■ ECTOPIC TESTICLE
The testicle may lodge itself somewhere in the lower abdomen. It may be felt in the groin, at the base of the penis, or even the upper thigh. Surgical correction is recommended to preserve fertility.

LUMPS IN THE TESTICLE OR SCROTUM

A firm structure felt at the back of the testicles is the epididymis. Small lumps within the skin of the scrotum are common, being minor infections or yellow fat-filled cysts.

See also PAIN IN TESTICLES, page 372.

PROBABLE
VARICOCELE
EPIDIDYMAL CYST

POSSIBLE
CANCER OF TESTICLE

RARE
SYPHILIS
TUBERCULOSIS

PROBABLE

■ VARICOCELE
A harmless swelling caused by enlarged veins, 'like a bag of worms', felt behind the testicle. *See also page 373.*

■ EPIDIDYMAL CYST
Another harmless swelling, arising from the epididymis.
* Commonest in elderly men.
* Often, cysts on both sides of the scrotum.
* The swelling feels separate from the testicle.

Once confirmed, nothing need be done about a cyst unless it is causing discomfort.

POSSIBLE

■ CANCER OF THE TESTICLE
This is a rare cancer, but is the most common one to affect men between 15 and 40 years of age. Twice as many now develop it each year, compared with 25 years ago.

Just as women examine their breasts for lumps, men should check their testicles every month for any signs of changes.
* A lump in a testicle is cancer until proven otherwise.
* Feels hard.
* A feeling of heaviness.
* Often also a swollen scrotum.
* Pain is unusual.

The treatment depends on the precise kind of tumour, but carries a very positive outlook, particularly if any changes are spotted early.

Don't delay — report any changes in your testicles to your doctor immediately.

RARE

■ SYPHILIS
May still arise in Third World countries.
* A slowly growing lump.
* Previous features of syphilis; *see page 324.*

■ TUBERCULOSIS
Also uncommon, though increasing among the poor and homeless.
* A painless lump.
* May discharge like an abscess, but without throbbing.
* Other features of tuberculosis, such as cough, malaise, sweats, weight loss.

PAIN IN TESTICLES

In boys and young men, pain equals torsion (*see below*) until proven otherwise. In adults there is a wider range of possible diagnoses.

PROBABLE
EPIDIDYMITIS
TORSION

POSSIBLE
INJURY
VARICOCELE
STONE
HERNIA

RARE
MUMPS ORCHITIS
PANCREATITIS

PROBABLE

■ EPIDIDYMITIS
The epididymis is a structure involved in the transport of sperm from the testicles, and can normally be felt at the back of the testicle. Inflammation usually occurs for no obvious reason, but

if there is also a discharge from the penis, a doctor must test for venereal disease and non-specific urethritis (NSU).

Epididymitis is an unsafe diagnosis to make for a boy before puberty, in whom torsion is far more likely.

* Pain, initially behind testicle, builds up over a few hours.
* Swelling of testicle and scrotum which are exquisitely tender.
* Fever, nausea.

Antibiotic treatment is needed, plus rest, for a couple of weeks.

■ TORSION

The testicles hang on a cord which can twist. Other structures near the testicles can also twist, giving a similar condition. Deciding which has happened con only be done during an operation.

* Sudden, severe pain in one testicle.
* Nausea, vomiting.
* Affected testicle swells and is tender.

An urgent operation is nearly always needed to untwist the testicle, and to anchor it into place to prevent recurrence. It is usual to operate on the other testicle also: if one has twisted, the other is likely to do so in the future. Neglected torsion will inevitably lead to death of the affected testicle, with future effects on fertility.

POSSIBLE

■ INJURY

* A definite history of injury to the scrotum, such as a kick in the crutch.
* Modest pain and tenderness.
* Normal urinary stream and no blood.

Support and time to heal are the only remedies.

■ VARICOCELE

Rather like a varicose vein, this is a sheath of enlarged veins, felt at the back of the testicle.

* Increasingly common with age.
* You notice an ache, not pain.
* Aching slowly increases over months.

No treatment is needed unless the varicocele is affecting fertility.

■ STONE

A stone in the urinary system gives rise to:

* Pain of rapid onset, lasting an hour or so.
* Pains recur over days and weeks.
* Appears to radiate from the low back (kidney region) to the testicles, or to the tip of the penis.
* Nausea, vomiting.
* Blood in urine.

Often a stone will pass; if it sticks, surgical removal is needed.

■ HERNIA

See INGUINAL HERNIA, page 325.
This frequently gives an ache, felt generally around the scrotum or testicles.

RARE

■ MUMPS ORCHITIS

Mumps is an increasingly rare disease which in a very few cases gives rise to inflammation of the testicles, called orchitis.

* Mumps causes swellings, like

hamster cheeks, just in front of the jaw joint.
* After three to four days, one or both testicles may swell.
* Fever, pain.

The risk of orchitis is much less than once thought. Although sterility may follow, it appears that this, too, is much less of a risk than was once feared.

■ PANCREATITIS
See page 150.

SMALL TESTICLE

Testicles vary slightly in size and the left testicle usually hangs lower than the right one. Alcoholism, and drugs used in treating cancer of the prostate, may cause previously normal testicles to decrease in size.

PROBABLE
PREVIOUS INJURY OR INFECTION

POSSIBLE
HORMONE DISORDERS

RARE
GENETIC DISORDERS

PROBABLE

■ PREVIOUS INJURY OR INFECTION
Likely if:
* Only one testicle is small.
* Previous pain.
* Previous swelling.

Possible causes include twisted testicle and orchitis. *See PAIN IN TESTICLES, pages 372-4.*

POSSIBLE

■ HORMONE DISORDERS
* Both testicles are small.
* Individual is often very tall.
* Absent or decreased body hair.
* Breast development.
* Infertility.

Hormone testing is needed to pinpoint the root cause.

RARE

■ GENETIC DISORDERS
A fascinating, highly complex area, touching on 'intersex' and ambiguous sexual development.
* Testicles and penis may be abnormally formed.
* Man is likely to be abnormally tall or short.
* Infertility.

SWOLLEN TESTICLE OR SCROTUM

This means swelling without any obvious lump. For lumps in the testicle or scrotum, see the appropriate section. Swellings may be due to an underlying cancer, and should always be medically examined.

Don't delay in reporting to your doctor any changes you notice in your testicles — early treatment has a very significant effect on the likelihood of affecting a complete cure.

PROBABLE
HYDROCELE
ORCHITIS

POSSIBLE
HERNIA

RARE
FILARIASIS

PROBABLE

■ HYDROCELE
An accumulation of fluid around the testicle.
* Tense, swollen testicle.
* Pain may or may not be present.
* If chronic, can be very large.
* In children, often accompanies a hernia.
* Not uncommon at or soon after birth.

Specialist opinion should be sought, since there may be an underlying cause such as infection or cancer of the testicle.

■ ORCHITIS
A general term for a swollen, inflamed testicle.
* Pain builds up over a few hours.
* Scrotum usually also swells with fluid.

Underlying causes include injury, infection and mumps. *See MUMPS ORCHITIS, page 373.*

An acutely painful testicle may be twisted, with a risk of future sterility. Medical attention is essential, especially for children.

POSSIBLE

■ HERNIA
When the bowel bulges through a weakness in the wall of the abdomen.
* Usually just a lump in the groin.
* In children, commonly extends into the scrotum, which appears to be swollen.
* Less common in adults.
* Swelling may disappear after lying flat.

See page 325.

RARE

■ FILARIASIS
A parasite which blocks the drainage of tissue fluids, leading to swelling of the affected region.
* A disease of the Far East.
* Repeated inflammation of the testicles, epididymis.
* After several infections, the scrotum remains permanently swollen.

Advanced disease needs surgical treatment.

The Brain and Nervous System

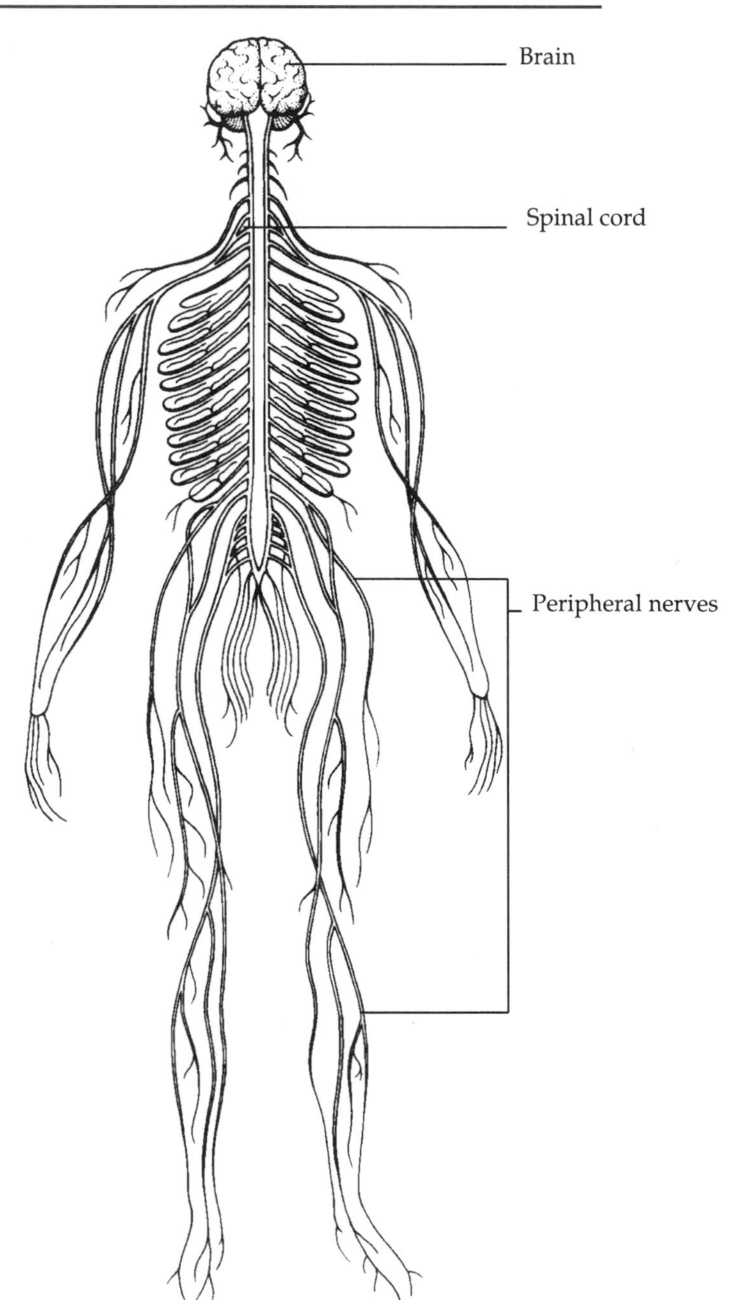

Symptoms in this section do not follow the order adopted elsewhere: they are arranged alphabetically.

ANXIETY

Anxiety can be quite well defined as a state of worry and fear. Mild degrees of anxiety are normal and increase the individual's readiness to deal with problems of life.

Anxiety becomes abnormal when it is out of proportion to the situation or when one problem or event becomes the focus of severe worry and starts to interfere with daily life *(see OBSESSIONS AND PHOBIAS)*. The symptoms are multiple and include:

* A feeling of tension mingled with apprehension.
* Headache.
* Sweating: hands, armpits and forehead are particularly affected.
* Palpitations.
* Dry mouth.
* Tremor.

But many other symptoms occur, too, such as overbreathing, impotence, diarrhoea, dizzy turns, restlessness.

PROBABLE

ANXIETY STATE

POSSIBLE

OTHER PSYCHOLOGICAL DISEASE
OVERACTIVE THYROID GLAND
DRUG AND ALCOHOL EFFECTS

RARE

LOW BLOOD SUGAR
PHAEOCHROMOCYTOMA

PROBABLE

■ ANXIETY STATE

Worry comes naturally to human beings, to some more naturally than to others; heredity plays a part. Every society has its own anxieties: the worry of choosing perfectly matched table decorations does not, on the face of it, compare with the worry of a sabre-toothed tiger intent on repossessing your cave. But who are we to judge? Childhood experiences, repressed sexual urges, the depersonalization of modern society: all are theoretically reasonable explanations of anxiety, suggested by some of the wisest minds. One thing is certain: there is more and more of it about.

Diagnosing anxiety is usually straightforward, based on the symptoms given above; sympathetic discussion will usually reveal an underlying cause of stress. Physical symptoms as alarming as breathlessness may need investigating before the individual can accept that the symptom is psychological in origin. Treatment ranges from drugs for acute, disabling anxiety to explanation via counselling or psychotherapy.

THE BRAIN AND NERVOUS SYSTEM

POSSIBLE

■ OTHER PSYCHOLOGICAL DISEASE
Possible when anxiety:
* Appears in a previously stable personality.
* No obvious source of stress.
* Other disturbance of mood, thought, or concentration.

Possibilities which are dealt with separately, and should be followed up, include *DEPRESSION, DEMENTIA* and *SCHIZOPHRENIA* *(the latter on page 386)*.

■ OVER-ACTIVE THYROID GLAND
Gives all the symptoms of anxiety, but there are suggestive additional features:
* Fine tremor.
* Weight loss.
* Increased appetite.
* Intolerance of heat.
* Rapid pulse.
* Bulging eyes.
* Swelling in neck.

Where there is doubt, a blood test will help to confirm diagnosis.

■ DRUG AND ALCOHOL EFFECTS
Withdrawal of many abused drugs and of alcohol may cause:
* A coarse tremor.
* Anxiety.
* Sweating.

There may be other features of drug abuse such as:
* Neglected appearance.
* Hallucinations.
* Needle marks on limbs.

Specialized clinics are available to help with these problems.

RARE

■ LOW BLOOD SUGAR
Commonest in diabetics on treatment with pills or insulin.
* The symptoms appear rapidly.
* Light-headedness.
* Sweating.
* Hunger.
* Drowsiness.

All diabetics should recognize the warning symptoms, keeping some glucose at hand in an easily absorbed form (for example, boiledsweets or sugar tablets).

■ PHAEOCHROMOCYTOMA
A tumour which produces a hormone that causes high blood pressure. The level of hormone can rapidly increase, causing:
* Sudden anxiety, sweating, palpitations.
* Pallor.

When an attack is in progress, blood pressure will be very high.

COMA

A precise medical term meaning a state of unrousability and unresponsiveness to stimuli. At its most severe there is :
* No response to pain.
* No movement.
* No speech.

Stupor is less severe: the individual can be roused by painful stimuli. The causes are the same. There are many stages in between the two, such as sleepiness and confusion and there may be some delirium, too.

Cases of coma require urgent hospital admission in order to search for the many possible causes. You will be providing extremely useful information to the hospital if you can report on:
* A history of diabetes; any drowsiness and confusion in the preceeding hours.
* Drug or alcohol abuse; evidence such as bottles, syringes.
* Epilepsy, with details of previous fits and of medication.
* A head injury in the previous few weeks.
* Previous strokes; treatment for high blood pressure.
* Depression and suicidal intent: empty pill containers.

PROBABLE
STROKE
HEART ATTACK
DRUGS OR ALCOHOL

POSSIBLE
EPILEPSY
INFECTION
METABOLIC DISEASE
INJURY

RARE
HYPOTHERMIA
OTHER CAUSES

PROBABLE

■ STROKE
Usually in the elderly.
* Sudden collapse.
* One-sided paralysis *(see PARALYSIS, RAPID ONSET).*

■ HEART ATTACK
See page 229.
Coma following:
* Chest pain.
* Breathlessness.
* Sweating and blue lips.

■ DRUGS OR ALCOHOL
Diagnosis tends to depend on a knowledge of the person's habits and other pointers, such as the smell of alcohol. Drug abuse is a strong possibility if there are:
* Deep, shallow breathing.
* Pinpoint-sized pupils.
* Signs of intravenous injections (red marks on the arms or thickened hard veins).

POSSIBLE

■ EPILEPSY
After a severe convulsion someone suffering from epilepsy may be comatose for a few minutes. *See page 384.*

■ INFECTION
Although any severe infection may cause coma through shock *(see page 472)*, meningitis is the most likely, especially in babies. It should be suspected in any infant showing otherwise unexplained:
* Irritability, drowsiness.
* Increasing drowsiness.

* Purple rash on body.
* In a baby, a bulging soft spot on the skull.

In adults there may also be:
* Neck stiffness.
* Aversion to bright lights.

An emergency. Take the individual to hospital without delay.

■ METABOLIC DISEASE
Most probably kidney or liver disease or diabetes, usually already known.
* Diabetics may have developed another illness or missed injections.
* Urine output either greater or much less than usual.
* Deep, heavy breathing.
* Possibly jaundice.

The coma can often be reversed, especially with diabetics.

■ INJURY
A head injury is the commonest injury causing coma, usually following an accident. The diagnosis will be obvious. Stupor or coma occuring a few weeks after a serious head injury may be due to a blood clot on the brain resulting from that injury. Surgical removal of this blood clot usually allows full recovery.

RARE

■ HYPOTHERMIA
A profound drop in body temperature, most common in the elderly, in winter, following a fall or a stroke. *See page 451.*

■ OTHER CAUSES
A book could be written about the other causes of coma, since it can be the final scenario of any serious upset to the body's working. Rare causes can only be diagnosed after investigations, blood tests and medical examination.

LACK OF CONCENTRATION

Peoples' attention span is very variable and depends on factors such as mood, conditions of work and stress. There is rarely any serious reason for this symptom. Children have a much shorter attention span than adults, as measured scientifically by the "but you've only just had an ice cream" test.

PROBABLE
TIREDNESS
HYPERACTIVITY

POSSIBLE
ANXIETY

RARE
MINIMAL BRAIN DISORDER

PROBABLE

■ TIREDNESS
May affect adults and children.
* Normally sound health and adequate concentration.

* Obvious lack of rest or overwork.
* Concentration returns after rest.

■ HYPERACTIVITY
Doctors disagree as to whether such a specific condition exists in children and, less commonly, in adults. It is true, however, that some children exhibit:
* Inability to settle down to a task.
* Rapid loss of interest in one activity.
* Frequent movement and restlessness.

Social circumstances and food ingredients such as colourants have both been blamed for this condition. It is likely that a number of factors is responsible. There may be an overlap with minimal brain disorder *(see below)*.

POSSIBLE

■ ANXIETY
See page 377.
* Tension.
* Sweating.
* Palpitations.

RARE

■ MINIMAL BRAIN DISORDER
A somewhat controversial childhood diagnosis.
* Child shows abrupt changes in behaviour.
* Poor learning ability.
* Disruptive behaviour.

Treatment is very difficult, and such children often need special schooling.

THE BRAIN AND NERVOUS SYSTEM

CONFUSION

A combination of disorientation and emotional upset. Gradual confusion is most likely to occur in the elderly *(see also DEMENTIA)*. Sudden confusion at any age may have an acute underlying cause and will probably need investigation.

PROBABLE
SENILE CONFUSION

POSSIBLE
DIABETIC COMPLICATIONS
DRUGS OR ALCOHOL
HEART FAILURE
INFECTIONS
MINOR STROKE
RESPIRATORY FAILURE
HYPOTHERMIA

RARE
UNDER-ACTIVE THYROID GLAND
METABOLIC FAILURE
SUBDURAL HAEMATOMA

PROBABLE

■ SENILE CONFUSION
There is a breakdown of memory for recent events. Confusion follows as the individual forgets why they are where they are and what

for. At its worst, it develops into *DEMENTIA*, But for many elderly people confusion is just a nuisance.
* General health normal for age.
* No confusion or problem with familiar tasks and journeys.
* Can cope by using notes, lists.
* Deterioration occurs only gradually, but major changes in lifestyle, for example, a holiday, may bring it on.

POSSIBLE

■ DIABETIC COMPLICATIONS
Confusion can be caused by either too little or too much sugar.
* Onset over hours or minutes and may progress to *COMA* *(see page 472).*
* Irritability, drowsiness.
* Deep, sighing breathing, thirst.
* Hunger, light-headedness.

Diabetics should be aware of the early signs and take appropriate action — increasing their dose of insulin, or taking glucose.

■ DRUGS OR ALCOHOL
This diagnosis tends to rely on knowledge of a previous history of drug abuse or alcoholism. In alcoholics, an acute state of confusion needs urgent medical attention.

■ HEART FAILURE
Confusion as a symptom of heart failure is most likely to affect the elderly.
* Breathlessness, swollen ankles.
* Inability to lie flat.
* Recent chest pain or tiredness could signal a heart attack.

■ INFECTIONS
In the elderly, any acute infection may worsen a tendency to confusion. There may or may not be a fever.
* Cough.
* Need to pass urine frequently suggests a bladder infection

In a younger person, the combination of:
* Confusion,
* Headache,
* Aversion to light,

suggests meningitis, needing emergency hospital care.

■ MINOR STROKE
* Sudden confusion.
* Sudden slurring of speech or difficulty finding words.
* Face may droop on one side.
* Possibly loss of function of an arm or leg.

Recovery from such minor strokes is often rapid. It is advisable to have them followed up by a doctor.

■ RESPIRATORY FAILURE
Most likely in someone with chronic bronchitis or emphysema *(see page 222).*
* A chest infection may be the trigger.
* Blue lips and tongue.
* Warm hands.
* Breathlessness.

Needs hospital treatment.

■ HYPOTHERMIA
Confusion is a common early symptom of low body temperature. Usually affects the elderly.

RARE

■ UNDERACTIVE THYROID GLAND
* Weight gain; sluggishness; intolerance of cold; yellowish, puffy appearance.
* Slow pulse.

■ METABOLIC FAILURE
This includes liver and kidney disease.
* Liver disease suggested by previous history of alcoholism; jaundice; easy bruising; red palms; swollen ankles.
* Kidney disease suggested by either very high or very low urine output; anaemia; malaise; yellow tinge to skin.

■ SUBDURAL HAEMATOMA
A collection of blood, which has built up following an injury to the skull and which puts pressure on the brain.
* Symptoms emerge over several weeks.
* History of head injury.
* A fluctuating degree of confusion and abnormality of behaviour.
* One-sided weakness of arm and leg may develop.

Though uncommon, a subdural haematoma is a treatable form of confusion, now relatively easy to diagnose, thanks to brain scans.

CONVULSIONS

The features of a convulsion, also known as a fit or epileptic attack, are:
* Possibly a warning of an impending attack, called an aura; it may be a feeling, a visual disturbance, a smell, a headache.
* The individual may cry out, then collapse unconscious.
* Remains stiff; may turn blue around the lips for about 30 seconds.
* Arms and legs then begin to jerk in a coordinated manner.
* Possibly incontinence of urine, frothing at mouth.
* Afterwards, drowsiness, confusion, before return to normal.

Not all convulsions are as dramatic. One form of convulsion is no more than a brief absence of consciousness, which may be misinterpreted as a blank look.

A convulsion is different from a simple faint, where there is no aura, no incontinence, no shaking of limbs. Investigations are needed if there is any doubt.

PROBABLE

EPILEPSY
FEBRILE FIT

POSSIBLE

ECLAMPSIA OF PREGNANCY
ALCOHOL RELATED
MENINGITIS

THE BRAIN AND NERVOUS SYSTEM

RARE
METABOLIC DISORDER

PROBABLE

■ EPILEPSY
Epilepsy is caused by abnormal electrical discharges in the brain. Most cases are of unknown origin, but it can result from previous brain injury, for instance a stroke, a head injury or cerebral palsy. Anyone having a fit for the first time needs careful assessment since occasionally it may be a symptom of brain disease, such as a tumour or abnormal blood vessels.

Most epileptics can lead a full life, taking care to avoid situations which would be dangerous if they had a fit, such as climbing ladders, driving or using hazardous machinery.

■ FEBRILE FIT
A convulsion in a child who is feverish. Anyone with a high enough temperature may go into convulsions: but children's brains are more sensitive to relatively minor fevers. It is to reduce the chances of a fit that children with fevers should be given para–cetamol and kept cool.

Febrile fits are common, occuring in some 10 per cent of all children, and do not mean that the child will grow up epileptic. A child having a febrile fit for the first time needs immediate medical attention: often admission to hospital will be advised to test for meningitis. Children who have recurrent febrile fits can be managed at home, as long as the parents know how to give an anti-convulsant if the fit becomes prolonged. They are uncommon after the age of five.

* Child is feverish, typically with a cold or ear infection
* Sudden stiffness, rolling of eyes, breathing stops.
* Then, coordinated jerking, of limbs and possibly incontinence.
* May last five to ten minutes.
* Child becomes responsive, but remains drowsy for a few hours.
* The fit usually occurs early on in the fever, as the temperature rises.

In children below six months or older than five years, it is not safe to make a diagnosis of febrile fits and other causes must be considered by a professional.

POSSIBLE

■ ECLAMPSIA OF PREGNANCY
A risk of later pregnancy: the blood pressure suddenly rises too high and the mother starts to have a convulsion. The situation should be avoided by routine antenatal checks. Warning symptoms are:

* Fingers and feet swell rapidly.
* Headache, flashing lights.

Tests will also detect protein in the urine (besides the high blood pressure). This is an emergency, calling for urgent reduction in blood pressure to reduce risks to mother and baby.

■ ALCOHOL-RELATED
Both excess alcohol and sudden

abstention from it can bring on fits, the diagnosis usually being obvious from previous knowledge of the individual. Alcoholics are as likely as anyone else to develop true epilepsy, so the usual full assessment should be made.

■ MENINGITIS
An infection around the brain possible at all ages but an especial worry in childhood. *See also DROWSINESS.*

RARE

■ METABOLIC DISORDER
This usually means breakdown in the function of the kidneys or liver and should be detected on routine investigation of epilepsy.

DELIRIUM

Meaning the rapid appearance of:
* Confusion.
* Restlessness.
* Hallucinations.
* Incoherent speech and thought.
* Often worst at night.

Often, the confusion fluctuates, with severe symptoms interspersed with relatively normal phases.

The causes are those given under *CONFUSION,* but with an added urgency because of the greater risk of serious underlying illness, and with a higher chance of an infection being the cause.

The elderly are more likely to become delirious during an otherwise moderately serious illness. In children, delirium frequently accompanies a harmless feverish illness and should be treated by bringing the temperature down. If there is any suspicion of:
* Headache,
* Aversion to light,
* Neck stiffness,

meningitis may be involved, and immediate medical attention is needed.

DELUSIONS

There is no reliable definition of a delusion: conventionally, it is a belief which appears not to be founded in reality — reality as judged by a reasonable group of people sharing the same cultural background — which gives scope for gross abuse of the term. It has, indeed, been a convenient way of labelling as mentally ill those who have held such shocking beliefs as liberty, democracy and freedom.

Nevertheless, there are individuals who hold beliefs so bizarre that they are taken as prime signs of mental illness: the unshakeable conviction, for instance, that you are Napoleon Bonaparte or that if your left knee itches your wife is being unfaithful. The deluded person may then act on that belief, so that what appears to be a motiveless crime proves to have been the logical outcome of delusions. With appropriate caveats, psychiatrists therefore take delusions seriously.

THE BRAIN AND NERVOUS SYSTEM

PROBABLE
SCHIZOPHRENIA

POSSIBLE
EARLY DEMENTIA
DEPRESSION

PROBABLE

■ SCHIZOPHRENIA
A common mental illness in which the sufferer experiences a breakdown of reality and a disintegration of personality. About 1 per cent of the population is schizophrenic or goes through an episode of schizophrenia. A 'schizoid state' is a less serious condition and describes individuals who have an abnormal set of emotional responses and relationships with others and are frequently loners.

Schizophrenia is not the 'split personality' of popular myth, although it is true that a schizophrenic may appear unremarkable until you happen to touch upon his or her particular delusion. Most specialists believe that schizophrenia is the result of disorders of the chemistry of the brain. Treatment based on this view is quite successful, allowing many schizophrenics to lead quiet, undemanding, but self-sufficient lives.

* Delusions ranging from single ideas to whole networks of belief about the nature of reality.
* Hallucinations.
* Mood is often flat and emotionless.
* Apathy, self-neglect.
* Onset may be slow or rapid.

Treatment is with medication, often for years on end.

Schizophrenics often need long-term support and supervision: the toll on their families, forced to witness the disintegration of a personality, can be appalling.

POSSIBLE

■ EARLY DEMENTIA
See DEMENTIA, below. In the early stages, memory loss may result in giving delusional explanations for events, whose cause the individual has forgotten: for example, believing that a mislaid handbag has actually been stolen.

■ DEPRESSION
Those with severe depression may come to hold delusions about their own health or that of their families — for example, they may think that a loved one has an incurable disease. People in deep depression have tragically murdered their own children in the delusional belief that they were giving relief from a terrible illness.

DEMENTIA

General breakdown of the mind, with the basic defect being loss of memory. Dementia becomes more common with age. About 20 per cent of those over 80 suffer from it.

* Memory loss an early feature.
* Personality change.
* Forgetfulness about who you are, where you are and 'when you are'.
* Self-neglect.
* Depression and anxiety accompany early awareness of deterioration.
* Memory for childhood events is preserved.
* Gradually increasing confusion.

Despite this picture, the individual appears fully conscious, with no drowsiness. Although most cases are incurable, there are few treatable causes which blood tests and brain scans can detect, and of which everyone should be aware.

PROBABLE
ALZHEIMER'S DISEASE

POSSIBLE
DRUG EFFECTS
ALCOHOLISM
MULTIPLE STROKES

RARE
HUNTINGTON'S CHOREA
HYPOTHYROIDISM
HYDROCEPHALUS
LIVER OR KIDNEY DISEASE
MENINGIOMA
BRAIN HAEMATOMA
B12 DEFICIENCY
SYPHILIS
AIDS

PROBABLE

■ ALZHEIMER'S DISEASE
This term is replacing the old ones of senile and pre-senile dementia, especially as more is learned about the changes in the brain that cause dementia. However, there is at present no treatment and the outlook is progressive decline to a state needing nursing care.
* The symptoms are those of dementia, as above.
* Deterioration occurs steadily.

POSSIBLE

■ DRUG EFFECTS
Might be suspected if:
* Dementia appears rapidly and fluctuates.
* The individual is on multiple treatments, especially common with tranquillizers and drugs to treat Parkinson's disease.

The test is to stop treatment and to see what happens.

■ ALCOHOLISM
Gives rise to a distinct form of dementia, due to lack of B vitamins.
* Profound loss of memory for recent events.
* A tendency to make up excuses to cover up for memory loss.
* Disorders of eye movements, for instance, jerking.
* Unsteady gait.

This condition is treatable.

■ MULTIPLE STROKES
Dementia follows when a series of small strokes destroys more and

more of the brain.
* Dementia worsening as a series of small, abrupt steps.
* Often specific weakness of an arm or leg.
* Mood swings rapidly from tears to laughter.

Occasionally, investigation detects a treatable source of the strokes.

RARE

■ HUNTINGTON'S CHOREA
* Family history.
* Dementia with coarse tremor of limbs begins in the 30s or 40s.
* Physical and mental deterioration is progressive and inevitable.

■ HYPOTHYROIDISM
A severely under-active thyroid gland.
* Apathy, sluggishness; weight gain.
* Slow thought, intolerance of cold, slow pulse.
* Rarely, a yellowish tinge to skin.

Treatment with thyroid hormone will reverse this condition.

■ HYDROCEPHALUS
An uncommon condition of increased pressure within the brain, but found much more often now that brain scans are widely available. Treatable.
* The degree of confusion fluctuates.
* Urinary incontinence.
* Unsteady gait.
* Clumsiness.

■ LIVER AND KIDNEY DISEASE
Should be detected on routine screening. *See under METABOLIC FAILURE, page 383.*

■ MENINGIOMA
A very slowly growing brain tumour. Apart from dementia, dependent on its position, it may cause:
* Epilepsy.
* Weakness of an arm or leg.
* Progressive headache.
* Loss of sense of smell.

Diagnosis will be confirmed by a brain scan.

■ BRAIN HAEMATOMA
A blood clot on the brain, following a head injury. A possibile cause of dementia of rapid onset. *See SUBDURAL HAEMATOMA, page 383.*

■ VITAMIN B12 DEFICIENCY
Pernicious anaemia.
* Pallor from anaemia.
* Tingling in hands and feet.

Another rare but treatable cause of dementia.

■ SYPHILIS
In its final stages, many years after first infection, syphilis can cause dementia, plus:
* Unsteady gait.
* Drooping eyelids.
* Delusions, often of grandeur.
* Small, irregular pupils.

Blood tests will confirm the diagnosis and antibiotic treatment can then halt, though not reverse, the condition.

■ AIDS
A diagnosis to be considered in a younger person developing dementia. Other pointers include:

being in a high-risk group — homosexuals, bisexuals, intravenous drug-abusers; unusual chest infections; weight loss; persistently enlarged glands.

DEPRESSION

When is it an illness? And when is it a natural response to life's trials? Depression ensuing from bereavement used to be considered something different from severe depression arising by itself. Now it seems less likely that there is a clear-cut distinction. All forms of depression may benefit from treatment with anti-depressants, although these drugs need to be used with caution.

Everyone has a duty to be aware of depression as a severe illness in its own right. Growing out of unhappiness, or perhaps just from long-term 'knocks', 'clinical depression' goes beyond unhappiness and carries the real risk of suicide.

Mood, appearance and speech are usually enough to make a firm diagnosis of severe depression. The symptoms, familiar to all, are:

* Loss of enjoyment.
* Lack of energy and poor concentration.
* Loss of sexual desire, or impotence.
* Sadness.
* Tearfulness.
* Frequently, headaches, like a band around the head.

Severe depression gives rise to:

* Loss of appetite.
* Constipation.
* Early-morning waking from sleep.
* Self-disgust.
* Delusions of disease.
* Suicidal thoughts.

Telling people to pull themselves together is as useless as telling someone with appendicitis to snap out of it. The elderly deserve particular attention, as does anyone who has attempted suicide; also women experiencing severe depression after childbirth. Treatments range from counselling to anti-depressants to hospital admission for electro-convulsive therapy.

Other causes of depression to be considered are:

POSSIBLE
POST-VIRAL SYNDROME
EARLY DEMENTIA
EARLY SCHIZOPHRENIA

RARE
HYPOTHYROIDISM
PARKINSON'S DISEASE
HORMONE DISORDERS

POSSIBLE

■ POST-VIRAL SYNDROME

* Follows a vague illness with aches, pains.
* Mild depression and easy tiring.
* Most cases clear up within a few weeks.
* Occasionally becomes prolonged, with profound weakness and

THE BRAIN AND NERVOUS SYSTEM

tiredness.

The cause of post-viral syndrome is controversial. There are no tests to monitor the condition. The basic treatment is rest, but sometimes a low dose of an anti-depressant helps. Improved treatments may be available in due course.

■ EARLY DEMENTIA
See DEMENTIA, In the late middle-aged or elderly.
* Memory loss is marked.

Depression is probably the result of the individual's awareness that his or her mind is going. Some idea of how this must feel can be found in the film 2001, where, in a scene of great poignancy, the circuits which give the super-computer HAL its 'mind' are stripped away, one by one.

■ EARLY SCHIZOPHRENIA
See page 386.
* A possibility in a young person with depression.
* Possibly delusions and hallucinations.

RARE

■ HYPOTHYROIDISM
A severely under-active thyroid gland may give a state simulating depression. *See page 383.*

■ PARKINSON'S DISEASE
In the elderly.
* Tremor of hands.
* Stiff, shuffling gait.
* Impassive appearance.

This can be helped by drugs
.

■ HORMONE DISORDERS
Might be considered in someone with rapid onset of depression who appears otherwise unwell, especially with:
* Rapid weight gain or weight loss.

DIZZINESS

A common symptom, but rather difficult to define since it can mean different things. For some, it appears to be an inability to concentrate, with feelings of lightheadedness; for others, it is true vertigo with giddiness. You will find that your doctor will try hard to pin down just what you mean by dizziness.

DIZZINESS WITH VERTIGO

There is giddiness, unsteadiness and the room spins when you turn your head.

PROBABLE
VESTIBULITIS

POSSIBLE
MÉNIERE'S SYNDROME

RARE
DISEASE OF BRAIN OR SPINAL CORD

PROBABLE

■ VESTIBULITIS
A harmless infection of the inner ear giving rise to:
* Abrupt onset of giddiness.
* Worse when turning head.
* No pain or ringing in ear.
* Lying flat, you feel completely well.

Though alarming, the symptoms fade over a few days, with the help of anti-nausea drugs. Usually caused by a viral infection.

POSSIBLE

■ MENIERE'S SYNDROME
A gradual process of degeneration in the ear.
* Ringing (tinnitus) is an early feature.
* Gradually worsening deafness.
* Sudden attacks of vertigo, in which the above symptoms worsen for a few minutes.

Treatments include drugs, and devices to mask the tinnitus.

RARE

■ DISEASE OF BRAIN OR SPINAL CORD
Although highly unlikely as a cause of a few episodes of sudden dizziness, there are several such diseases which can cause dizziness in combination with:
* Unsteady gait.
* Tingling or numbness of hands or feet.
* Visual disturbances such as double vision.
* Weakness of an arm or leg.

A neurologist's opinion will be needed.

DIZZINESS WITHOUT VERTIGO

The crucial clues are: in what circumstance the dizziness occurs; at what time of day; for how long; how often; and how you feel before and afterwards.

PROBABLE
CAUSE UNKNOWN
EMOTIONAL FACTORS

POSSIBLE
ANAEMIA
LOW BLOOD PRESSURE
LOW BLOOD SUGAR

RARE
HEART AND CIRCULATION PROBLEMS
POLYCYTHAEMIA
TEMPORAL LOBE EPILEPSY

PROBABLE

■ CAUSE UNKNOWN
Accounts for the great majority of cases. A safe conclusion as long as:
* You are otherwise well.
* Attacks of dizziness are not prolonged or recurrent.

A medical check-up may be

THE BRAIN AND NERVOUS SYSTEM

reassuring; investigations are not needed.

■ EMOTIONAL FACTORS
Here dizziness is used to mean:
* Inability to concentrate.
* A 'band' around the head.
* Muddled thinking.
* Difficulty in making decisions.

Try to review what in your life is giving rise to unusual degrees of stress and worry.

POSSIBLE

■ ANAEMIA
* Pallor.
* Tiredness.
* Breathlessness.
* A lightheaded feeling when you stand up.

Unless the cause of the anaemia is obvious, for instance, very heavy periods, a prudent doctor will probably recommend some investigations.

■ LOW BLOOD PRESSURE
* Dizziness when you stand up.
* Passes off after a few seconds.

This is common in the elderly, whose circulation is less efficient at making the rather complex adjustment for standing up.

Occasionally, it is because treatment for high blood pressure has been over-effective and sometimes medication must be changed. It is also common in pregnancy. Some authorities hold that low blood pressure is a disease in itself — a matter of hot debate.

■ LOW BLOOD SUGAR
As experienced by anyone missing a meal, and especially a risk for diabetics.
* Rapid onset.
* Difficulty concentrating.
* Irritability.
* Sweating.

Symptoms are quickly relieved by eating.

RARE

■ HEART AND CIRCULATORY PROBLEMS
These can really only be confirmed by medical examination. They become commoner with age, and pointers include:
* Palpitations.
* A pulse rate that feels unusually fast, unusually slow, or irregular.
* Breathlessness.
* Chest pains.
* Dizziness when looking up.
* Symptoms of a minor stroke, with temporary limb weakness, disturbed speech or vision.

The underlying problem may be abnormal heart rhythms or narrowed valves of the heart, conditions which can be treated. Most likely, arteries to the brain have become 'furred up'. It is a matter of adjusting your lifestyle to allow for the complaint.

■ POLYCYTHAEMIA
The opposite of anaemia, in which there is an over-concentration of blood. Commonest in those with chronic lung problems such as bronchitis and emphysema; *see page 222.*
* A red complexion.
* Headaches.
* Itchiness of skin.

Treatment depends on the underlying cause.

■ TEMPORAL LOBE EPILEPSY
Difficult to diagnose if dizziness is the only reported feature. Other symptoms may include:
* A warning sensation (an aura) preceding the dizziness.
* Awareness of unusual smells, tastes or visual disturbances just before the dizziness.
* Associated drowsiness.

DROWSINESS

Drowsiness caused simply by lack of sleep or by excess alcohol is not covered here.

Drowsiness in someone otherwise expected to be alert is an important symptom, and in children unusual drowsiness is a warning symptom which always needs medical assessment.

PROBABLE
DRUG EFFECTS
NON-SPECIFIC INFECTION

POSSIBLE
HEAD INJURY
ENCEPHALITIS

RARE
BRAIN TUMOUR
NARCOLEPSY
SLEEP APNOEA SYNDROME

PROBABLE

■ DRUG EFFECTS
* Most likely in the elderly.
* Commonly those on sleeping tablets, night sedation.
* Drowsiness clears during the day.

The dose may need adjustment, or a shorter-acting drug may be appropriate.

■ NON-SPECIFIC INFECTION
Drowsiness commonly accompanies the early stages of many illnesses, especially viral ones. There may also be:
* Muscular aches and pains.
* Fever.
* Aching eyes.

The infection soon shows itself, typically, as a cough or sore throat.

POSSIBLE

■ ENCEPHALITIS
A non-specific irritation of the brain, commonly caused by mild viral infections, but which may accompany meningitis.
* Severe, persistent drowsiness.
* Confusion.
* Headache.
* Bright lights hurt the eyes.
* As it worsens, convulsions, coma, paralysis of limbs.

If you suspect encephalitis in a child, get medical advice; adults should also see a doctor unless the above combination of symptoms is very mild.

■ HEAD INJURY
Drowsiness occuring after a blow

to the head may signify bleeding within the skull. Other warning signs are:
* Confusion.
* Nausea and vomiting.
* Loss of use of a limb.
* Double vision.
* Slow pulse.

A neuro-surgical opinion is needed urgently.

RARE

■ BRAIN TUMOUR
Brain tumours really are rare and when they do occur have usually spread to the brain from a tumour elsewhere, typically the lung or breast. The features of a brain tumour are:
* Progressively worsening headache, more painful at night.
* Change of personality.
* Double vision.
* Later, loss of use of one side of the body.

Treatment depends on the type of tumour.

■ NARCOLEPSY
* Sudden sleepiness, totally out of the blue.
* For a while, the individual cannot be roused.

This unusual illness tends to run in families. It is treated with amphetamines.

■ SLEEP APNOEA SYNDROME
A condition now recognized more widely than before. During sleep, breathing becomes very shallow and stops altogether for brief periods. The resulting disturbed sleep causes marked daytime drowsiness.
* In the grossly overweight.
* Usually, in those with chronic bronchitis or emphysema.

EMOTIONAL INSTABILITY

In the context of previous emotional stability may be significant if there are also:
* Changes in personality.
* Irritability.
* Mood swings.

In some highly-strung people, apparent emotional instability is merely an exaggeration of the normal. They have abrupt swings of mood, often intensified by alcohol. They are not 'ill' as long as:
* Emotional states do not interfere with work, social and domestic life.
* The individual retains insight into his or her personality.
* General health and thought processes appear normal – for instance, no delusions.

However trying such people may be, they are often useful and creative.

That leaves relatively few underlying causes of emotional instability:

PROBABLE
ANXIETY

POSSIBLE
MENTAL ILLNESS
EARLY DEMENTIA

RARE
BRAIN TUMOUR
BRAIN DISEASE

PROBABLE

■ ANXIETY
Anyone, whatever their previous personality, will become emotional under conditions of stress and tension.
* Difficulty concentrating.
* Tension headaches.
* Abrupt outbursts.

They will be aware of the change and they will retain insight into their personality.

POSSIBLE

■ MENTAL ILLNESS
When emotional instability really does appear to exceed the norm, psychiatrists will look for:
* Delusions.
* Hallucinations.
* Loss of insight into behaviour.
* Severe depression.
* Manic, irresponsible behaviour.

Underlying diagnoses include manic depression, severe depression and schizophrenia.

■ EARLY DEMENTIA
See page 386. With breakdown of mental function, there is a loss of emotional control.

RARE

■ BRAIN TUMOUR
See page 394.
Highly unusual:
* Widespread changes in personality.
* Ill health.
* Headache.

■ BRAIN DISEASE
Numerous conditions can affect emotional control and are covered under *DEMENTIA.*
Suspected if there is:
* Memory loss.
* Disturbances of speech, gait, use of limbs.

FAINTING

A momentary interruption in the flow of blood to the brain will cause lightheadeness; any longer pause is very likely to become a faint. Serious causes are unusual, unless fainting is recurrent or abrupt.

PROBABLE
HARMLESS CAUSES

POSSIBLE
LOW BLOOD PRESSURE

RARE
HEART PROBLEMS
BLEEDING
EPILEPSY
MINOR STROKE

PROBABLE

■ HARMLESS CAUSES
The great majority of causes are trivial: standing too long in the heat, missing a meal, over-tiredness. Fainting is common in pregnancy, after emotional shock and in reaction to severe pain.
* Recovery occurs within moments.
* No convulsions or incontinence.

POSSIBLE

■ LOW BLOOD PRESSURE
See page 392.
* Recurrent lightheadeness on standing.
* Most likely if you are diabetic, or if you take drugs which affect your blood pressure.

RARE

■ HEART PROBLEMS
Worth considering if there is:
* Faintness on exertion.
* Palpitations.
* Slow, rapid or irregular pulse rates.

Most of the heart problems that will lead to fainting are treatable.

See also pages 193-204.

■ BLEEDING
Faintness, in combination with injury or pain, may be a symptom of serious blood loss.
* Sweating.
* Pallor.
* Thirst.

Careful examination will reveal the source of the bleeding. If you suspect internal bleeding, for example, after a car accident, seek medical help immediately.

See also page 426.

■ EPILEPSY
Look for:
* Convulsions.
* A warning aura.
* Urinary incontinence.

See page 384.

■ MINOR STROKE
* Possibly temporary loss of speech, or of the use of a limb.

See page 404.

HALLUCINATIONS

An experience without any basis in reality: a vision, a sound, a sensation. Dreams are 'normal' hallucinations. Hallucinations occuring in clear consciousness are symptoms of major mental disease.

PROBABLE
DELIRIUM
CONFUSIONAL STATES

POSSIBLE
DRUG OR ALCOHOL ABUSE
SCHIZOPHRENIA
DEPRESSION

RARE
TEMPORAL LOBE EPILEPSY

PROBABLE

■ DELIRIUM
The hallucination occurs against a background of restless confusion.

■ CONFUSIONAL STATES
In this context, hallucinations are part of a general breakdown of personality. *See DEMENTIA.*

POSSIBLE

■ DRUG OR ALCOHOL ABUSE
* Bizarre behaviour.
* Unresponsive.
* Tremor suggests alcoholism.

■ SCHIZOPHRENIA
Hallucinations, wound into a web of delusion, are prime symptoms of schizophrenia. *See DELUSIONS.*

■ DEPRESSION
Very severe depression may give rise to hallucinations of abusive, mocking voices. *See page 386.*

RARE

■ TEMPORAL LOBE EPILEPSY
* Hallucinations of smell and taste are commonest.
See page 393.

HYPERACTIVITY

Typically a childhood problem (in adults, *see MANIA)* combining:
* Restlessness.
* Inability to settle down to an activity.
* Destructive, aggressive behaviour.
* Poor concentration.

It is unclear whether this is a result of disease or an exaggeration of normal personality traits.

PROBABLE
CHILDHOOD HYPERACTIVITY
PSYCHOLOGICAL CONFLICT

POSSIBLE
NORMAL CHILD

RARE
FOOD ALLERGY
MINIMAL BRAIN DAMAGE

The Brain and Nervous System

PROBABLE

■ CHILDHOOD HYPERACTIVITY
Doctors disagree as to whether such a specific condition exists in children. It is true, however, that some children exhibit:
* Inability to settle to one task.
* Rapid loss of interest in the current activity.
* Frequent movement and restlessness.

Social circumstances and food additives such as artifical colourings have both been blamed for this condition. It is likely to be due to many factors acting together, and it may overlap with minimal brain damage (*see below*).

■ PSYCHOLOGICAL CONFLICT
A possible diagnosis where the close family displays:
* Emotional conflict.
* Alcoholism.
* Mental illness.

POSSIBLE

■ NORMAL CHILD
Some parents have a low tolerance for normal childhood behaviour. Thirty seconds' exposure in a crowded surgery usually makes or (literally) breaks this diagnosis.

RARE

■ FOOD ALLERGY
A highly controversial diagnosis, which can only be proven after careful dietary experiment.

■ MINIMAL BRAIN DAMAGE
Most likely if there is also:
* Clumsiness, difficulty in completing simple manual tasks.
* Severe learning difficulties.

Such children often need special schooling. This syndrome is new and not fully defined. Not all doctors agree on its cause or how best to manage affected individuals.

HYSTERIA

The popular definiton of hysteria is wild, reckless, exaggerated behaviour. The (more precise) medical definition is:
* Symptoms that have no physical basis, which appear to arise without conscious desire to deceive.

It can be difficult, if not impossible, to prove that the behaviour is not motivated by a need to deceive.

Hysterical symptoms include blindness, paralysis of a limb, lack of speech. Women, usually between the ages of 30 and 50, are more commonly affected than men.

PROBABLE
PSYCHOLOGICAL FACTORS

POSSIBLE
UNDETECTED PHYSICAL DISEASE

RARE
BRAIN DISEASE

PROBABLE

■ PSYCHOLOGICAL FACTORS
This diagnosis has some validity when physical disease can be excluded and gains strength if:
* There is a demonstrable psychological bonus from the behaviour: typically, attention or enhanced status.
* The hysteric is indifferent to symptoms a 'normal' person would find devastating — say, blindness.

Treatment is extremely difficult. It requires the hysteric to recognize that the cost of his or her behaviour outweighs the short-term psychological gain. In most cases recovery occurs within a year or so.

POSSIBLE

■ UNDETECTED PHYSICAL DISEASE
Even the most blatantly hysterical symptoms should be given the benefit of the doubt, and a search should be made for physical disease.

RARE

■ BRAIN DISEASE
Hysteria may be an early symptom of dementia or a brain tumour. If symptoms specific to these diseases accompany the hysteria, seek medical advice. *See DEMENTIA,* and *page 394.*

INSOMNIA

Sleep is still a mystery; that we all need it is certain, but how much is astonishingly variable. Imagined insomnia is often a mismatch between how much sleep someone thinks they need and how much their body really needs. It is often worth asking the individual's partner how much sleep they are getting.

PROBABLE
TEMPORARY DISTURBANCE OF SLEEP PATTERNS

POSSIBLE
REDUCED NEED FOR SLEEP

RARE
DEPRESSION

PROBABLE

■ TEMPORARY DISTURBANCE OF SLEEP PATTERNS
Worries, pain, discomfort cause insomnia which frequently persists once these problems have passed. Stimulants such as coffee and alcohol may be to blame, as may day-time snoozes.
* A cause is usually obvious — after a little reflection.
* Day-time drowsiness.
* Sleep eventually comes — because you are exhausted.

THE BRAIN AND NERVOUS SYSTEM

It is best to tackle insomnia by not going to bed until you feel tired, then following a set routine leading to bed. Sleeping tablets have a role only in the short-term treatment of insomnia.

POSSIBLE

■ REDUCED NEED FOR SLEEP
For many people, 'eight hours' sleep and a daily bowel movement' is Life's Golden Rule. Many individuals often cannot accept that they need far less of either, and the rules of the institutions where they may find themselves may reinforce this opinion.
* No obvious worries.
* No day-time drowsiness.

Chronic insomniacs should accept that they have gained extra hours in their day; that nature is telling them to do the ironing at 3.00 am... and to leave the extra daylight hours for better things.

RARE

■ DEPRESSION
Insomnia is an important symptom of depression.
* Sleep comes easily.
* You awaken early, then lie worrying for hours. *See page 389.*

IRRITABILITY

Greater than normal anger and hostility. No one need be in any doubt about normal irritability: it is a simple response to the 'F' words of workaday life:
* Fatigue.
* Frustration.
* Being fed-up.

Hunger and lack of sleep often make people extra-irritable. The more sinister causes of irritability are:

POSSIBLE
ANXIETY

RARE
EARLY DEMENTIA
HEAD INJURY
MENINGITIS

POSSIBLE

■ ANXIETY
See page 377.
* Irritability out of proportion to circumstances.

RARE

■ EARLY DEMENTIA
See page 386. As memory fades, irritability emerges in reaction to an increasingly bewildering world.

■ HEAD INJURY
An injury severe enough to cause unconsciousness is frequently followed by:
* Irritability.
* Difficulty in concentrating.
* Swings of mood.

■ MENINGITIS
* Anger at being touched or moved.
* In babies, crying at any contact; bulging soft spot on skull.
* Aversion to light.
* Headache.
* Stiff neck.

A rare but extremely serious possibility, which frequently cannot be excluded without further tests in hospital.

MANIA

Manic behaviour includes:
* Frantic activity, insomnia.
* Sudden switches of direction of thought.
* Ideas spilling out, but barely connected, grandiose.
* Rapid speech.
* Nervous, jittery activity.
* Hallucinations.

Full-blown cases of mania are rare. The milder hypomanic state is commonest.

PROBABLE
EMOTIONAL STRESS

POSSIBLE
OVER-ACTIVE THYROID GLAND
DRUG EFFECTS
DEMENTIA

RARE
MANIC DEPRESSION
SCHIZOPHRENIA

PROBABLE

■ EMOTIONAL STRESS
See also ANXIETY.
A hypomanic state:
* Not going as far as self-neglect.
* Understandable sources of stress.

POSSIBLE

■ OVERACTIVE THYROID GLAND
See page 378. It is as if the body's 'thermostat' has been turned up.
* Tremor.
* Weight loss. * Bulging eyes.

■ DRUG EFFECTS
Mania occuring in a previously sound personality may result from abuse of amphetamines or cannabis. Steroids, used widely in rheumatic disorders and asthma, may cause mania in some people with a sensitivity to these drugs.

■ DEMENTIA
Mania arises from the loss of inhibition. A distressing combination. *See page 386.*

RARE

■ MANIC DEPRESSION
Mania and depression are opposite extremes; manic depressives swing between both moods.
* Recurrent mania.
* Recurrent depression.
* A combination of both.

Often needs hospital admission (for the individual's own safety), followed by long courses of medication.

■ SCHIZOPHRENIA
See page 386. Acute schizophrenia may begin as a manic state, together with characteristic
* Delusions;
* Hallucinations.

POOR MEMORY

It is common to have an excellent memory for some types of information, for instance, names, but a poor memory for others, such as phone numbers.

PROBABLE
NORMAL AGEING PROCESS
ANXIETY

POSSIBLE
ALCOHOLISM
HEAD INJURY
STROKE

RARE
DEMENTIA

PROBABLE

■ NORMAL AGEING PROCESS
Every day, 10,000 of our brain cells die, more than 250 million over a 70-year lifetime. A dense web of additional cells and rich interconnections mask the effects of this loss; but eventually it catches up with us, and we notice our memories worsening.
* Memory for long-past events remains good.
* Difficulty learning new tasks.
* Personality generally unchanged.

There is some evidence that using your mind does preserve its function.

■ ANXIETY
Interferes with concentration and memory. *See page 377.*

POSSIBLE

■ ALCOHOLISM
Affects memory by causing vitamin deficiencies. *See page 387.*

■ HEAD INJURY
See page 393.
* Poor memory.
* Irritability.
* Mood swings.

■ STROKE
See also CONFUSION, and page 404.
Sudden loss of memory together with:
* Loss of use of a limb.
* Interference with speech.

There is often recovery from a minor stroke over several months.

RARE

■ DEMENTIA
If the personality remains intact, it is very unlikely that memory loss is due to early dementia, *page 386.*

MENTAL IMPAIRMENT

A general lack of intelligence, as shown by:
* Poor learning ability.
* Difficulty in coping with complex situations.
* Poor language skills.
* Clumsiness.

Past illness and injury may be to blame, but many cases remain unexplained.

PROBABLE
CEREBRAL PALSY
CONGENITAL
STROKE

POSSIBLE
DEMENTIA
HEAD INJURY

RARE
DEGENERATION OF THE BRAIN
VITAMIN DEFICIENCIES
METABOLIC DISORDERS
SYPHILIS

PROBABLE

■ CEREBRAL PALSY
Injury or infection of the brain at birth.
* Child is floppy.
* Fails to thrive; *see page 412.*
* Spastic limbs.

■ CONGENITAL
A similar picture to that of cerebral palsy, *above*, but with specific features, giving a recognized condition such as Down's syndrome.

■ STROKE
See page 404. A reason for sudden deterioration in a previously normal intellect.

POSSIBLE

■ DEMENTIA
See page 386. General deterioration of brain function.

■ HEAD INJURY
See page 393. Has much the same effect as a stroke.

RARE

■ DEGENERATION OF THE NERVOUS SYSTEM
Can happen in several ways. Possible if:
* Intellect was previously normal.
* Gradual deterioration of thought processes.
* Associated tremors, weakness and paralysis.

Diagnosis is for a specialists.

■ VITAMIN DEFICIENCIES
Affects the growing child and is a tragic cause of impaired intellect in undeveloped countries.
* Poor growth.
* Swollen belly, poor bone formation.
* Loss of hair, patchy pigmentation of skin.

Vitamin deficiencies are also

found in alcoholics, the mentally ill and the poor.

■ METABOLIC DISORDERS
Such as liver and kidney disease. *See page 383.*

■ SYPHILIS
Can cause a general deterioration of brain function years after first infection. *See page 388.*

PARALYSIS, RAPID ONSET

Usually the inability to use an arm or leg, but less commonly affecting muscles of the eyes, swallowing and breathing. The manner of onset gives a clue to the cause.

Urgent medical attention is always needed.

PROBABLE
STROKE
SUBARACHNOID HAEMORRHAGE
INJURY

POSSIBLE
ARTERIAL DISEASE

RARE
HYSTERIA

PROBABLE

■ STROKE
This is the overwhelmingly likely cause, being interference with blood flow to the brain usually from a burst — or suddenly blocked — blood vessel. Normally in the middle-aged or elderly.
* Often a history of high blood pressure.
* Paralysis affects one side of the body.
* Face may droop.
* Speech is slurred.
* Confusion of variable degree, even coma.

Treatment consists of nursing and intensive physiotherapy, plus attention to underlying causes, such as high blood pressure or heart disease. In many cases a return to near-normal function is achieved. Occasionally, investigations show up a brain tumour or abscess.

■ SUBARACHNOID HAEMORRHAGE
A special type of stroke, caused by a bleeding blood vessel on the surface of the brain.
* Relatively common in those aged 55-60 but possible at any age.
* Sudden, severe headache, 'like being hit in the back of the head'.
* Collapse, neck stiffness, aversion to light.

Surgical intervention is sometimes necessary to stop bleeding from the vessel and to prevent further occurrences.

■ INJURY
* A severe blow to the head.
* Probably coma and one-sided paralysis.

POSSIBLE

■ ARTERIAL DISEASE
Sudden paralysis of one leg, less commonly an arm, may be due to blockage of an artery if there is also:
* Sudden pain.
* Sudden pallor of the limb, developing into blueness. The limb is extremely cold.

To save the limb, the obstruction must be rapidly removed.

RARE

■ HYSTERIA
See page 398. In exceptional cases, sudden apparent paralysis is a possible feature.

PARALYSIS, SLOW ONSET

PROBABLE
COMPRESSION OF A NERVE

POSSIBLE
BRAIN TUMOUR
MULTIPLE SCLEROSIS
VITAMIN B12 DEFICIENCY

RARE
GUILLAIN-BARRE SYNDROME
MOTOR NEURONE DISEASE
POLIOMYELITIS

PROBABLE

■ COMPRESSION OF A NERVE
Common sites are the neck, affecting the arms; or a slipped disc in the back, affecting a foot.
* Persistent pain and tingling confined to one part of one limb.
* Partial weakness of the affected limb.
* Health otherwise sound.

Investigations will show a reason for the compression and exclude general disease of the nervous system. Treatment depends on the cause, for example, traction of the neck.

POSSIBLE

■ BRAIN TUMOUR
* Slow, progressive weakness of one side of the body.
* Headache.
* Change of personality.

The slow progression makes diagnosis difficult, but brain scans have improved the chance of reliable diagnosis.

■ MULTIPLE SCLEROSIS
A slowly degenerative disease of the young to middle-aged.
* Often begins with a sudden loss of vision in one eye.
* Numb patches, tingling, weak-

THE BRAIN AND NERVOUS SYSTEM

ness of limbs, clumsiness.
* Symptoms come and go over months and years.

The outlook is very variable, often with years of relatively good health. An unfortunate minority become severely disabled.

■ VITAMIN B12 DEFICIENCY
* Pallor.
* Tingling of hands and feet.
* Smooth, sore tongue.
* Stiff, weak legs.

The commonest cause is pernicious anaemia (*see page 421*), easily treated with injections of Vitamin B12.

RARE

■ GUILLAIN- BARRE SYNDROME
A rare inflammation of the spinal cord that may follow a minor viral illness.
* Initially, tingling in the hands and feet.
* Paralysis of the limbs rapidly appears.
* May spread to involve muscles of swallowing and breathing.

This serious condition needs intensive nursing care and assistance with breathing and feeling. Although recovery may take months, 80 per cent of sufferers recover completely.

■ MOTOR NEURONE DISEASE
An exceptionally rare, tragic disease of deterioration of muscle function in middle age.
* Begins with loss of bulk of the muscles of the hands.
* Muscle-wasting spreads more generally, with resulting paralysis.
* Widespread twitching of the muscles.
* Mental function remains intact.

There is no known cure.

■ POLIOMYELITIS
Rare, thanks to vaccination programmes.
* Mild, viral symptoms of sore throat, diarrhoea, muscle aches.
* Then symptoms of meningitis; *see page 444.*
* Then increasing muscle ache.
* Followed by paralysis, especially of leg and shoulder muscles.

Recovery can take a year; residual paralysis is common.

CHANGE OF PERSONALITY

PROBABLE
PSYCHOLOGICAL DISORDER(S)

POSSIBLE
ALCOHOL OR DRUG ABUSE
HEAD INJURY
STROKE

RARE
BRAIN TUMOUR

PROBABLE

■ PSYCHOLOGICAL DISORDER(S)
It is hardly surprising that

psychological factors underlie most changes of personality, since personality is the sum of our emotional state, mood and intellectual outlook and reflects our upbringing and experiences. Any psychological disease can affect personality.

Noticeable features include:
* Anxiety.
* Emotional instability.
* Irritability.
* Aggression or passivity.
* Delusional thought.
* Self-neglect.

These symptoms have to be judged against the background of:
* General health.
* Relationships.
* Pressures at work and at home.
* Age.
* Drug and alcohol consumption.

The symptoms are covered elsewhere in this section under individual headings. Stress and minor anxiety states will most often be to blame.

POSSIBLE

■ ALCOHOL OR DRUG ABUSE
Usually a self-evident diagnosis, suggested by:
* Self-neglect.
* Tremor; emotional instability.
* Memory loss.

■ HEAD INJURY
See page 400.

Personality change is a common consequence, together with:
* Irritability.
* Poor memory.

■ STROKE
See page 404. The resulting brain damage can cause erratic behaviour, irritability and emotionally instability.

RARE

■ BRAIN TUMOUR
Although a rare reason for personality change, doctors bear it in mind if rapid change in personality is combined with:
* Recent severe headaches, which wake the individual at night.
* Double vision.
* Fits suddenly occuring in adult life.
* Weakness of one side of the body.

Most brain tumours are secondary cancers, arising from cancer elsewhere, typically, but not exclusively, lung or breast. Brain scans have revolutionized diagnosis. Treatment depends on the exact type of tumour and may only be decided at the time of operation.

OBSESSIONS AND PHOBIAS

Meaning morbid fears or a recurrent train of thought. Mild obsessions are common: for example, fear of spiders, or checking you have locked a back door three times before going on holiday. Severe forms can dominate your life: for example, agoraphobia, a fear of open spaces. Probably these symptoms reflect an inner insecurity, though often there is no obvious cause.

Obsessions and phobias feed on themselves: what you have avoided in the past, you fear to meet in the future.

PROBABLE
PSYCHOLOGICAL FACTORS

POSSIBLE
SCHIZOPHRENIA

PROBABLE

■ PSYCHOLOGICAL FACTORS
In this situation, external factors causes stress, which leads to exaggerated feelings. These then become an obsession or phobia.
* Rest of personality and thought is normal.
* The individual has insight into the problem.

It is only when the particular focus of your obsession and phobia starts to make life unnecessarily difficult or impossible that you need professional help.

POSSIBLE

■ SCHIZOPHRENIA
* Bizzare obsessions.
* Hallucinations, delusions.

Presumably the obsession makes sense within the schizophrenic's distorted world-view.

SHOCK

In medical language, 'shock' means a massive and rapid fall in blood pressure with its accompanying effects, and is a very serious condition that requires rapid treatment. This is totally different from the layman's use of the term in which shock is the emotional reaction to a serious psychological blow, such as awful news or witnessing a serious acccident. Nonetheless, the symptom is considered here in the context of the brain and nervous system because shock can appear to be a nervous reaction — indeed, the nervous system is in part responsible for its occurrence.

Anyone thought to be in shock needs emergency help as quickly as possible.

See also BLUISH SKIN, page 424, and COLLAPSE WITH SHOCK OR COMA, page 472.

Critical features of medical shock are the rapid appearance of:
* Collapse.
* Sweating.
* Pallor.
* Weak, thready pulse.
* Confusion.

EMOTIONAL SHOCK
Features following a severe 'fright reaction' include:
* Pallor.
* Numbness of thought.
* Difficulty in concentrating.
* Life seems trivial.
* Nothing matters except the event.
* Tearfulness.

* Feelings of guilt.
* Loss of confidence.

Continuous support from relatives and friends is important. Talking about the event and crying aloud are helpful and necessary.

PROBABLE
BLOOD LOSS
HEART ATTACK

POSSIBLE
SERIOUS INFECTION
DEHYDRATION

RARE
ALLERGIC SHOCK (ANAPHYLAXIS)

PROBABLE

■ BLOOD LOSS
The source may be obvious, for example, after a stab wound; less obvious sources are:
* Black vomit.
* Black, tarry-looking motions following a severe blow to the abdomen.
* Ectopic pregnancy *(see page 355)*.
* After severe back ache (*see AORTIC ANEURYSM, page 164*).

■ HEART ATTACK
A combination of:
* Chest pain.
* Collapse.
* Breathlessness.

See page 329.

POSSIBLE

■ SERIOUS INFECTION
Danger arises when infection spreads into the bloodstream. Commonest in babies or the elderly.
* Usually a pre-existing illness, commonly of the chest or of the skin.
* Fever, sweats and rigors.
* Rapid collapse.
* Purple spots may appear on the skin.

■ DEHYDRATION
Loss of fluid from the body eventually causes:
* Thirst.
* Restlessness.
* Dry mouth, lax skin.
* Reduced output of urine.

Those especially at risk are babies and diabetics.

RARE

■ ALLERGIC SHOCK
Medical term anaphylaxis.
This is an unpredictable reaction to, say, a bee sting, an injection, or some foods.
* Face and lips swell within minutes.
* Breathing rapidly becomes wheezy.
* Collapse, possibly within a few minutes.

Those who know they are at risk should carry an antidote. (In some cases this is adrenaline.)

'General' Symptoms

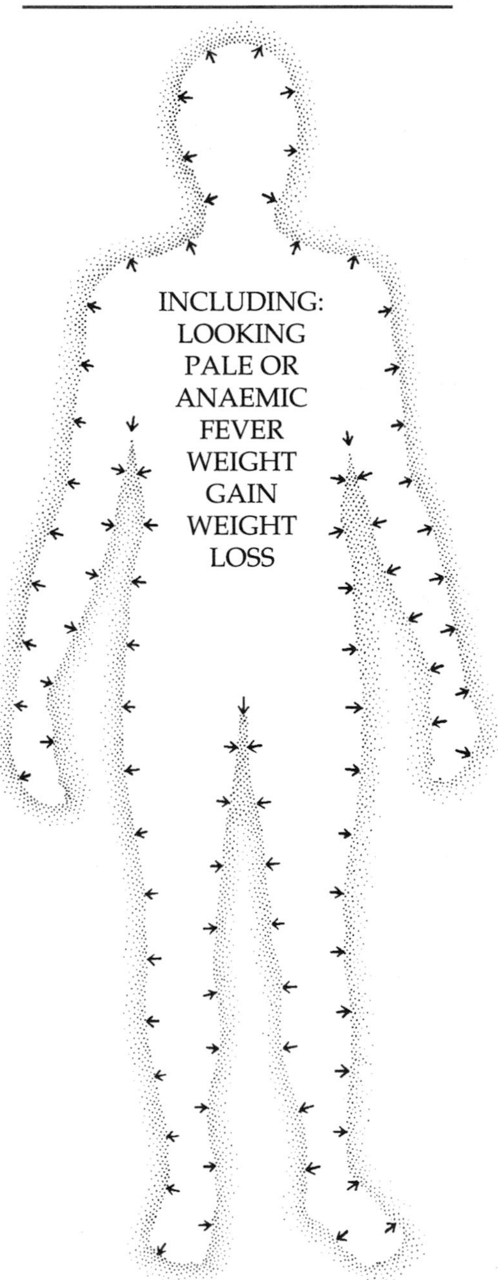

ABNORMALLY LIGHT BABY

Defined as less than 5lb (2.5 kg) birth weight. The incidence nationwide is a fundamental reflection of the general standards of living in a country. Such babies tend to:
* Have difficulty feeding.
* Become jaundiced, with the possibility of effects on brain development.
* Have breathing problems immediately after birth.

Routine antenatal care aims to detect and to control problems in the mother such as high blood pressure or smoking which might result in a premature or a low birth weight baby. Frequently the reason for low birth weight is unknown and the baby goes on to develop into a normal child.

PROBABLE
DISADVANTAGE
SMOKING IN PREGNANCY
PREMATURE BIRTH

POSSIBLE
MULTIPLE PREGNANCY
MATERNAL ILLNESS IN PREGNANCY
ABNORMALITY OF THE BABY

RARE
INFECTION IN THE MOTHER

PROBABLE

■ SOCIO-ECONOMIC DISADVANTAGE
The birth weight of a baby is linked to the mother's standard of living, presumably reflecting her general nutrition and self-care during pregnancy.

■ SMOKING
Babies born to mothers who smoke are, on average, about 1/2lb (0.25 kg) lighter than babies of mothers of similar social class who are non-smokers. The reason is uncertain; the message is clear. If you really cannot stop smoking in pregnancy, try to cut down.

■ PREMATURITY
That is, a baby born before 37 weeks gestation, for any reason. Sometimes doctors find it difficult to judge whether a baby is premature or has a low birth weight. The diagnosis depends on the overall appearance and behaviour of the baby.

POSSIBLE

■ MULTIPLE PREGNANCY
The average birth weight of babies decreases in each pregnancy after the first three or four births. It may also be affected if there are twins, triplets and so on.

■ MATERNAL ILLNESS IN PREGNANCY
The most common in developed countries is high blood pressure. Worldwide, severe malnutrition is the major scourge.

'GENERAL' SYMPTOMS

■ ABNORMALITY OF THE BABY
Many congenital abnormalities cause low birth weight, especially cerebral palsy, commonly known as brain damage.

RARE

■ INFECTION DURING PREGNANCY
Rubella is the commonest and is avoidable through vaccination.

No one can be certain of the long-term consequences of low birth weight, but there is strong evidence that babies born small can remain smaller than average at least up to puberty, and sometimes into adult life.

BABY OR CHILD UNABLE TO PUT ON WEIGHT OR TO GROW ADEQUATELY

The medical term for this symptom is failure to thrive, and applies to babies and young children who fail to reach the accepted milestones of development for their age. The search would be on for physical reasons, but it is well recognized that emotional neglect can also contribute to failure to thrive.

PROBABLE
FEEDING PROBLEM
LOW BIRTH WEIGHT
NEGLECT

POSSIBLE
VOMITING
MALABSORPTION
INFECTION

RARE
HYPOTHYROIDISM

PROBABLE

■ FEEDING PROBLEMS
No neglect is implied, but simple problems such as:
* Feeds prepared incorrectly.
* Teat openings too small to allow adequate intake.
* An over-rigid feeding schedule.
* The baby rapidly catches up once the problem is identified.

■ LOW BIRTH WEIGHT
Severely premature babies, with low birth weight, may not to grow as well as normal babies at first. Babies born small but on time can be expected to grow at a normal rate, although they remain smaller compared to other children.

■ NEGLECT
This includes emotional neglect, as well as food deprivation.
* A withdrawn, unresponsive child.
* Fearful of strangers.
* Other signs of neglect such as injuries, bruising, dirtiness.

POSSIBLE

■ VOMITING
All babies vomit, some more than

others. It is usually a passing feature and the baby's weight soon catches up. Pyloric stenosis is a not uncommon reason for persistent vomiting. It is caused by a blockage in the stomach and relieved by a minor operation:
* Much commoner in boys than girls.
* Vomiting begins after the first few weeks of life.
* The baby feeds normally, then vomits forcefully — so-called projectile vomiting.
* The baby is ravenous.

■ MALABSORPTION
The child has a normal intake of food, yet fails to grow. Suspicious symptoms would include:
* Chronic diarrhoea, especially with bulky, greasy, smelly stools.
* Recurrent chest infections.

The commonest causes of malabsorbtion in developend countries are *CYSTIC FIBROSIS, page 146* and *COELIAC DISEASE, page 146.*

■ INFECTION
Repeated infection over time slows down growth. The most common culprit is a urinary infection, causing fevers and tummy pain. However, urinary infections may cause no symptoms at all, other than poor growth. They need to be individually investigated.

RARE

■ HYPOTHYROIDISM
An underactive thyroid gland. Appears in the first few weeks of life. Sometimes this goes undetected. If severe, symptoms could include:
* Prolonged jaundice in the days after birth.
* A lethargic baby, tending to constipation and poor feeding.
In some areas there are routine screening tests for this easily treated condition.

BIRTH ABNORMALITY PLUS FAILURE TO GROW

If the causes of failure to grow on *pages 412-3* have been excluded, malformation might be suspected. Specialists will test for: interference with swallowing, perhaps due to a cleft palate; cerebral palsy; heart disease; a *CHROMOSOMAL ABNORMALITY (see page 415)*; or (rare), a metabolic disorder or kidney failure. See relevant sections for further details.

DISTRESSED OR CRYING BABY

First, know your child. All mothers know that a child will cry in different ways, depending on whether he or she is hungry, angry or in pain. Daily experience of your child qualifies you to recognize when the child is crying in an unusual way. When this happens, check through the common causes. Remember also that a usually placid baby or child can become irritable in response to your own mood, or even to the way you handle it.

'General' Symptoms

PROBABLE
HUNGER OR THIRST
DISCOMFORT
DESIRE FOR COMFORT

POSSIBLE
COLIC
INFECTION
PAIN

RARE
MENINGITIS

PROBABLE

■ HUNGER OR THIRST
* Due for a feed?
* Roots for the teat.
* Sucks eagerly.

■ DISCOMFORT
* A dirty nappy?
* Too hot? Flushed, sweating.
* Cold: blue hands, cold to the touch.
* Noise, bright lights, smoke?

■ DESIRE FOR COMFORT
* Excited when you appear.
* Crying stops when cuddled, recurs when put down.

POSSIBLE

■ COLIC
* After a feed or in the evening.
* Draws up legs, whimpers.
* Relieved by winding or, in the case of evening colic, the problem simply stops after a few weeks.

■ INFECTION
* Snuffles, a *COLD* (*see page 454*) or a cough.
* Other signs of infection: increased sleepiness, fever, rash, off food.

■ PAIN
* Rubbing ear; teething?
* More of a scream than a cry.
* Only briefly relieved by comforting.

RARE

■ MENINGITIS (*see page 444*). An infection of the brain which can appear in hours in a previously well baby or child. It is rare, but potentially so serious that anxiety is understandable. Difficult to diagnose in very young babies: much depends on how ill the child looks. Because of the difficulty of diagnosis, see a doctor immediately if you suspect meningitis. He or she may well admit the child to hospital for investigation.
* The baby or child is initially irritable.
* Increasingly drowsy, lethargic.
* Vomiting.
* Soft spot of skull may be bulging.
* High-pitched, animal cry.
* Fine purple skin rash.

SHORT STATURE

This is generally defined as height which is in the lowest 3 per cent of the population for age. Although parents worry about it, regular measurements at three-monthly intervals will show whether a child is small, but growing at a normal rate, in which case the child is almost certainly short because he or she is made that way.

PROBABLE
FAMILY PATTERN
SMALL FOR DATES BABY

POSSIBLE
CHROMOSOMAL DISORDER
CHRONIC DISEASE
HYPOTHYROIDISM
ACHONDROPLASIA

RARE
GROWTH HORMONE DEFICIENCY

PROBABLE

■ FAMILY PATTERN
Short parents have children who will be short, although genetic mechanisms ensure that, on average, the children end up taller than the parents. There are formulae, based on parental height, which can help to predict the final height of a child.

■ SMALL-FOR-DATES BABY
See LOW BIRTH WEIGHT, page 412. Babies born small may remain small throughout life.

Achondroplasia

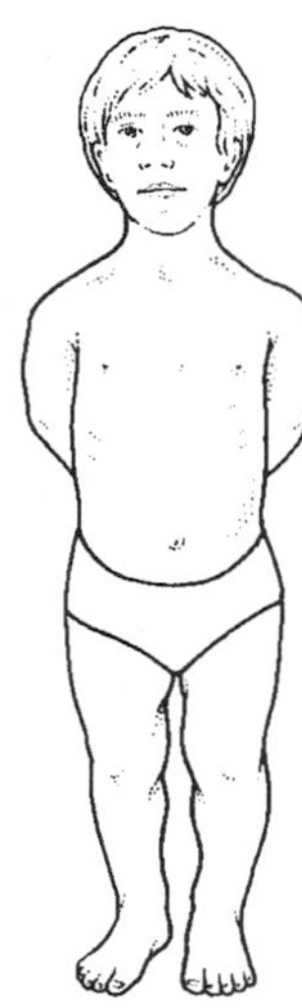

POSSIBLE

■ CHROMOSOMAL DISORDER
Common disorders are DOWN'S SYNDROME, with characteristic flat face; large hands; fold of skin on inner part of eyeball and other abnormalities. Another is TURNER'S SYNDROME; two symptoms of this condition are:
* Webbed neck.
* Infertility in later life.

■ CHRONIC DISEASE
Any long-term disease will stunt growth. Common culprits are kidney disease and heart disease.

■ HYPOTHYROIDISM
An under-active thyroid gland. *See page 461.* Many babies are screened for this condition. Treatment enables growth to resume at a normal rate.

■ ACHONDROPLASIA
A genetic disorder. The child is very small:

* Very short limbs.
* Large head, normal trunk.
* Normal intelligence.

RARE

■ GROWTH HORMONE DEFICIENCY
This unusual condition is now treatable by giving injections of the missing hormone.
* The child is normal, but grows slowly.
* Tendency to be overweight.
Mental development is normal.

BLUISH-COLOURED SKIN

See BLUISH SKIN, page 424.

BODY SIZE

See ACROMEGALY, page 275 and TALLNESS, page 428.

BRUISING

PROBABLE
ACCIDENT
PHYSICAL ABUSE

POSSIBLE
BLOOD DISORDER
SCURVY

PROBABLE

■ ACCIDENT
Bruises on exposed areas, such as shins or elbows, which come and go.

■ PHYSICAL ABUSE
Suggested in particular if there is a history of family difficulties.
* Multiple bruises of varying ages, some old, some fresh.
* Inadequate explanation.
* Appearance of neglect — dirty, ill-fed.
* Bruising around ankles or wrists.
* The characteristic bruising of bite marks is not unusual on abused children.

POSSIBLE

■ BLOOD DISORDER
Severe anaemias and serious blood disorders.
* Purple spots or patches appear on skin.
* Spontaneous bleeding from gums, nose.
* Rapid onset in an already ill person.

A blood test is essential and should be taken as soon as possible. *See also BLEEDING — SPONTANEOUS AND GENERAL, page 426.*

■ SCURVY
Caused by lack of Vitamin C. *See page 426.*

PALE APPEARANCE, COMING ON SLOWLY

Some people are naturally pale, so the best way to check for pallor is to look at the areas where blood flows close to the surface, for example beneath the fingernails and under the eyelids.

Pallor alone is an unspecific symptom: medical investigation is usually needed to establish the cause.

PROBABLE
ANAEMIA

POSSIBLE
HYPOTHYROIDISM

RARE
HYPOPITUITARISM

PROBABLE

■ ANAEMIA
See also page 419. Inadequate supply of essential nutrients in the diet to make normal blood.

General features include:
* Tiredness; being easily fatigued.
* Breathlessness — gradual onset.
* Dizziness, especially on standing up.

In addition, there may be symptoms suggesting the underlying cause, such as:
* Weight loss.
* Self-neglect.
* Sores on skin and bruising.
* Heavy periods.
* Jaundice.

POSSIBLE

■ HYPOTHYROIDISM
See also page 461. An under-active thyroid gland causes a slow-down in all aspects of body function over several months. As well as pallor, which is due both to a mild anaemia and to changes in the skin, you may notice:
* Sensitivity to the cold.
* Gruff voice, coarse skin, thinning hair.
* Constipation, slowness of thought.

This condition is readily treatable by taking thyroid tablets once the diagnosis has been established by a doctor.

RARE

■ HYPOPITUITARISM
A failure of the pituitary gland in the brain, crucial to controlling many hormones — the body's 'chemical messengers'. Pallor can be a striking feature of this condition, plus other symptoms, such as:
* Hypothyroidism, as above.
* In women, periods cease; loss of sexual drive.
* Reduction of pubic hair, and hair in armpits.
* Lack of stamina.

Usually treatable to some degree.

PALE APPEARANCE, COMING ON RAPIDLY

Over days, hours or minutes. Unless the individual has simply fainted, this may well signify a problem which requires urgent medical attention. The likeliest reason is blood loss.

PROBABLE
A FAINT
INTERNAL BLEEDING

POSSIBLE
HYPOGLYCAEMIA
HEART RHYTHM DISORDER
GASTRIC UPSET
HEART ATTACK

RARE
ACUTE BLOOD DISORDER

PROBABLE

■ A FAINT
The many well-recognized causes of fainting include missing a meal; emotional shock; prolonged standing; excessive heat; pregnancy.
* Otherwise sound health.
* Initial lightheadedness, sweating, dizziness.
* Collapse to ground or on to furniture.
* Cold, clammy skin; thin, slow pulse.

It is essential to leave someone who has fainted lying flat until they recover, which generally takes just a few minutes.

■ INTERNAL BLEEDING
Often there is a previous history of abdominal discomfort. The blood loss may be obvious:
* Bloody or black stools.
* Blood in urine.
* Vomit containing blood or with specks looking like coffee grounds.
* Excessive vaginal bleeding, especially after a delayed period.

Early symptoms are similar to those of anaemia, *see page 419*, but of more rapid onset. As blood loss increases there will be:
* Severe giddines.
* A feeling of being cold, plus cold, clammy extremities.
* Low urine output.
* Rapid breathing.
* Eventually, drowsiness and unconsciousness.

There will probably be pointers to the cause of the bleeding. Previous dyspepsia (indigestion) suggests a duodenal or gastric problem. Bowel disturbance may signify inflammation of the bowel, a tumour or a perforation (hole) in the intestine. Aspirin and other anti-arthritic drugs can also cause bleeding into the bowel.

POSSIBLE

■ HYPOGLYCAEMIA
A problem for diabetics, especially those on insulin, who must learn to recognize the early symptoms:
* Hunger, irritability, lightheaded-

ness, progressing to:
* Sweating, confusion, slurring of speech, unconsciousness.

Taking sugar or glucagon gives relief in minutes.

■ HEART RHYTHM DISORDER
Very rapid, slow or irregular heart rhythms mean that blood is pumped around the body with reduced efficiency. Commonest in the 50-plus age group.
* You may be aware of a thumping or a fluttering in your chest.
* Onset is usually abrupt; symptoms often end abruptly, too.
* Pallor, breathlessness, dizziness.

■ GASTRIC UPSET
The early stages of a severe attack of gastroenteritis may be ushered in with:
* Nausea, vomiting, sweating, griping abdominal discomfort.
* Pallor.
* Diarrhoea follows within a few hours.

■ HEART ATTACK
Pallor will probably not be the only, or even the main, symptom. The classic picture is:
* Crushing pain in the central chest, arising suddenly.
* Breathlessness, sweating, pallor.

Heart attacks, especially in the elderly, may not be so clear-cut, causing just pallor, fatigue and breathlessness.

RARE

■ ACUTE BLOOD DISORDER
Including leukaemia and any breakdown in the blood's clotting mechanism. Commonest in children and young adults.
Suggested by:
* A bad sore throat, vague malaise, then pallor.
* Nose bleeds, bleeding gums, blood in bowel or urine.
* Spontaneous bruising.

LOOKING PALE OR ANAEMIC

When the body's red blood cells fall below the necessary level, or if haemoglobin, the oxygen-carrier in red blood cells, is somehow impaired or reduced, anaemia develops. It results in:
* Paleness or pallor — an important sign of anaemia, but often a misleading one, since many people are naturally pale. Best judged by looking at parts of the body where the blood runs close to the surface, typically the undersurface of the eyelids or under the fingernails.
* Feeling tired much of the time.
* Fatige on exertion.
* Faintness (in severe cases).
* Flat fingernails.

There is a vast range of possible causes of anaemia, but in practice the appearance of the red blood cells under a microscope, together with the patient's history and an examination, usually confirm the diagnosis.

'GENERAL' SYMPTOMS

PROBABLE
BLOOD LOSS IN MENSTRUATION
PREGNANCY
RAPID GROWTH (in childhood)
POOR DIET

POSSIBLE
PERNICIOUS ANAEMIA
CHRONIC BLEEDING

RARE
CANCER
CHRONIC DISEASE
THALASSAEMIA
WORM INFESTATIONS

PROBABLE

■ BLOOD LOSS IN MENSTRUATION
The 70 to 80 mls of blood lost in normal menstruation is replaced by the body within a day or two. However, anaemia is a risk if:
* Periods are very heavy, with clots.
* Periods are very frequent.
* Periods are prolonged, or there is inter-menstrual bleeding.
* If you have a poor diet.

■ PREGNANCY
Anaemia in pregnancy should be detected by routine blood tests. In fact, it is so common in pregnancy that some degree of anaemia is considered normal.
Iron supplements are not always given to pregnant women: your doctor will advise you if he or she thinks it is necessary. While you are pregnant, iron must only be taken in conjunction with folic acid.

■ RAPID GROWTH
During childhood growth spurts, the body's need for iron and vitamins may outstrip the supply. The result can be slight anaemia, just enough to make the child tire easily. A balanced diet should overcome this effect, so vitamin and iron supplements only make sense if your child's diet really is poor. If you have doubts or worries, a formal dietry assessment is advised.

■ POOR DIET
That is, a diet deficient in iron or in the vitamins needed to make haemoglobin. The elderly, alcoholics or those on low incomes are at risk.
* Lack of meat, eggs or green vegetables such as peas.
* Cracked skin at corners of the mouth.
* Easy bruising, bleeding gums.

Leaving vegetables to soak, or boiling them for a long time, will destroy their vitamin and iron content. Steaming vegetables is preferable to boiling them.
Dark leaf vegetables, fish, eggs, liver, meat and cereals are sources of iron.

POSSIBLE

■ PERNICIOUS ANAEMIA
Caused by lack of Vitamin B12, because of failure to absorb the vitamin.
* Gradual onset, sometimes leading to very low levels of haemoglobin.
* Often, a family history.
* Sore, smooth tongue.
* Tingling, numbness of limbs.
* Unsteady walk.
* A hint of jaundice is possible.

■ CHRONIC BLEEDING
Caused by disease, such as a bleeding peptic ulcer, or by drugs, of which aspirin and certain anti-inflammatory agents are the commonest culprits. Also, don't underestimate the effect of chronically bleeding haemorrhoids.
* Passage of bloody or black stools.
* Blood in vomit.
* Excessive or prolonged menstrual bleeding (*see above*).
* Features of underlying disease, weight loss, anorexia, alteration of bowel habit.

RARE

■ CANCER OR OTHER CHRONIC DISEASE
Anaemia is unlikely to be the only symptom, except for cancers causing internal bleeding (*see CHRONIC BLEEDING above*). The same is true of chronic diseases such as kidney failure or rheumatoid arthritis.

■ THALASSAEMIA
Occurs because of a failure of the mechanism which produces normal haemoglobin. It runs in families.
* Generally causes a mild, chronic anaemia, though more serious forms exist.

■ WORM INFESTATIONS
For example, hookworm; rare in the West, but common causes of anaemia in tropical countries. Detected from stool samples.

LOOKING PALE OR ANAEMIC PLUS SKIN PROBLEMS

Rashes, sores and skin changes can be a feature of anaemia, but usually only if the anaemia is especially severe or if it is one of the rarer types which are a side effect of some other underlying disease.

PROBABLE
IRON DEFICIENCY ANAEMIA

POSSIBLE
PERNICIOUS ANAEMIA

RARE
DRUG SIDE EFFECT
AUTO-IMMUNE DISEASE

PROBABLE

■ <u>IRON DEFICIENCY ANAEMIA</u>
See also anaemia, page 419. General features of anaemia, plus:
* Painful cracked skin at corners of mouth.
* Sore smooth tongue.

POSSIBLE

■ <u>PERNICIOUS ANAEMIA</u>
* Can cause a sore, smooth tongue. *See anaemia, page 419*, for more details.

RARE

■ <u>DRUG SIDE EFFECT</u>
Any drug which causes anaemia may also cause skin rashes, blotches, bruises and a sore mouth.

■ <u>AUTO-IMMUNE DISEASE</u>
A range of diseases in which the body attacks its own components resulting in general effects of malaise, rashes, joint pains.
* A butterfly-shaped rash across the cheeks is characteristic of *SYSTEMIC LUPUS ERYTHEMATOSIS, page 448.*

LOOKING PALE OR ANAEMIC, PLUS LOSING WEIGHT

This is a worrying combination, especially in the middle-aged and elderly. There is the possibility of underlying disease causing internal bleeding or possibly affecting the ability of the body to absorb the food, iron and vitamins needed to make red blood cells. In children, the combination is more likely to suggest poor food intake or a malabsorption condition.

PROBABLE
NEGLECT
MALABSORPTION

POSSIBLE
CHRONIC DISEASE
CANCER OF THE BOWEL
CANCER OF THE STOMACH

RARE
ANOREXIA NERVOSA
CHRONIC MYELOID LEUKAEMIA

PROBABLE

■ <u>NEGLECT</u>
Typically self-neglect, with a diet so poor that individuals are literally starving themselves. In developed countries, it is usually

only seen in those who are either very poor, living alone, or too frail to provide adequately for themselves. It is sometimes found in alcoholics and, rarely, in drug abusers.

In children, there may be other signs of neglect by their guardians, such as:

* Unexplained bruising.
* Dirty appearance.
* Withdrawn behaviour.
* No food in the house.

■ MALABSORPTION

The term covers a range of conditions which undermine the digestive tract's ability to absorb nutrients. The possibilities are wide and what is probable in children is rare in adults. Some clues which suggest malabsorption as the underlying cause of anaemia and weight loss are:

* Gradual appearance of symptoms
* Change in bowel habit, with persistent, loose stools or diarrhoea.
* An apparently adequate intake of food.
* Appetite healthy until later stages of the illness.
* Co-existing, recurrent chest infections

Bowel cancer is common. In the United States, routine, annual bowel examinations are increasingly used to test for cancer. A number of screening tests are available in the United Kingdom. You can ask your doctor for a stool examination: the presence of blood in a sample is a crude check for cancer.

Family history

A family history of bowel cancer means that you run a significant risk of developing the condition. Ask your doctor for regular checks once you reach the age of 40 — or earlier, if your relative developed cancer early.

POSSIBLE

■ CHRONIC DISEASE

Several chronic diseases, such as tuberculosis or long-term infection, can cause this combination of symptoms. The nature of the underlying disease will not necessarily be clear. Seek help from your doctor if any symptoms persist.

■ CANCER OF THE BOWEL

This common cancer has an excellent outlook if diagnosed sufficiently early. Besides anaemia and weight loss, the other warning signs are:

* Persistent change of bowel habit — for instance, the bowels open daily whereas they used to be open less often, or vice versa.
* Blood in stools.
* Mucus or slime from back passage.
* A feeling of not completely emptying the bowel.

■ CANCER OF THE STOMACH

Again, the earlier this is diagnosed, the better the outlook.

* Indigestion and acidity as a new symptom in middle-age.
* Loss of appetite.
* Pains in upper abdomen.

* Vomiting of blood or passage of black motions.

RARE

■ ANOREXIA NERVOSA
Although associated with young women, it is sometimes seen in men. Those with anorexia are often good athletes or high achievers at school. The signs are:
* Obsession with body image: the individual is convinced that she or he is obese.
* Appearance may vary from very slim to outright starved.
* In women, monthly periods cease.
* An excess of fine body hair may appear.
* Bouts of binge eating (bulimia).

■ CHRONIC MYELOID LEUKAEMIA
A disease of gradual onset in middle-age.
* Enlarged liver.
* Enlarged spleen.
* Diagnosis made on blood tests.

BLUISH SKIN

Otherwise known as cyanosis: a bluish-purple colouring, visible especially where blood flows close to the surface, for example the lips, the tongue and under the finger-nails. It arises when blood becomes 'stale' — unable to discharge waste carbon dioxide, or to take on fresh oxygen from the lungs. Fingers commonly show cyanosis in cold weather due to sluggish blood flow. In more serious cases, the lips and tongue also become blue.

PROBABLE
TEMPORARILY POOR CIRCULATION

POSSIBLE
CHRONIC BRONCHITIS OR EMPHYSEMA
INHALED FOREIGN BODY
HEART FAILURE

RARE
CONGENITAL HEART DISEASE (CHILDREN)
DRUG OVERDOSE

PROBABLE

■ TEMPORARILY POOR CIRCULATION
Common at any age:
* Results from a drop in temperature.
* A slight degree of cyanosis confined to fingers and toes, which feel cold and numb.
* Disappears rapidly on warming the limb.
* Worse in winter, better in summer.

Occasionally, a blood clot may block the circulation to part of a limb, usually the lower leg or toes. This gives a quite different set of symptoms, typically found in an elderly person with pre-existing

circulatory disease.
* Sudden onset of pain, coldness, numbness and paralysis of the limb.
* Limb may at first look pale, cyanosis setting in over a few hours.

This is an emergency: seek urgent medical help.

POSSIBLE

■ CHRONIC BRONCHITIS/EMPHYSEMA
See page 222. These are lung diseases causing persistent cough, wheeze and breathlessness. It is only after many years of disease that cyanosis becomes a regular feature, by which time the sufferer has long suffered breathlessness on the slightest exertion.
* Cyanosed nail beds, tongue and lips.
* Hands and feet can feel surprisingly warm. Caused by high concentrations of carbon dioxide in the blood.

■ INHALED FOREIGN BODY
The rapid appearance of cyanosis in someone who is breathless suggests a sudden obstruction to airflow. In children it may be caused by inhaling a small object.
* Typically occurs when eating steak or similar chunky food.
* Clutching at the throat, trying to gasp; clearly very distressed.

The Heimlich manoeuvre is a useful first aid procedure designed to relieve such obstructions.

■ HEART FAILURE
Mild heart failure is actually quite common, caused usually by diseased coronary arteries. It is readily and effectively treatable. Only in severe cases is cyanosis a prominent symptom together with:
* Constant breathlessness.
* Swollen legs.
* Breathlessness on lying flat.
* Coughing frothy fluid.

RARE

■ CONGENITAL HEART DISEASE (CHILDREN)
Following conception, the human embryo's heart and great blood vessels develop via a complex process open to error at all points, and it is remarkable that so few serious congenital heart conditions occur. If they do, the result may be a 'blue' or cyanosed baby, in whom the blood is not pumped properly through the lungs.

Symptoms show at or very soon after birth.
* Breathlessness on feeding.
* Baby looks anxious.
* The baby fails to gain weight normally during the first few weeks and months of life.
* Dizziness, headache and fatigue.
* Thromboses (blood clots).

■ DRUG OVERDOSE
Suspected in an otherwise well young person who is:
* Unconscious.
* Breathing reduced to a point at which cyanosis appears.

'GENERAL' SYMPTOMS

BLEEDING

Everyone experiences surprise bleeding from time to time: blood on the tooth brush or perhaps bleeding from the back passage. Follow up these symptoms in detail under the relevant sections for the part of the body involved.

APPETITE, LOSS OF

See NO APPETITE, page 474.

BLEEDING — SPONTANEOUS AND GENERAL

Covered here is spontaneous bleeding from the gums or the nose; blood in the urine, in stools and from the vagina. It will almost certainly be accompanied by widespread bruising. The symptoms point to a general breakdown of the blood clotting process.

PROBABLE
SCURVY

POSSIBLE
ANTICOAGULANT OVERDOSE
THROMBOCYTOPENIA

RARE
HAEMOPHILIA
SEVERE INFECTIONS

PROBABLE

■ SCURVY
Results from a diet lacking vitamin C, which is contained in fresh fruit and vegetables. So the problem is usually one of the elderly or the poor.
* Chronic feeling of being ill.
* Bleeding, especially from between the teeth.
* Sore gums, loose teeth.
* Easy bruising.

Readily treated by vitamin C supplements.

POSSIBLE

■ ANTICOAGULANT OVERDOSE
The drug warfarin is widely used for certain heart disorders, and also for thrombosis in a limb. Regular blood tests help to check that the dose is correct, but overdosage can happen easily.

See your doctor immediately if you begin bleeding unexpectedly while taking warfarin. Nosebleeds can be the first sign of excessive dosage, which in some cases can even be fatal.

■ THROMBOCYTOPENIA
A general term for a fall in the numbers of platelets in the bloodstream. Platelets are crucial to blood clotting, so if they are in

short supply, widespread bleeding occurs. Many serious general illnesses can cause thrombo–cytopenia, the cause usually being obvious after just a few investigations, for example:
* Aplastic anaemia, with rapid appearance of weakness, pallor and malaise.
* Childhood leukaemia, as with aplastic anaemia, but also sore throat.
* Adult leukaemias: a slower onset than childhood leukaemias, enlarged lymph nodes, sweats.
* Bone cancers, with pain, malaise, weight loss.

Thrombocytopenia can also be drug-induced. There is also a benign form, affecting children, which cures itself spontaneously. Treatment is aimed at the underlying cause, if known.

RARE

■ HAEMOPHILIA
A bleeding disorder, caused by an inherited abnormality in the blood clotting system. Almost exclusively in males.
* A family history is common: two-thirds of cases are hereditary.
* Early symptoms are prolonged bleeding from, say, a small cut; spontaneous bruising; bleeding into joints, giving joint pain and swelling.

■ SEVERE INFECTION
Many serious infectious diseases cause chaos in the blood clotting system. These include septicaemia (blood poisoning), malaria and typhoid fever.
* Sweats and chills while the patient is also
* Generally very ill.

BLOOD SLOW TO CLOT

You may notice this as easy bruising; bleeding from the gums and teeth; blood in the urine or stools; or unusually heavy periods.

POSSIBLE
SCURVY
EXCESS OF ANTI-COAGULANT DRUG

RARE
HAEMOPHILIA

POSSIBLE

■ SCURVY
Vitamin C deficiency, associated with diets low in fresh fruit.
* Widespread, spontaneous bruising.
* Sore gums, loose teeth.
* Vague ill health.

Vitamin C treatment reverses the condition.

■ EXCESS OF ANTI-COAGULANT DRUG
See page 426.

'GENERAL' SYMPTOMS

RARE

■ HAEMOPHILIA
See page 427.

TALLNESS

Meaning (for a given age) height greater than that of the tallest 3 per cent of the population. Only rarely is tallness due to disease.

PROBABLE
NATURAL TENDENCY
EARLY PUBERTY

POSSIBLE
HYPERTHYROIDISM
GENETIC ABNORMALITY

RARE
EXCESS GROWTH HORMONE
MARFAN'S SYNDROME

PROBABLE

■ NATURAL TENDENCY
Tall parents have tall children. There are formulae which can predict a child's height, based on the heights of the parents.

■ EARLY PUBERTY
The complex hormonal changes of puberty can make a child leap up in height. In later puberty, growth slows, so the child who was unusually tall may finish smaller than his or her peers who reach puberty later. The familiar signs of puberty are:
* Growth of body hair around genitalia, armpits.
* Breast development.
* Deepening voice.

POSSIBLE

■ HYPERTHYROIDSM
This will enhance growth in childhood. *See page 479.*

■ GENETIC ABNORMALITY
The commonest (it affects one in 500 males) is Klinefelter's Syndrome.
* Tall and thin with a female body shape, small testicles and breast development.
* Usually infertile.

RARE

■ EXCESS GROWTH HORMONE
In children, this causes excessive height and size. In adults it causes acromegaly with progressively coarse, heavy features.
* Enlargement of hands and feet.
* Protrusion of lower jaw.
* Possibly heavy sweating and diabetic symptoms.

■ MARFAN'S SYNDROME
This interesting hereditary condition affects about two people per 100,000; it causes:
* Long thin bones, spider-like fingers and toes.

* An unusually high arch to the palate.
* Heart valve problems, which may cause breathlessness.
* Visual disturbance through dislocation of the lens of the eye.

SWOLLEN BODY

Three categories of disorder cause generalized body swelling: heart failure, kidney disease and low-protein states.

The mechanics of swelling are complex. Because fluid sinks to the lowest level of the body, the early signs are swollen ankles or a puffy face in the morning. As more fluid accumulates, swelling spreads up the legs and builds up inside the abdomen and chest.

PROBABLE
PRE-MENSTRUAL SWELLING
PRE-ECLAMPSIA
HEART FAILURE

POSSIBLE
NEPHRITIS
LIVER DISEASE
MALNUTRITION
MALABSORPTION

RARE
NEPHROTIC SYNDROME
VITAMIN B1 DEFICIENCY

PROBABLE

■ PRE-MENSTRUAL SWELLING
Hormone changes in the few days before a period cause a mild degree of fluid retention:
* A regular pattern each month; health otherwise normal.
* Breasts, abdomen, ankles all become slightly enlarged.
* Weight gain of a few pounds.
* Disappears within days of the period beginning.

■ PRE-ECLAMPSIA
Rapid swelling due to fluid retention in late pregnancy. Checks may also show a rise in blood pressure and protein in the urine. One of the few conditions exclusive to pregnancy. Monitoring women for the problem is one of the key reasons for ante-natal care. Requires hospital treatment. Commonest in first pregnancies.
* Rapid weight gain over a few days.
* Swollen fingers and feet.
* Headaches, dizzy spells, nausea.
Treatment of pre-eclampsia is necessary to prevent progression to eclampsia — dramatic rise in blood pressure, epileptic fits, danger to the baby.

■ HEART FAILURE
A common cause of persistent swelling of the legs in later life.
* Often high blood pressure, angina or other heart disease.
* At first, swelling of ankles, tiredness.
* Later, breathlessness on exertion, or when lying down (causing

inability to lie down).
* Paroxysms of breathlessness at night, coughing frothy sputum.

Modern drugs can usually provied effective treatment, although the swelling may not clear completely.

POSSIBLE

■ NEPHRITIS
Actually a group of diseases, all of which involve some degree of inflammation of the kidneys. This causes swelling of the body, partly due to loss of protein in the urine and partly due to failure to excrete sufficient urine. In children, nephritis presents with:
* Sudden onset, often after a minor throat infection.
* Low urine output.
* Blood in urine.
* Puffiness, especially of the face.
The outlook for recovery is good. In adults it tends to present more slowly, with:
* Progressive swelling of the legs.

Assessment involves blood tests and biopsy of the kidney, after which the outlook can be judged, depending on the type of nephritis.

■ LIVER DISEASE
One of the liver's many functions is to make proteins. These circulate in the blood stream, and if their levels fall, body swelling follows.
* Often a history of alcohol abuse, hepatitis, drugs toxic to the liver.
* Easy bruising, blood-stained vomit.
* Tiredness, loss of sexual drive, clubbed fingers.
* Tiny, spider-like red veins on face, upper body.
* Red palms.
* Swelling of the abdomen, with fluid.
* Jaundice is a late symptom, as is confusion, coma.

■ MALNUTRITION
Globally, this is a major cause of swelling in children:
* Swollen abdomen.
* Patchy pigmentation of body.
* Apathy, coarse skin, lack of resistance to infection.

■ MALABSORPTION
A possibilty in those with chronic bowel disease, for example coeliac disease or ulcerative colitis — which interfere with absorption of nutrients. Some general symptoms include:
* Failure to thrive (children); diarrhoea, smelly, greasy stools.
* Bleeding from bowel.
* Chronic abdominal pain.
* Recurrent, severe chest infections.
* Clubbing of finger nails.

RARE

■ NEPHROTIC SYNDROME
The term describes generalized swelling associated with low blood protein and heavy loss of protein in the urine. There are many causes, including drugs and chronic infections, as well as kidney disease. In childhood it is commonest in boys of two to four years, giving a characteristic, gradually developing picture of:
* Puffy face, swollen eyelids.

* Abdomen distended with fluid.
* Breathlessness, tiredness.

Recovery depends on the cause. Children usually recover completely.

■ VITAMIN B1 DEFICIENCY
Otherwise called beri-beri. Vitamin B1 (thiamine) is found in whole-grain cereals including rice, and in liver. In developed countries, the deficiency is likely only through severe deprivation.
* Early symptoms are tender calves and vague weakness.
* Then swelling of legs, palpitations.
* Eventually, general swelling, exhaustion, rapid pulse.

B1 deficiency can take other forms, particularly in children. Treatment with B1 gives dramatic improvement within hours. Many manufactured foods and cereals contain added levels of this vitamin.

SWOLLEN PART OF BODY

PROBABLE
INJURY
INFECTION
DEPENDENT OEDEMA

POSSIBLE
LYMPHATIC OBSTRUCTION
VENOUS THROMBOSIS

RARE
ALLERGY
FILARIASIS
CANCER

PROBABLE

■ INJURY
Tissue swelling is the normal reaction to any modest injury, together with reddened, warm skin.

■ INFECTION
Including insect bites and minor cuts.
* Throbbing pain, redness.
* Swelling of local lymph glands.
* Pus may be visible.

■ DEPENDENT OEDEMA
Older people who are inactive frequently notice this, one of the commonest reasons for a mild degree of ankle swelling.
* General health good.
* Swelling lessens if activity is increased.

No need for treatment unless it is a nuisance.

POSSIBLE

■ LYMPHATIC OBSTRUCTION
Also known as lymphoedema. Results from interference with the lymphatic channels, which drain away tissue fluid. Commonest after surgery in the groin or armpit — typically to treat breast cancer. In rare cases it can be congenital.

'GENERAL' SYMPTOMS

* Gross swelling of limb.
* Swelling becomes hard; does not 'pit' when pressed.

■ VENOUS THROMBOSIS
Acute swelling of a limb, nearly always a leg, suggests thrombosis. It occurs when clotted blood obstructs a blood vessel.
* Acute onset of pain in calf.
* Swelling and warmth of calf.

If confirmed, needs anti-coagulants to reduce the risk of a pulmonary embolus *(see page 225)*.

RARE

■ ALLERGY
In reaction to an insect bite or injection.
* Limb swells dramatically in a few seconds.
* Swelling may spread to body, lips, throat.
* At worst, difficulty breathing, collapse *(see page 468)*.

■ FILARIASIS
A tropical worm infestation capable of causing massive swelling of limbs (elephantiasis).

■ CANCER
Suspected in otherwise unexplained swelling of a limb. Long bones are the likeliest sites.
* Persistent pain, tenderness.
* Enlarged local lymph nodes.

Cancer may also obstruct the drainage of fluid from a limb: for example, pelvic cancers may cause swelling in the legs.

WEIGHT LOSS WITH ANAEMIA

See LOOKING PALE OR ANAEMIC, PLUS LOSING WEIGHT, page 422.

WEIGHT LOSS AND LACK OF APPETITE

See NO APPETITE, LOSING WEIGHT, page 475.

WEIGHT LOSS — PROGRESSIVE

Persistent, progressive weight loss ranks as one of the major symptoms of disease.

People with weight loss usually seek help at an early stage, when other features of disease may not be prominent.

Obtaining the individual's full background story usually reveals other symptoms, for example, abdominal pain, and these may lead to tentative diagnosis.

The following are some of the possibilities for which there are few other symptoms to point the way. Many of these possibilities are considered in more detail elsewhere in the book.

PROBABLE
DIABETES MELLITUS
ANXIETY
CANCER OF THE STOMACH

POSSIBLE
CHRONIC INFECTION
ANOREXIA NERVOSA
HYPERTHYROIDISM
PYLORIC STENOSIS
TUBERCULOSIS
CANCER — GENERAL

RARE
MALABSORPTION
PARASITE INFECTION
KIDNEY DISEASE
HIV INFECTION/AIDS

PROBABLE

■ DIABETES MELLITUS
In young adults and children, the onset of diabetes tends to be dramatic: rapid weight loss is prominent, alongside thirst and excessive urine output. *See page 485.*

■ ANXIETY
A modest, slow weight loss could reasonably be put down to anxiety in the absence of other symptoms, and where there is no other clear cause for concern. Anxiety should not divert attention from the significance of a steady weight loss, particularly in adults, where other causes must be excluded.

■ CANCER OF THE STOMACH
Early detection of this cancer gives the best hope of cure. For this reason, the possibility is considered in any adult with weight loss, especially if there is also:
* Loss of appetite.
* Blood in vomit or in motions.
* Pain in upper abdomen.
* Feeling of fullness after eating only a small amount.
* Indigestion appearing for the first time in someone over the age of 40.

POSSIBLE

■ CHRONIC INFECTION
This includes chronic abscesses — *see page 447.*

■ ANOREXIA NERVOSA
Excessive dieting, usually in young women who have a distorted image of their true size. *See page 424.*

■ HYPERTHYROIDISM
Weight loss alone is unusual, unless the accompanying tremor and sweating have been overlooked. The full picture is described on *page 479.*

■ PYLORIC STENOSIS
A childhood condition: part of the intestine is obstructed, causing profuse vomiting and rapid weight loss a few weeks after birth. *See page 144.*

■ TUBERCULOSIS
The poor, alcoholics and people from underdeveloped countries might have this serious but curable infection. *See page 447.*

■ CANCER — GENERAL
Laymen and doctors think of cancer to explain weight loss in

the 40-plus age group. It is by no means the only explanation, yet it remains true that, occasionally, an advanced cancer, which has spread around the body, produces only vague symptoms until a late stage. So, be aware of your body: report to your doctor any unusual changes such as bleeding, swellings, weight loss, pain or prolonged cough.

RARE

■ MALABSORPTION
This causes weight loss by preventing the absorption of food. Associated symptoms are:
* Difficulty in swallowing.
* Anaemia.
* Recurrent abdominal pains, intermittent diarrhoea, greasy stools.
* Bleeding into stools.

Underlying causes include cancer of the gullet, which causes very rapid weight loss, ulcerative colitis, Crohn's disease, coeliac disease and chronic pancreatitis.

■ PARASITE INFECTION
Not a usual cause of weight loss. Diagnosis is confirmed by identifying cysts in stools.

■ KIDNEY DISEASE
At the early stage of causing weight loss, this needs to be confirmed by blood tests.
See page 467.

■ HIV INFECTION/AIDS
Now to be considered in any case of vague ill-health, weight loss, fevers and cough, particularly when an individual is at increased risk: homosexuals, bisexuals, intravenous drug users.

Heterosexuals, too, are increasingly affected by the HIV virus.

LOSING WEIGHT PLUS JAUNDICE

The combination points to disease of the liver and related parts of the digestive system. Appearance in adults must trigger a careful search for a primary cancer, which may have spread to involve the liver. The jaundice results from obstruction to bile flow from the liver.

PROBABLE
CANCER OF THE PANCREAS
SECONDARY CANCER OF LIVER

POSSIBLE
CANCER OF THE STOMACH
PERNICIOUS ANAEMIA

RARE
CANCER OF GALL BLADDER

PROBABLE

■ CANCER OF THE PANCREAS
The pancreas lies at the back of the abdomen, partly surrounding the

bile duct. The tumour blocks the bile duct, producing jaundice.
* Initially, vague upper abdominal pain.
* Weight loss.
* Painless jaundice.

■ SECONDARY CANCER OF LIVER
Cancers of many kinds can spread around the body from their original site. The liver is a common secondary site. The primary cancer is likely to have shown itself already, with symptoms such as:
* Weight loss.
* Pain.
* Swelling.
* Unusual bleeding.

POSSIBLE

■ CANCER OF STOMACH
See STOMACH DISEASE, page 164.

■ PERNICIOUS ANAEMIA
The combination of anaemia and a yellow tinge to the skin gives an impression of jaundice. The diagnosis is based on blood tests. *See page 421*. Treatment reverses symptoms.

RARE

■ CANCER OF GALL BLADDER
A disease of the elderly, causing symptoms similar to gall stones.
* Recurrent pains in the right upper abdomen.
* Jaundice.

POSTURE APPEARS STIFF AND HUNCHED

PROBABLE
AGEING

POSSIBLE
ANKYLOSING SPONDYLITIS
PARKINSON'S DISEASE
PAGET'S DISEASE

RARE
TUBERCULOSIS OF THE SPINE
RICKETS

PROBABLE

■ AGEING
With age, bone density is lost and there is shrinkage of the discs between the vertebrae — the bones which link together to form the spine. In some post-menopausal women, rapid thinning of bone, or osteoporosis, takes place, leaving the vertebrae somewhat delicate and liable to collapse.
* Posture becomes hunched over several years.
* Collapse of a vertebra causes a sudden change of posture plus pain.

Calcium and hormone replacement therapy are being used increasingly to help delay and alleviate this process.

'General' Symptoms

POSSIBLE

■ ANKYLOSING SPONDYLITIS
A disease that begins in early adult life, especially affecting men. Over many years, the normal joints and ligaments of the spine are replaced by inflexible bone. Genetically transmitted.
* Initially just back pain, and morning stiffness of the spine.
* The back becomes increasingly rigid, with a stooped posture.
* Eventually, spine movements are severely restricted.

The stooped posture, though not totally avoidable, need not be as severe a problem as in the past, thanks to improvements in treatment.

■ PARKINSON'S DISEASE
See page 438. A neurological disease rarely present before the age of 50. The main symptoms are:
* Tremor of the hands at rest.
* Stooped, inflexible posture.
* Shuffling gait.
* Immobile facial expression.

■ PAGET'S DISEASE
A disorder of bone formation, quite common in a mild form in later life and frequently causing no symptoms.
* Pain in bones.
* Legs becomes bowed, back stoops; head may enlarge (hat size may increase).
* Deafness.

Advanced cases are generally easy to recognize, but usually X-rays and blood tests are needed to confirm the diagnosis.

RARE

■ TUBERCULOSIS (TB) OF THE SPINE
This used to be common. The infection destroys bone.
* Increasing pain and stiffness in part of the spine.
* Other features of TB such as malaise, weight loss, cough, night sweats.

■ RICKETS
A bone disease caused by a disturbance in the way calcium is incorporated. Other symptoms include some bone pain, bow legs and weakness. Associated with poor diet and living conditions. Cured by taking vitamin D.

LOOKING OLD BEFORE YOUR TIME

POSSIBLE
SMOKING
HYPOTHYROIDISM
SUN DAMAGE (HOT CLIMATES)

RARE
HEREDITARY CAUSES

POSSIBLE

■ SMOKING
This is known to accelerate lining of the face and coarsening of the skin.

■ HYPOTHYROIDISM
See page 461. This common condition makes the skin thicken and coarsen.

■ SUN DAMAGE
In hot, sunny climates, such as that of Australasia, sun damage is the most common cause of a prematurely aged appearance.

RARE

■ HEREDITARY CAUSES
With one exceptionally rare condition, progeria, growth ceases by about three years of age, and the child becomes mentally retarded, bald and develops a beaked nose.

BODY SIZE, SHRINKING

PROBABLE
OSTEOPOROSIS

RARE
PAGET'S DISEASE OF BONE

PROBABLE

■ OSTEOPOROSIS
See page 276.

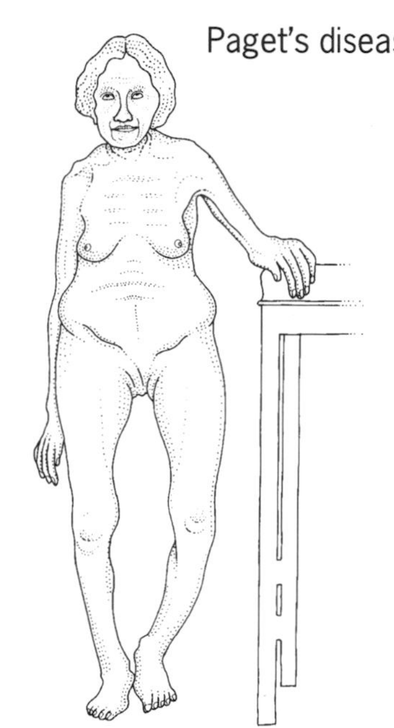

RARE

■ PAGET'S DISEASE OF BONE
Also known as osteitis deformans. Abnormal turnover of bone causing thickening and deformity of bones, particularly the skull, and the long bones. The bone, despite appearing thicker, is weaker than normal bone. The disease affects men and women equally, but rarely affects people from Asia, Africa and the Middle East. It normally appears after the age of 40. Although often symptom-free, there may be:
* Bony deformities. The skull may appear large; often, only one bone is affected.
* Fractures.
* Kyphosis (*see page 288)* causing apparent height loss.
* Heart failure, due to increased workload on heart.

'GENERAL' SYMPTOMS

* Vision and hearing deteriorate as deformed bone damages nerves.

Diseased bone can, very rarely, develop into a malignant bone tumour — osteosarcoma. Diagnosis is confirmed by blood tests.

TREMBLING OR SHAKING

PROBABLE
NATURAL PHYSIOLOGICAL CAUSE
BENIGN ESSENTIAL TREMOR

POSSIBLE
HYPERTHYROIDISM
PARKINSON'S DISEASE

RARE
BRAIN DISEASE
SYPHILIS

PROBABLE

■ NATURAL PHYSIOLOGICAL CAUSE
How steady are your hands? Everyone has tremor to a greater or lesser degree.
* Mostly causes no interference with delicate manual activities.
* Worsened by anxiety, alcohol, stimulants such as coffee, some drugs.

■ BENIGN ESSENTIAL TREMOR
An exaggerated form of normal tremor and an embarrassment rather than a disease.
* Hereditary.
* Slow tremor, affecting upper limbs and head.
* Gradually worsens with age.

POSSIBLE

■ HYPERTHYROIDISM
See page 433. An over-active thyroid gland causes an exaggeration of normal tremor.

■ PARKINSON'S DISEASE
Trembling movements of the thumb and forefinger:
* An early symptom is loss of normal swinging of arms when walking.
* Limbs held rigid, slowing of all movements.
* Tremor at rest, diminishing on activity.
* Immobile, 'mask-like' facial appearance.
* Handwriting becomes increasingly small.

There are now many useful treatments for this common disorder.

RARE

■ BRAIN DISEASE
Brain tumours, strokes, multiple sclerosis and head injuries may all cause tremors. Associated symptoms might include:
* Paralysis of one side of the body.
* Progressive headache, blurring of vision.

* Change of personality.
* Deterioration of memory, slurring of speech.
* Noticeable flicking movements of the eyes.
* Difficulty in walking.

■ SYPHILIS
Though syphilis is now rare, its effects can appear many years after infection, so it is still routinely considered as a possible cause of dementia.
* Dementia.
* Tremor of the head and the lips.
* Stiff legs.

TWITCHING

Uncontrollable, short-lived muscle jerks. The gulf between the common twitches and those with a serious cause is so wide that there should rarely be any reason to suspect disease in the absence of other symptoms.

PROBABLE
HABIT
SPASMODIC TORTICOLLIS

POSSIBLE
BENIGN FIBRILLATION
EPILEPSY

RARE
CHOREA
GILLES DE LA TOURETTE SYNDROME
MOTOR NEURONE DISEASE
KIDNEY FAILURE

PROBABLE

■ HABIT
Blinking and similar grimaces, normal in everyone to a degree, which sometimes become excessive. Deserves sympathy even in grubby, twitching schoolboys, in whom it disappears gradually.
* Typically young boys or nervous adults.
* Frequency increases under stress.

No satisfactory treatment and, please remember, sufferers really cannot help it.

■ SPASMODIC TORTICOLLIS
Recurrent jerking of the neck to one side.
* A disorder of the middle-aged.
* The individual is otherwise perfectly well.

Treatment with botulinum toxin looks promising.

POSSIBLE

■ BENIGN FIBRILLATION
A part of a muscle that twitches spontaneously; the thigh is a common site, probably because it is easily noticed.
* Other muscles unaffected.

* Muscle strength normal.
* Disappears after a few days.

■ EPILEPSY
Spasmodic jerking of limbs is a feature of most forms of epilepsy:
* Same limb is affected each time.
* Brief warning before the jerking episode starts.
* May progress to a generalized fit, with loss of consciousness, incontinence, foaming at mouth.
There is usually very little doubt that epilepsy is the cause.

RARE

■ CHOREA
Irregular movements of limbs. Rheumatic fever was once a common cause; *see page 448.* Other neurological conditions with twitching as a feature include Huntington's chorea:
* A strong family history.
* Disintegration of personality in middle-age.
* Eventually, dementia, epilepsy, paralysis.

■ GILLES DE LA TOURETTE SYNDROME
A disorder with a reputation out of all proportion to its rarity.
* Onset in adolescence.
* Multiple tics.
* Abrupt swearing, grunting.
* Echoing other people's words.

■ MOTOR NEURONE DISEASE
Exceptionally rare, tragic disease causing deterioration of muscle function in middle-age.
* Begins with loss of bulk of muscles in hands.
* Muscle-wasting spreads generally.
* Widespread twitching of muscles may be seen.
* Mental function remains intact.
* Eventually, paralysis.

■ KIDNEY FAILURE
A late symptom in someone already known to have kidney disease:
* Nausea, vomiting.
* Twitching of muscles.
* Clouded consciousness.
* Spontaneous bleeding.
* Low urine output.

FEVER, INTRODUCTION

Just why the body produces fever in response to illness is still not fully understood. Presumably it helps in some way to fight illness, but exactly how is still surprisingly controversial.

Since ancient times, fever has been recognized as a key signal that someone is unwell. Fevers tell us much about the illness itself: not only is it important to take account of its severity, but also of its variation during the day, and over the course of the illness.

Modern medicine offers diagnosis and treatment of most prolonged fevers, replacing the long, anxious period of observation until the fever breaks.

WHEN TO START WORRYING?
With the decline of serious infections, at least in developed countries, the onset of fever should not cause alarm. In the

very young and in the elderly, fever still calls for a careful assessment of health; but in older children and for much of adult life a day or two of raised temperature will usually be the prelude to one of the minor illnesses considered in the following pages. Of course, there are more sinister causes, but they are rare, and fever alone is unlikely to raise even the professional's suspicions.

Before worrying about serious disease, look at the individual's overall condition, assessing:

* Risk factors for unusual disease, for example, foreign travel, poor sanitation, epidemics.
* Rapid onset of a high fever — greater than 40°C/104°F.
* Severe headache or delirium.
* Pain.
* Night sweats.
* A rapid pulse or fast breathing, remembering that:
* Pulse rate rises by about ten beats per minute for every 0.5 degree Centigrade rise in temperature.
* A baby's normal pulse rate is about 120 per minute, even at one year of age.

TAKING TEMPERATURE

An adult's normal temperature is conventionally taken to be 37°C/ 98.4°F, based on a mouth reading. You may have a temperature half a degree either way and be perfectly well. In children, temperature can be measured under the armpit, in which case 36.5°C/97.7°F is the norm.

Take into account:

* Mouth breathers, whose mouth temperature is lower than normal.
* The amount of clothing worn may raise or lower temperature.
* Warm or cold drinks alter temperature in the mouth for about 15 minutes.

Feeling the brow offers comfort, but is not very reliable, especially if there is a low-level fever, with sweat on the forehead that cools the skin.

FEVER: THE POSSIBILITIES

To list all the hundreds of possible reasons for fever would simply be confusing. Instead, we look, on the following pages, at fevers of different durations. We believe that this is how you will usually meet the problem.

The possibilities listed are those expected in a developed country. There is a separate section (*see page 450*) on tropical diseases. We remind you again that fever in the very young and very old demands special attention, and that in any case, concern about a person's overall condition means you must get professional advice, even if the fever itself is minor.

FEVER, THE FIRST 48 HOURS, page 442.
FEVER, 3 TO 14 DAYS, page 444.
FEVER LASTING TWO WEEKS OR MORE, page 446.
FEVER, RECURRENT ATTACKS, page 449.
FEVER IN OR AFTER VISITING THE TROPICS, page 450.

FEVER, THE FIRST 48 HOURS

See also FEVER, INTRODUCTION page 440. Along with the fever there will be some combination of chills, muscular aches, sweating, a mild headache and fatigue.

PROBABLE
VIRAL ILLNESS
EAR INFECTION
TONSILLITIS
CHEST INFECTION

POSSIBLE
URINARY INFECTION
CHICKENPOX
RUBELLA
MUMPS
SCARLET FEVER

RARE
MENINGITIS

PROBABLE

■ VIRAL ILLNESS
Including the build-up to a common cold; *see page 454.*
* Mild sore throat.
* Symptoms oscillate between mild and irritating within hours.
* Sniffing and sneezing begins after a couple of days,
* Or the illness fades away leaving you, and your doctor, none the wiser.

Mumps

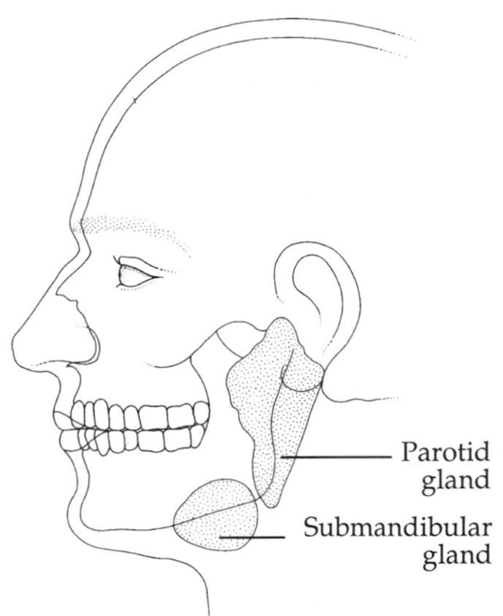

■ EAR INFECTION
Very common in children, sometimes with no other symptoms.
* Typically, the child already has a cold.
* Abrupt onset of pain in ear.
* Babies just begin crying and will not settle, even with comforting. They may shake their head, or rub an ear.
* Occasionally progresses to a burst ear drum, causing a green/yellow, possibly bloodstained discharge for a few days. Healing over a couple of weeks is the norm.

Painkillers will help the symptoms. The role of antibiotics is controversial: currently they are advised.

■ TONSILLITIS
The picture presented is usually unmistakeable:
* Pain in the throat, worse on swallowing.

* Swollen neck glands.
* Nasal twang to speech.
* Breath smells foul.
* White spots on the tonsils.

■ CHEST INFECTION
Again, the picture is usually clear.
* Cough. * Phlegm.
* Chest pain when breathing deeply.

POSSIBLE

■ URINARY INFECTION
* Pain or burning sensation when passing urine.
* A need to pass urine frequently.
* Aching over the kidneys.
* In severe cases, rigors, blood in the urine.
* In babies, there may be no symptoms other than fever and irritability, hence the need to test urine in a feverish infant.

■ CHICKENPOX
A viral illness causing small blisters over the body, in the mouth and in the scalp. Usually occurs in epidemics. Incubates for about 14-21 days after contact with another carrier.
* Itchy rash appears within 48 hours of fever.
* Rash lasts for two or three weeks.

The rash consists of spots, which tend to appear in crops and soon become blisters; they dry out and become scabs.

Usually a mild, though miserable, illness calling for plenty of care and attention.

■ RUBELLA — GERMAN MEASLES
Mild in itself but notorious because of the risk it poses to the developing baby if the mother catches it during early pregnancy. For this reason there are public health vaccination programmes which have made the disease less common.
* A fine, red-brown rash appearing after 24-48 hours of fever.
* Rash with no particular pattern to its spread appears all at once.
* Swollen tender glands at the back of the skull.
* In adults, commonly accompanied by mild arthritis lasting for some weeks.

■ MUMPS
An infection of the salivary glands, increasingly uncommon thanks to vaccination programmes. The incubation period is two to three weeks.
* Non-specific fever and chills for 24-48 hours..
* Then the salivary glands enlarge at the angles of the jaw and just in front of the ears.
* The illness settles in five to ten days.
* Complications can give pain in the testicles and the abdomen, and cause deafness, but these are rare.

■ SCARLET FEVER
Onset is sudden with high fever, sore throat or even tonsillitis; *see above*.
* A very fine generalized red rash after 24-48 hours.
* The rash spares the area around the mouth, giving it a contrasting, white appearance.
* Furred tongue goes from whitish to raw over a few days.

Scarlet fever was once much

feared because it could cause rheumatic fever *(see page 448)* and nephritis *(see page 430)*. These complications are now extremely rare. However, penicillin is still necessary if scarlet fever is diagnosed.

RARE

■ MENINGITIS
Mentioned here as a reminder that it should be considered in any feverish child, especially if the child shows:
* Drowsiness.
* Stiff neck.
* A wish to avoid bright lights.
* Sudden appearance of a fine purple rash.
* And, in a baby, a bulging soft spot (fontanelle) on the top of the head.

If suspected, this is a medical emergency and help must be sought.

FEVER, 3 TO 14 DAYS

See also FEVER, INTRODUCTION page 440. Minor viral illness is still likely to underlie this symptom, just as with fever lasting 48 hours *(see page 442)*. However, the need to consider less common illnesses arises.

PROBABLE
VIRAL ILLNESS
MEASLES
ROSEOLA

POSSIBLE
GLANDULAR FEVER
PNEUMONIA
ABDOMINAL INFECTION
INFECTIOUS HEPATITIS
ROSS RIVER FEVER AND Q FEVER

RARE
TYPHOID/PARATYPHOID FEVER
SEPTICAEMIA
ENDOCARDITIS

PROBABLE

■ VIRAL ILLNESS
No rash, no progression, and no other symptoms apart from sweats, aches and generally feeling unwell. But although the cause is probably a virus, it is prudent to review the diagnosis every few days, considering the possibility of any of the following:

■ MEASLES
'Measles is misery' sums up this childhood illness, now avoidable thanks to vaccination. It usually occurs in epidemics, with an incubation period of 10 to 14 days from being infected by another carrier.

* A miserable, snuffly, coughing child with bloodshot eyes who wants to avoid bright lights.
* Delirium at night is common.
* White spots may be seen in the mouth by the back teeth.
* A blotchy red rash appears after four days of fever, spreading downwards, from face via chest to the limbs.
* The child continues feverish for several more days as the illness subsides.

Measles is a serious problem in underdeveloped countries, but in developed countries its complications, such as pneumonia or encephalitis, are rare.

■ ROSEOLA
A fairly common, harmless viral illness which can fool doctors into suspecting measles.
* High fever for three to four days; the child is snuffly.
* A pinkish rash appears over the body.
* The fever stops, and the child perks up.

POSSIBLE

■ GLANDULAR FEVER *(see also page 462).*
* Bad sore throat or tonsillitis.
* Fever and fatigue persisting for weeks or months.

The problem usually clears up.

■ PNEUMONIA
Certain forms of pneumonia are known for causing fever alone, without the other, more dramatic symptoms of pneumonia.
* Slight cough.
* Feeling vaguely unwell; fatigue, night sweats.

A chest X-ray confirms the diagnosis and treatment is straightforward.

■ ABDOMINAL INFECTION
Suspect this if fever starts soon after abdominal surgery, or after abdominal pain. Prolonged fever can signal an abscess in any of the abdominal organs, the commoner ones being:

The appendix, preceded by a few days of pain, which may start centrally but then settles low down on the right.

The large intestine: pain in the left lower side, possibly bleeding from the back passage, intermittent diarrhoea.

Infected ovaries or fallopian tubes: lower abdominal pain, vaginal discharge.

■ INFECTIOUS HEPATITIS
This is now known to be caused by several different viruses, hepatitis B being the dangerous form, spread by shared needles used for intravenous drug abuse and unprotected homo- and hetrosexual intercourse. The incubation period of hepatitis A is a few weeks, of hepatitis B a few months.
* Fever, chills, joint pains, back aches; generally feeling unwell for a week.
* Jaundice — yellowish discolouration of the skin — first spotted in the whites of the eyes; then the skin turns yellow.
* Darkening of urine, light stool colour.

There is no treatment other than

rest. With hepatitis B there is a risk of long-term liver damage. Those at risk, including people exposed to blood in their work, should be vaccinated against hepatitis B.

■ ROSS RIVER FEVER
A mosquito-borne infection that occurs in Australia's Ross River and Murray River areas, and elsewhere in the south-west Pacific.
* 3 to 14-day incubation.
* Fever, joint pains, enlarged lymph nodes.
* Tingling in the hands and feet.
* A rash.
Recovery takes about a month.

■ Q FEVER
A tick-borne infection spread through contact with cows and sheep, hence its association with Australia — though it occurs elsewhere.
* Incubation period up to two or three weeks.
* Abrupt high fever, muscle aches, headache.
* A cough, due to a kind of pneumonia.
The diagnosis relies on chest X-ray and blood tests. Full recovery is usual, though it may take several weeks.

RARE

■ TYPHOID OR PARATYPHOID FEVER
Infections spread via food and water in conditions of poor sanitation. Profuse diarrhoea is a major feature.
* Fever, gradually rising to a peak over a couple of weeks.
* Cough, headache, limb pains.
* After a week, a non-itchy rash appears on the stomach, chest and lower back. In typhoid, it is sparse and rapidly fading; in para–typhoid, more widespread.
* Diarrhoea begins after a week or so, becoming profuse.
Typhoid is still a very serious illness, despite modern antibiotic treatment. Paratyphoid, though less serious, is nevertheless very unpleasant.
Immunization is recommended for many parts of the world.

■ SEPTICAEMIA
This means infection spreading in the blood stream. It is usually a rapidly developing illness causing chills and collapse.

■ ENDOCARDITIS
See page 463. An infection of the valves of the heart, causing chronic illness including fever, anaemia and clubbed finger nails.

FEVER LASTING TWO WEEKS OR MORE

See also FEVER, INTRODUCTION., page 440. By now, fever is a diagnostic challenge. It is likely that someone who is ill as well as feverish for as long as this would be admitted to hospital for investigation.

However, in some people, fever shows itself only with the feeling of being vaguely unwell (malaise) together with night sweats and other symptoms pointing to nothing in particular. Causes now include not only infections, but also rheumatic diseases, connective tissue disease, cancers and drug side effects. But remember that many of the illnesses noted in *FEVER, 3 TO 14 DAYS, page 444,* could still be suspected, along with the following:

PROBABLE
CHRONIC INFECTION
TUBERCULOSIS

POSSIBLE
ULCERATIVE COLITIS
CANCER, LEUKAEMIA
HODGKIN'S DISEASE
RHEUMATOID ARTHRITIS
RHEUMATIC FEVER
SYSTEMIC LUPUS ERYTHEMATOSIS (SLE)

RARE
SYPHILIS
DRUG SIDE-EFFECT
BRUCELLOSIS
AIDS

PROBABLE

■ CHRONIC INFECTION
This is still the likeliest reason for prolonged fever. Recent surgery, together with abdominal pain, could be pointers. Less common causes might include:

Prostatitis *(see page 362*: in men, pain between the legs, burning urine.

Osteomyelitis *(see page 475)*: pain and tenderness in a bone; usually in children. The long bones, typically of the leg, are most commonly involved.

Bronchiectasis *(see page 223)* causing persistent cough, sweats, possibly breathlessness, finger clubbing.

■ TUBERCULOSIS
A significant possibility, causing chronic illness, weakness and infection:
* A low-grade fever.
* Weight loss.
* Cough.
* Night sweats.
* Possibly bloodstained sputum.

POSSIBLE

■ ULCERATIVE COLITIS
A chronic inflammation of the bowel. The early symptoms can be limited to:
* Persistent diarrhoea.
* Low-grade fever.
* Vague malaise.

Once suspicion is aroused, this illness can be rapidly confirmed and treated.

■ CANCER, LEUKAEMIA
Fever otherwise unexplained and lasting for months brings these to mind. There may well be other suspicious symptoms such as:
* Weight loss.
* Unusual pains.
* Unusual bleeding from bowel, bladder, vagina, stomach.
* Chronic cough.

These symptoms may allow the

'GENERAL' SYMPTOMS

cancer to be tracked down. Blood tests will screen for leukaemia. Cancer of the kidney is one tumour well known to cause persistent fever.

■ HODGKIN'S DISEASE
Young people are at most risk of this disease of the lymph glands. As well as fever there will be:
* Persistently swollen, painless glands in the neck, groin or armpits.
* Night sweats.
* Anaemia.
The sooner it is diagnosed, the greater the chance of a complete cure.

■ RHEUMATOID ARTHRITIS
Persistent fever and vague malaise can continue for several weeks. *See page 279.*

■ RHEUMATIC FEVER
Thankfully, a rarity in developed countries but, sadly, common elsewhere. A disease which 'licks the joints but savages the heart'.
* Usually begins after a sore throat.
* Fleeting pains in knees, ankles, elbows.
* Rashes can occur.
* Jerkiness of movement, involuntary movements.
The heart valves are damaged, leaving the child prone to future heart disease.

■ SYSTEMIC LUPUS ERYTHEMATOSIS (SLE)
One of a group of connective tissue disorders in which the body reacts against its own tissues. It can be a very vague illness at first. Commonest in women aged between 30 and 50.
* Rashes, joint pains, malaise.
* A butterfly rash across the cheeks is typical.
Early diagnosis is important to prevent progression to the kidneys or the brain.

RARE

■ SYPHILIS
Characteristically, 6 to 12 weeks after the initial infection, syphilis causes:
* A rash over hands and feet, including the palms and soles.
* Malaise, fever, enlarged lymph nodes; aching joints.
* Wart-like swellings around genitalia and back passage.
Readily treatable.

■ DRUG SIDE-EFFECT
When all else fails, drugs may be suspected as the cause of a persistent fever.

■ BRUCELLOSIS
A disease spread through cow's and goat's milk, and therefore a risk for workers in the dairy industry.
* Gradual onset, with fevers, joint pains, cough, anorexia, night sweats.
* Bouts of fever every few days or every few weeks.
* Often cures itself.

■ AIDS
A risk mainly for drug abusers and homosexuals; but also worryingly present in the heterosexual population.

* Weeks or months of fever and night sweats.
* Diarrhoea, slight swelling of lymph nodes.
* Loss of weight.

The change from being HIV positive to developing AIDS may be signalled by many different symptoms. Prolonged fever is just one of these.

FEVER, RECURRENT ATTACKS

See FEVER, INTRODUCTION, page 440. Apart from brucellosis, most of these infections are somewhat unusual in developed countries. Their symptoms return after a period of apparent recovery. This is in contrast to the far more conventional pattern of infections in which there is fever by day or by night, whose disappearance can be taken as a reliable sign of recovery.

POSSIBLE
BRUCELLOSIS
MALARIA
TYPHOID

RARE
DENGUE
RELAPSING FEVER
TRYPANOSOMIASIS
YELLOW FEVER

POSSIBLE

■ BRUCELLOSIS
A disease spread through unpasteurised milk or cheeses, or through contact with cows and goats. It gives rise to bouts of fever for days at a time, which appear to settle, only to recur after weeks or months. *See also page 446.*

■ MALARIA
See page 453. Anyone who has returned from abroad, and who has been in an area where malaria is present, and who develops a high temperature and chills should be suspected of having this dangerous illness particularly if they have not been taking anti-malaria tablets. Depending on the type of malaria, the episodes of fever and shaking return every three or four days.

The fever may recur some months after foreign travel.

■ TYPHOID
A feverish illness causing severe diarrhoea, spread through poor sanitation or contaminated water, or food — mainly shellfish products. *See page 446.* The illness takes three to four weeks to run its course.

RARE

Meaning rare in developed countries. Elsewhere these are fairly common diseases, but they pose a relatively small risk for tourists. Enquire locally about areas where these diseases might be a hazard. If you develop feverish illness soon after returning from a danger area, report it to a doctor without delay, being ready with details of where you have been.

■ DENGUE
A mosquito-borne infection of south-east Asia and Africa.
* Begins with sudden fever, aches and rash.
* Severe pains in the bones are particularly characteristic.
* Improvement over about a week.
* Relapse after another few days, with a more widespread rash.
Recovery takes several weeks.

■ RELAPSING FEVER
Spread by ticks. Common in Africa, India, South America and parts of the Mediterranean.
* Abrupt high fever and confusion lasting for about a week.
* Then apparent recovery, followed by relapse after another week or so.
* Several further relapses may occur.
Effective treatment exists.

■ TRYPANOSOMIASIS
Sleeping sickness. Different forms exist in Africa and South America. Treatment, started early, is quite effective. After an insect bite there is typically:
* Painful swelling at the site of the bite.
* Then relapsing fevers, enlarged lymph nodes.
* Eventually, after months or years, lethargy, continuous mild confusion, headaches, drowsiness.

■ YELLOW FEVER
Especially prevalent in Africa, Central and South America. There is no specific treatment for this serious illness, but vaccination is effective.
* Abrupt fever, rigors, jaundice.
* Signs of improvement by fourth or fifth day.
* Relapse during the next week with more fever, jaundice.

FEVER IN OR AFTER VISITING THE TROPICS

Tropical disease should always be considered in someone who becomes feverish soon after returning from a 'Third World' country or, indeed, certain developed countries where they are a known risk. The following are the commoner examples, rather than an exhaustive catalogue, of these many dangerous diseases. If suspected, seek help urgently: you will probably be sent to a specialist centre.

Protective measures and vaccinations exist for many of these diseases and anyone likely to be at risk should see their doctor to arrange these before travelling. Some of the measures require time to become effective.

The most likely tropical disease is malaria, common in Africa, India, the Far East. Symptoms include high fever, drenching sweats and rigors. *See page 453.*

Among the rarities are:
PLAGUE: Far East, Africa, India, South America. It is a flea-borne illness, with dramatic onset, high

fever, delirium and tender, swollen lymph nodes (glands) in the groin.

RELAPSING FEVER: South America, Africa, India, Near East. Sudden high fever, rigors, delirium. Liver and spleen enlarge.

SLEEPING SICKNESS: tropical Africa. Spread by the tse-tse fly. At first fever, enlarged lymph nodes, anaemia. Later (months, years), drowsiness, tremors, fits.

TYPHUS FEVER: a term covering several diseases, named for the areas where they are found, for example, Rocky Mountain spotted fever. Fever increasing over several days, with headache, red eyes, rash, delirium.

YELLOW FEVER: Africa, especially West Africa and South America. Fever with rigors and jaundice. Effective vaccination exists.

ABNORMALLY LOW TEMPERATURE

Defined as a fall in 'core' body temperature to below about 35°C/95°F when measured via the rectum (rear passage). Technical term: hypothermia. Below about 32°C/89.5°C, there will be drowsiness, apathy, coma and eventually death.

Those at risk are the elderly without adequate heating and the new-born. Cold new-born babies do not shiver: they become lethargic, with cold limbs.

Hypothermia is an emergency, requiring immediate warmth and warm fluids. Severe hypothermia requires gradual, carefully monitored rewarming. Rapid heating up is dangerous.

Elderly people who suddenly become confused in the winter may be suffering from hypothermia.

It is not advisable to give alcohol to an elderly person whom you suspect is suffering from hypothermia. It may worsen their condition.

PROBABLE
EXPOSURE TO COLD

POSSIBLE
EXCESS ALCOHOL

RARE
HYPOTHYROIDISM
DRUG SIDE-EFFECT

PROBABLE

■ <u>EXPOSURE TO COLD</u>
* Shivering, feeling cold.
* Then apathy, slurred speech, difficulty in concentrating.
* Finally confusion, coma.

Remember, babies cannot control their temperatures as adults do. They are at risk in low temperatures, unless kept warm.

'GENERAL' SYMPTOMS

POSSIBLE

■ EXCESS ALCOHOL
By dilating blood vessels, alcohol increases heat loss. Add confusion (if not unconsciousness) following a heavy drinking bout, plus cold conditions, and there is potential for serious danger.

RARE

■ HYPOTHYROIDISM
A grossly underactive thyroid gland can cause severe hypothermia. It is rare nowadays for this degree of underactivity not to be noticed. *See page 461.*

■ DRUG SIDE-EFFECT
Anti-depressants and tranquillizers can make temperature drop. Usually this is a trivial effect, unless the drugs are taken in overdose or combined with self-neglect, alcohol and exposure to the elements.

SHIVERS OR CHILLS PLUS FEVER AND HEADACHE

In adults, this combination of symptoms, in a mild form, is not unusual and is often the earliest sign of a viral illness. In children this is by far the most likely reason, but other possibilities need to be considered, especially if the headache seems to be the major feature.

PROBABLE
COMMON COLD
INFLUENZA

POSSIBLE
CHEST INFECTION
INFECTION ELSEWHERE

RARE
MENINGITIS
WEIL'S DISEASE
MALARIA
OTHER TROPICAL DISEASE
TYPHUS

PROBABLE

■ COMMON COLD
See page 454.

■ INFLUENZA
See VIRAL ILLNESS, page 442.

POSSIBLE

■ CHEST INFECTION
These three symptoms in combination can be a feature of severe chest infections.

■ INFECTION ELSEWHERE
Any infection in the body may give this combination of symptoms. Parts of the body which might give rise to them when infected range from joints, through internal organs, to the skin.

Consider whether you have any other noticeable symptoms and look those up too.

RARE

The possibilities below are the less unusual rarities that someone in a developed country might encounter.

■ MENINGITIS
An infection of the brain and surrounding tissues. Meningitis is mainly a disease of childhood. The condition is checked for as a matter of routine if a baby appears to be seriously ill.
* The illness may develop rapidly over a few hours.
* Light hurts the eyes.
* Pain or stiffness in the neck on trying to lift the head.
* Nausea and vomiting.
* Drowsiness, delirium or coma.

Meningitis in the very young can occur in outbreaks, and on the face of it can seem identical to a simple viral illness. So, if you hear of meningitis in your locality, be on the look-out for:
* Excessive irritability, or worsening of an existing condition.
* Temperature rises higher than expected.
* Pain on being moved about.
* Inability to feed or drink adequately.
* Fine purple rash.

Always seek help or advice at an early stage. If later still in doubt, check again with your doctor. If suspected, immediate medical attention is required.

■ WEIL'S DISEASE
Rats spread this disease by infecting lakes, canals, sewers and mines. Swimmers, sailors and canoeists should be aware of this, as should sewage workers, miners or anyone working in a rat-infested area.
* Rapid onset of fever, headache and backache.
* Red eyes.
* A mild degree of jaundice is usual.
* Spontaneous bleeding from mouth, nose may occur.

■ MALARIA
Caused by a parasite spread by mosquitoes. A major risk in the tropics, where mosquitoes enjoy long periods of warmth and humidity. Modern air travel means that malaria can spread to anywhere in the world, so the possibility is worth considering in someone recently returned from Africa, Asia or India, even if they have been taking anti-malaria tablets.
* Attacks every two or three days.
* Attack begins with an hour or two of severe shivering and headache.
* High temperature starts as shivering finishes, and lasts for several hours.
* Heavy sweating.
* In between attacks, the infected person may feel quite well.

If malaria is suspected, seek medical help urgently.

■ OTHER TROPICAL DISEASE
If someone recently returned from the tropics becomes ill with high fever, it is safest to suspect tropical

disease first. Which one it is will depend on where they have been staying, and on the features of their illness. Seek medical help urgently.

■ TYPHUS
A general term for a variety of diseases spread by fleas and lice. Found not only in the Third World, but also in parts of America ('Rocky Mountain spotty fever') and in Britain (Lyme disease).
* Illness develops over 7 to 14 days.
* Tenderness and redness of the eyes is typical.
* A rash eventually appears.
* Joints may be painful.

The illness varies from mild to severe, depending on the cause.

A COLD?

Runny nose, itching eyes and aching across the face? Statistics say that you will suffer from this miserable, though trivial, illness two or three times a year. It is usually caused by an infection of the upper respiratory tract, which includes nose, larynx and pharynx. Hence the medical term for a common cold — upper respiratory tract infection, or 'URTI'. Any of more than 100 different viruses may be responsible.

However, a cold might be more than just a cold if the symptoms are recurrent or persistent.

PROBABLE
COMMON COLD

POSSIBLE
HAY FEVER
SINUSITIS
ALLERGY
FOREIGN BODY IN NOSE

RARE
HEAD INJURY COMPLICATION
NASAL TUMOUR

PROBABLE

■ COMMON COLD
A Nobel prize awaits the medical researcher who finds a cure for this condition.
* Begins with a sore or raw throat.
* Increasingly runny nose and sneezing with clear mucus.
* Mucus may turn yellow or green.
* Two or three days of loss of smell and taste.
* Occasionally progresses to a chest infection (*see page* 222).
* The illness runs its course over five to seven days, usually requiring no more than fluids, rest and warmth.
* Antibiotics reserved for those at risk of the cold progressing to a chest infection.

Upper respiratory tract

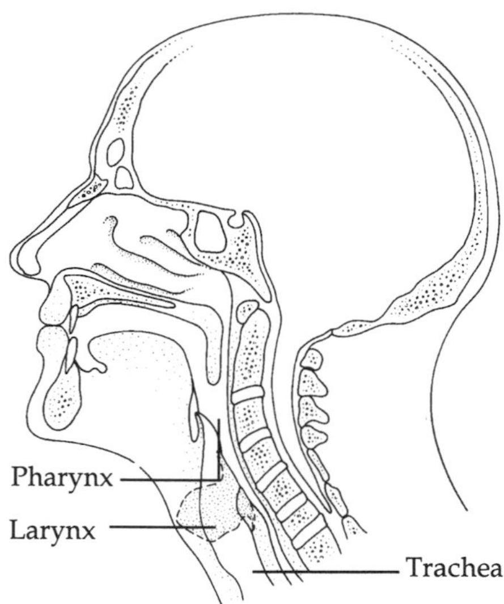

POSSIBLE

■ HAY FEVER
An allergic reaction of the lining of the nose in response to pollens, grass and other irritants.
* Sneezing in specific places or times of year.
* Persistent sniff and blocked nose.
* Itching, watery eyes.
* Sufferers frequently also have eczema or asthma.

■ ALLERGIC RHINITIS
A general term which includes hay fever and perennial rhinitis — 'allergic' runny or streaming nose.
* Reactions as for hay fever, but:
* Provoked by certain environments.

■ SINUSITIS
* Persisting common cold symptoms (*see above*).
* Passage of large quantities of yellow or green mucus.
* Aching across face, above and below the eyes, especially on leaning forward.
* Nasal tone of voice.

■ NASAL POLYPS
Common in people who suffer from allergic rhinitis.
* Visible as fleshy lumps inside the nostrils.
* Constant feeling of blocked nose.
* A peristent sniff with clear nasal discharge.
* Easily removed, but they frequently recur.

■ FOREIGN BODY IN NOSE
Peculiar to small children for whom small, round objects and body openings have a compelling interest.
* Persistent infected discharge from one nostril.
* Discharge may be blood streaked.
* The foreign body, typically a bead, is often visible.

RARE

■ HEAD INJURY COMPLICATION
Leakage of cerebro-spinal fluid, the liquid which surrounds the brain, might be suspected if, after a head injury, there is a persistent, clear watery discharge from the nose.

■ NASAL TUMOUR
* Persistent, one-sided bloody or foul-smelling discharge.

'GENERAL' SYMPTOMS

COLD SYMPTOMS PLUS FEVER

See FEVER LASTING 3 TO 14 DAYS, page 444.

SWEATING

Sweating is one of the body's ways of balancing heat loss against heat gain — an unglamorous, but nonetheless sophisticated mechanism. Normally, it goes on as a background activity with barely noticeable perspiration. Even apparently heavy sweating may not be abnormal if it is serving to regulate temperature.

PROBABLE
EXERCISE
FEVER
STRESS

POSSIBLE
EXCESS ALCOHOL
PAIN

RARE
DRUG-RELATED
TUBERCULOSIS
HIV INFECTION (AIDS)

PROBABLE

■ EXERCISE
It is of course normal that one should sweat when taking vigorous exercise. If you haven't taken any for a long time, and you are also overweight, you may be unpleasantly surprised at how much sweat you produce — but it is normal.
* Perspiration from brow, armpits and back.
* Clearly related to increased levels of exertion.
* Diminishes over a few minutes once exercise is stopped.

■ FEVER
Most fevers are accompanied by sweating. There will be the familiar symptoms of feverish illness such as:
* Aching muscles, headache, malaise, shivering.
* Commonly progressing to a sore throat, cough, earache.

Sweating as part of a feverish illness is less noticeable in the very old and the very young, whose temperature control mechanisms are less efficient than those of adults.

■ STRESS
Or anxiety, which can be described as long-term form of stress, or 'fear spread thin'.
* Sweaty palms, but dry mouth.
* Rapid heartbeat.
* Tension in neck muscles and across forehead.

Those who are prone to chronic anxiety will suffer chronic sweating.

POSSIBLE

■ EXCESS ALCOHOL
Strong drink dilates the blood vessels, and this often causes sweating across the brow.

■ PAIN
Any severe pain causes sweating through nervous reflexes that also cause:
* Pallor, restlessness.
* Rapid pulse.
* Collapse — in severe cases.

Thus sweating would be expected in any of the conditions causing *COLLAPSE (see page 468)*, including heart attacks and severe abdominal pain. But if there has been so much blood loss that the circulation is beginning to fail, clamminess replaces sweating.

RARE

■ DRUG-RELATED
Reactions due to abrupt withdrawal from alcohol or narcotic drugs cause sweating plus:
* Restlessness, muscle pains, drowsiness.
* Runny nose, dilated pupils, abdominal pains (narcotics).
* Tremor, disorientation, hallucinations (alcohol withdrawal).

Several other drugs, including antidepressants, can cause unusual sweating and need to be considered in otherwise unexplained cases.

■ TUBERCULOSIS
Frequent night sweats may well be the first indicator of this serious infection. You should seek a doctor's advice as soon as possible. *See page 447.*

■ HIV INFECTION (AIDS)
AIDS causes sweating as an early symptom. *See page 448.*

HEAVY SWEATING

Covered here are causes of sweating *other* than infectious diseases, for which *see FEVER, pages 440-51.*

PROBABLE
NATURAL TENDENCY

POSSIBLE
HYPERTHYROIDISM
MENOPAUSE

RARE
CARCINOID SYNDROME
PHAEOCHROMOCYTOMA
ACROMEGALY

PROBABLE

■ NATURAL TENDENCY
In other words, the way you are made. Though frequently just a nuisance, it becomes a significant problem if it ruins clothes, causes unpleasant body odour or interferes with manual activities such as draughtsmanship. The problem starts after puberty.

'General' Symptoms

* Hands, armpits or feet pour sweat.
* Symptoms tend to be unrelated to exertion, temperature.

Several effective roll-on and lotion treatments are now available. As a last resort, it is possible to cut the nerves near the spinal cord which control sweating of the hands or feet.

POSSIBLE

■ HYPERTHYROIDISM

See page 433. The thyroid gland could be described as the body's thermostat. Overactivity 'turns up' all aspects of body function. Profuse sweating plus:
* Hyperactivity, jitteriness.
* Bulbous, staring eyes.
* Weight loss, hunger, diarrhoea.
* Trembling hands.
* Fatigue, surprisingly, can be a prominent symptom.

Drug treatment is available. Tends to recur.

■ MENOPAUSE

Even before periods cease, women may be aware of flushes and sweating. Blamed, perhaps unfairly, for a wide range of middle-age symptoms.
* Usually in the 40 to 55 age range.
* Periods become infrequent, then cease.
* Associated with increased wrinkling (loss of elasticity) of skin, irritability or mild depression.
* Sudden sweats at any time, especially at night.
* Tiredness, headache, palpitations.

Modern treatment consists of hormone replacement therapy, which alleviates the symptoms and reduces thinning of the bones. All women should at least be offered the opportunity to consider taking hormone replacement therapy.

RARE

■ CARCINOID SYNDROME

Another hormone disorder. The nervous reactions that accompany changes in mood become grossly exaggerated. Caused by a hormone-secreting tumour in the intestine or liver. The full picture may take years to develop.
* Bouts of profuse watery diarrhoea with excessive bowel sounds.
* Facial flushing and sweating, especially after alcohol.
* Asthma.

■ PHAEOCHROMOCYTOMA

A tumour, which may occur near the kidneys, though not exclusively, causing high blood pressure and sudden, severe bursts of anxiety. It is curable, and though relatively rare, doctors quite often run tests for it if there are:
* High blood pressure, sometimes highly variable.
* Abrupt episodes of headache, sweating, pallor, palpitations.

Tracking the tumour down can be like detective work. Removed by surgery.

■ ACROMEGALY

See page 275.

HEAVY SWEATING AT NIGHT

If this goes on for a few days in an otherwise well person, don't worry. It is, however, a different matter if the symptoms are prolonged, especially if there has been recent illness, surgery or debility. Possibilities revolve around infectious diseases or collections of pus in the body.

PROBABLE
'FLU-LIKE ILLNESS

POSSIBLE
ABSCESS
SUBPHRENIC ABSCESS
ENDOCARDITIS

RARE
TUBERCULOSIS (TB)
BRUCELLOSIS
HODGKIN'S DISEASE
HIV DISEASE/AIDS

PROBABLE

■ 'FLU-LIKE ILLNESS
* Muscle aches.
* Mild headache.
* Sweating can be profuse.

After a few days, symptoms die away, with the possible emergence of a sore throat, cough or similar mild illness.

POSSIBLE

■ ABSCESS
An abscess is a collection of pus; it can form anywhere in the body and can cause mysterious symptoms. Although the symptoms should raise suspicion, blood tests are the only reliable proof of continuing infection. Pain or recent surgery may point to a probable site of infection. When all else fails, modern imaging techniques, such as ultra-sound scan or CT scan can pinpoint the abscess.

■ SUBPHRENIC ABSCESS
A collection of pus underneath the diaphragm. Could be a possibility after abdominal surgery or peritonitis. There may be no more than non-specific features, such as:
* Malaise, sweats, anaemia.
* Recurrent fever.
* Shoulder tip pain is a more tell-tale sign, caused by irritation of the diaphragm.

Treatment involves drainage and intensive antibiotic therapy.

■ ENDOCARDITIS
Infection of the valves of the heart. There is usually a previous history of heart valve problems. Both adults and children are suscept–ible. Onset can be gradual, with:
* Anaemia.
* Malaise, recurrent sweats.
* Eventually, clubbed finger nails, enlarged spleen.
* Splinter-like marks under the finger nails.

Treatment takes several weeks, with monitoring of the heart valves by ultrasound devices.

'GENERAL' SYMPTOMS

RARE

■ TUBERCULOSIS
Although previously a disease of underdeveloped countries, low-income groups and alcoholics, tuberculosis is increasing again after many years. All ages and all income groups can be affected.
* Cough, which may be blood stained.
* General malaise, weight loss, debility.

Modern treatments cure the disease if continued over several months.

■ BRUCELLOSIS
See page 448.

■ HODGKIN'S DISEASE
See page 490.

■ HIV DISEASE/AIDS
See page 448.

TIREDNESS

PROBABLE
OVEREXERTION
ANXIETY
ANAEMIA

POSSIBLE
POST-VIRAL SYNDROME
DEPRESSION
HYPOTHYROIDISM
HYPERTHYROIDISM
DIABETES

RARE
HEART DISEASE
CANCER
MALNUTRITION
KIDNEY DISEASE
OTHER: ADRENAL INSUFFICIENCY
MYASTHENIA GRAVIS

PROBABLE

■ OVEREXERTION
A few remarkable people never need relief from constant pressure and stress and can make do with short periods of sleep. But even they usually have some compensatory mechanism. The rest of us suffer from fatigue, which commonly goes with:
* Irritability.
* Tense feelings in neck and head.
* Diminished enthusiasm for life.

■ ANXIETY
One expert recently described this universal symptom as 'fear spread thin.' As well as the symptoms given above for overexertion:
* Palpitations, muscle tremors.
* Sweating.
* A constant fear that something unpleasant is going to happen.

At worst, anxiety is a truly disabling disorder needing treatment with a combination of psychological counselling and mild sedatives.

■ ANAEMIA
See page 419.

POSSIBLE

■ POST-VIRAL SYNDROME
After a viral illness such as influenza *(see page 442)*, it is common to get easily fatigued for a few weeks, occasionally for longer. Psychological support and an undemanding lifestyle are the best advice that doctors can offer at present.

■ DEPRESSION
Commonest in adult life, appearing over several weeks.
* Poor sleep.
* No enjoyment of anything, lack of motivation.
* Poor self-image.
* Crying.
* Changes in body weight.
* Poor concentration.

■ HYPOTHYROIDISM
This means an underactive thyroid gland. A disease of middle and later life, progressing so slowly that even the close family may not spot anything wrong, putting the symptoms down to ageing.
* The skin becomes dry and rough.
* You 'feel the cold'.
* Your voice becomes gruff, your features coarse.
* Weight gain, constipation, slow speech, slow thought.

It is important to recognize this combination of symptoms because the disorder is so easily treated.

■ HYPERTHYROIDISM
Surprisingly, an overactive thyroid gland can also cause tiredness. This is usually a rather dramatic disease appearing over a few weeks with:
* Nervousness, fine tremor of the hands.
* Sweating, weight loss, increased appetite.
* Muscle ache.
* Staring eyes.
* Diarrhoea.
* Rapid heart rate (tachycardia).

Again, treated easily.

■ DIABETES
Fatigue can be an early symptom of diabetes when there are no other obvious features. As diabetes is such a common disease, anyone with unusual fatigue should be tested for it. For more details, *see page 485.*

RARE

■ HEART DISEASE
In heart failure, especially in the elderly, fatigue may be the only early symptom. Look also for:
* Breathlessness on mild effort, and when lying flat.
* Swollen ankles.

■ CANCER
Fatigue is worrying if found together with other symptoms suggesting cancer, such as:
* Weight loss, loss of appetite.
* Unusual pains.
* Unusual swellings.
* Blood in phlegm, vomit, urine, motions or from the vagina (see under individual entries for these symptoms).

■ MALNUTRITION
Common worldwide. The fatigue

is due to lack of vitamins, protein and energy supplies. In the developed countries, may be seen in those with malabsorption *(see page 423)* or alcoholics who eat poorly.

■ KIDNEY DISEASE
Fatigue is an early symptom along, with the increased passage of urine day and night.

■ OTHER
Severe, unexplained fatigue also raises the possibility of two rare disorders: adrenal insufficiency and myaesthenia gravis, a disease of gradual onset in which muscles seem to work normally but rapidly tire, with exceptional weakness. Drooping eyelids are typical.

TIREDNESS AND LOOKING PALE

Anaemia is a common and significant cause of fatigue. Even mild anaemia can cause fatigue and may not be obvious. Those most likely to be affected are:
– Children during growth spurts.
– Women during the years of menstruation.
– Women during pregnancy.
– The elderly; people on low incomes with a poor diet, lacking iron and vitamins.

TIREDNESS PLUS FEVER

A minor degree of fatigue always accompanies feverish illness such as the common cold.

PROBABLE
VIRAL ILLNESS SUCH AS 'FLU

POSSIBLE
GLANDULAR FEVER
CHRONIC INFECTION

RARE
RHEUMATOID ARTHRITIS
ENDOCARDITIS

PROBABLE

■ VIRAL ILLNESS
Including influenza, the common cold and other minor illnesses common during the winter months.
* A sore throat for two or three days.
* Aching muscles.
* Mild headache, shivering.
* Cough, hoarseness.
* The illness runs its course over a week or so.

POSSIBLE

■ GLANDULAR FEVER
A viral infection which usually starts as a particularly bad sore

throat with excessive fatigue. The fatigue decreases over a few weeks, but can persist for months. Mainly an illness of young adults.
* A fine rash can be found.
* Can cause a mild degree of jaundice.

It is checked for with a simple blood test, called a 'monospot'.

■ CHRONIC INFECTION
Persistent fatigue and fevers would lead to a search for a smouldering infection in a common site such as the lungs, abdomen or urine; or a tooth abscess.

RARE

■ RHEUMATOID ARTHRITIS
This illness of the joints, most common in middle-aged women, can be preceded by a period of otherwise unexplained fever and fatigue along with:
* Transient aches and pains.
* Vague malaise.
* Varying stiffness and swelling of the small joints.

Eventually, the full-blown illness shows itself with severe pain and swelling of the joints.

■ ENDOCARDITIS
An infection of the valves of the heart, most likely in someone known to have a valve problem, caused, for example, by previous rheumatic fever.
* Anaemia.
* Clubbed fingernails.
* Tiny splinter-like streaks of bleeding under the nails.

TIREDNESS PLUS HEADACHE

This is such a common combi–nation of symptoms that only in exceptional circumstances need it raise a query about underlying disease. Almost always, the cause is tension.

PROBABLE
TENSION
PRE-MENSTRUAL TENSION

POSSIBLE
MIGRAINE

RARE
PITUITARY (OR OTHER BRAIN) TUMOUR
CARBON MONOXIDE POISONING
RAISED BLOOD PRESSURE

PROBABLE

■ TENSION
Ninety-eight per cent of headaches are caused by tension. This starts in the neck muscles and spreads across the scalp.
* Headache like a band around the head.
* Cause may not at first be obvious.
* Usually work or family-related pressures are to blame.

■ PRE-MENSTRUAL TENSION
This condition is a common prelude to the monthly period.

POSSIBLE

■ MIGRAINE
Prolonged tiredness can trigger a migraine. Full symptoms include feeling sick and, sometimes, visual disturbance. *See page 112.*

RARE

■ PITUITARY (OR OTHER BRAIN) TUMOUR
The pituitary gland is sited deep in the brain. If affected by a tumour, there is increased pressure inside the skull and interference with the hormones that control many body functions.

In women, this is reflected in irregular or absent periods. Other signs are related to the direct compression of the brain: you will notice primarily a reduction in your field of vision. *See also page 114.*

■ CARBON MONOXIDE POISONING
Probably more common than is recognized, and caused by fumes from inefficient gas appliances. The early symptoms are vague.
* Symptoms disappear rapidly once the individual breathes fresh air.
* Drowsiness or coma.

■ RAISED BLOOD PRESSURE
A popular myth blames raised blood pressure for headaches; actually, it causes no symptoms. However, severely raised blood pressure may, under exceptional circumstances, cause a headache.

FEELING WEAK OR FEEBLE

Weakness is such an unspecific symptom that few medical textbooks even recognize it as a topic in its own right. Nonetheless, people often go to their doctors saying that they feel weak, and expecting the doctor to discover associated symptoms that will point to a diagnosis.

If you are in search of symptoms associated with weakness, this book is full of them: perhaps the most significant are *BREATHLESSNESS, pages 207-19* and *FEVER, pages 440-51.*

In the following pages we concentrate on those conditions which can cause weakness without many other significant symptoms. The terms weakness and tiredness are used interchangeably.

WEAKNESS, RAPID ONSET

PROBABLE
OVERWORK
VIRAL INFECTION
ANXIETY

POSSIBLE
HEART RHYTHM IRREGULARITY
LOW BLOOD SUGAR
PREGNANCY

RARE
HAEMORRHAGE
HEART DISEASE
INFECTIOUS HEPATITIS
GUILLAIN-BARRE SYNDROME

PROBABLE

■ OVERWORK
This may be obvious to an outsider, but it is remarkable how often an overworked individual is simply unaware of the pressures on him or her. They become a habit. Very often, people overlook this cause of weakness and tiredness because they are so keen to find 'medical' reasons for the symptom. Try to take an honest look at your own life style and pressures. Is there a link between periods of maximum pressure and episodes of weakness?
* Tension in neck, shoulders.
* Slight headache.
* Irritability.
* Sheer fatigue.

■ VIRAL INFECTION
Tiredness or weakness frequently precedes infection by a day or two. You suspect that you are about to 'go down with something'. Soon there will be:
* Fever, muscle aches.
* Joint pains, headache.
* Cough, cold or sore throat.
See also POST-VIRAL SYNDROME, page 461.

■ ANXIETY
The source may be obvious: conflicting demands on your time, emotional stress, or anxiety may just be a feature of your personality. Simply recognizing this can defuse anxiety; otherwise, consider counselling, or try reading a book on relaxation technique. Your doctor will probably only want to prescribe tranquillizers as a last resort.
* Sweating; hand tremor.
* Inability to concentrate.
* A fear of something unpleasant always being near.

POSSIBLE

■ HEART RHYTHM IRREGULARITY
The heart goes into either a very rapid or a very slow rhythm. It pumps less efficiently, giving a sensation of weakness or breathlessness or, at worst, collapse. These irregularities can stop as abruptly as they begin, making diagnosis difficult between attacks.
* Thumping in chest.
* Lightheadness, faintness.
* Abrupt disappearance of symptoms.
* Coffee, tea, alcohol may set off attacks.

■ LOW BLOOD SUGAR
The brain runs on sugar and a dip in blood sugar levels between meals is common.

'GENERAL' SYMPTOMS

* Lightheadeness, difficulty in concentrating.
* Feeling cold.
* Symptoms rapidly relieved by a sweet drink or a snack.

■ PREGNANCY
Tiredness associated with early pregnancy can be a puzzle, since it can predate the first missed period, when diagnosis is easy.
* Tender breasts.
* Desire to pass urine frequently.

RARE

■ HAEMORRHAGE
External bleeding should be obvious, less so internal bleeding after an accident. Worth considering in someone who has had a heavy blow to the abdomen, fractured a long bone or had severe abdomnal pain; or has a history of peptic ulcers.
* Weakness, progressing to drowsiness, confusion.
* Swelling of the abdomen.
* Pallor, sweating, clammy skin.
* Rapid pulse, rapid breathing.

■ HEART ATTACK
Normally a dramatic event, but it can be quite unremarkable, especially in the elderly, causing:
* Sudden general deterioration.
* Weakness, breathlessness.
* Swollen ankles, breathlessness at night.

■ INFECTIOUS HEPATITIS
Remarkable for the unexplained tiredness that precedes the appearance of the jaundice:
* Fever, malaise, nausea, loss of appetite.
* Possibly tenderness under ribs on right.
* Jaundice appears after about seven days; then recovery is rapid.

■ GUILLAIN-BARRE SYNDROME
A neurological disorder of unknown cause, which leads to rapid development of muscle weakness. As it can affect the muscles involved in breathing, it needs hospital treatment. Recovery can take months.
* Typically accompanies a minor illness.
* Initial tingling of hands, feet, then numbness.
* Weakness rapidly involves the limbs.
* Muscles of breathing may be affected.

PROLONGED WEAKNESS

By its very nature, the cause of prolonged weakness is not likely to be clear from physical symptoms alone: investigation is needed. The following are a few of the commonest causes.

PROBABLE
POST-VIRAL WEAKNESS
ANAEMIA
THYROID DISEASE

POSSIBLE
HEART FAILURE
LOW BLOOD PRESSURE
KIDNEY DISEASE
MALNUTRITION

RARE
MUSCLE OR NERVE DISEASE
CANCER

PROBABLE

■ POST-VIRAL WEAKNESS
There is a major, continuing debate about whether this is a physical problem or a psycho–logical disorder. It is probably both. In its most prolonged form it is known as M.E. Glandular fever (*see page 462*) is the best-known infection associated with prolonged weakness. The best treatment is simply to avoid overexertion.
* Tiredness on expending effort.
* No physical findings.
* Rarely lasts for more than a few months.

■ ANAEMIA
See page 419. Mild anaemia causes a feeling of being 'below par'. Those at most risk are:
– Women during the years of menstruation.
– Children during growth spurts.
– The elderly and the poor, with diets lacking iron.
– Alcoholics.

■ THYROID DISEASE
Weakness is a feature of both over- and underactivity, either of which are easily treated. An underactive thyroid gland gives:
* Progressive pallor, constipation, coarse features.
* Sensitivity to cold.
* Slowing of thought.

An overactive thyroid is more dramatic, causing:
* Sweating, weight loss, hunger.
* Tremor, nervousness and bulging eyes.

POSSIBLE

■ HEART FAILURE
Weakness can be a feature before other symptoms of heart failure become prominent. Usually there is some warning of heart trouble, such as angina, high blood pressure, previous heart attack or alcoholism. Eventually there will be:
* Breathlessness on modest exertion.
* Ankle swelling, breathlessness at night.

■ LOW BLOOD PRESSURE
Only recently have doctors begun generally to accept low blood pressure as a cause of vague illnesss and weakness.

■ KIDNEY DISEASE
Very early symptoms are:
* Increased passage of urine, day and night.
* Vague weakness and tiredness.
* Later, anaemia, nausea.

'GENERAL' SYMPTOMS

■ MALNUTRITION
This should not be a problem in developed countries, even so, it is still seen in the poor, in alcoholics or in other cases of self neglect. The weakness results from a combination of protein and vitamin deficiencies.
* Easy bruising, bleeding from gums (vitamin C deficiency).
* Tender calves (vitamin B1 deficency); *see page 431*.
* In children, swollen wrists, stunted growth (vitamin D deficiency).

RARE

■ MUSCLE OR NERVE DISEASE
Diagnosis is a matter for specialists, since early changes are subtle and non-specific. Neurological disease might be suspected if there is:
* Progressive weakness of a group of muscles.
* Tingling, numbness or tremors of limbs.
* Unsteady gait.
Muscular disease in childhood affects boys:
* Thin thighs, but enlarged calves.
* Waddling gait, difficulty getting up from squatting position.
* In adults, twitching of muscles.

■ CANCER
It is unexplained why cancer can cause weakness before other, more obvious, symptoms. Suspicion would be aroused by unusual weakness in:
* Smokers.
* Someone who has had recent indigestion, or noticed change of bowel habit.
* Someone with loss of appetite, weight loss.
* Unusual bleeding from chest, bowel or vagina, or blood in the urine.

For further details, see specific entries for the symptoms listed.

COLLAPSE

Sometimes called prostration, and characterized by overwhelming weakness, thready pulse, pallor, sweating and confusion. Underlying most cases is low blood pressure, or toxic effects from serious infection or drugs. While sudden collapse suggests a stroke or a heart attack (*see COLLAPSE WITH SHOCK OR COMA, page 472*), less abrupt collapse can mean a more general disruption of body function, for instance diabetes. However, there is no clear-cut distinction. In any case, get medical help fast.

Recovery position
Anyone who collapses should be laid on their side, leaning forwards. Make sure their airway — neck and throat — is not obstructed. If possible, keep their head lower than, or at the same level as, their heart.

Always seek professional medical help immediately when anybody collapses.

PROBABLE
FAINT

POSSIBLE
SEVERE INFECTION
DRUG OVERDOSE
PULMONARY EMBOLUS
DEHYDRATION

RARE
PNEUMOTHORAX
SEPTICAEMIA
ADDISON'S DISEASE
SEVERE HYPOTHYROIDISM

PROBABLE

■ FAINT
Short-lived unconsciousness, caused by temporary reduction in blood supply to the brain. Caused typically by standing upright in warm or hot conditions. Lying flat will lead quickly to recovery. *See page 418.*

POSSIBLE

■ SEVERE INFECTION
The possibilities are considered in detail in *FEVER, pages 440-51.*

■ DRUG OVERDOSE
Including alcohol. Suspected in someone who collapses and is confused or unconscious, especially a young, otherwise fit person.
* Smell of alcohol, empty pill containers.
* Neglected appearance.
* Inflamed veins.
* Pupils may be widely dilated or pin-point sized.
* Puncture marks on skin, made by a needle, usually at front of elbow or on back of hand.

Blood and urine tests will be necessary.

■ PULMONARY EMBOLUS
See page 218.
A blood clot settles in the lung, cutting off blood flow.

■ DEHYDRATION
See page 483.

RARE

■ PNEUMOTHORAX
Collapse of a section of lung.
* Sudden, knife-like chest pain, worse on breathing in.
* Slight breathlessness.
* Serious cases progress to faintness, collapse and cyanosis.

■ SEPTICAEMIA
Infection in the blood, causing rigors and sweats. *See page 488.*

■ ADDISON'S DISEASE
Progressive, generalized weakness until some one-off stress causes collapse.*See page 488.*

■ SEVERE HYPOTHYROIDISM
An underactive thyroid gland is usually spotted well before the patient collapses. *See page 461.*

'GENERAL' SYMPTOMS

COLLAPSE WITH ABDOMINAL PAIN

Often hard to diagnose, because the reasons for abdominal pain differ with age. The following is the obvious, but not an exhaustive, list of illnesses that can cause collapse in adults. Neglect at this stage will lead on to shock and coma - *see page 472.*

PROBABLE
PEPTIC ULCER
PANCREATITIS
GALL BLADDER DISEASE
ECTOPIC PREGNANCY

POSSIBLE
SEVERE GASTRO-ENTERITIS
INFLAMMATORY BOWEL DISEASE

RARE
INTESTINAL OBSTRUCTION
INTESTINAL ISCHAEMIA

PROBABLE

The possibilities below all involve inflammation of internal organs, which can progress to rupture of the organ. It is frequently impossible to differentiate these causes without tests or surgery.

Gall bladder

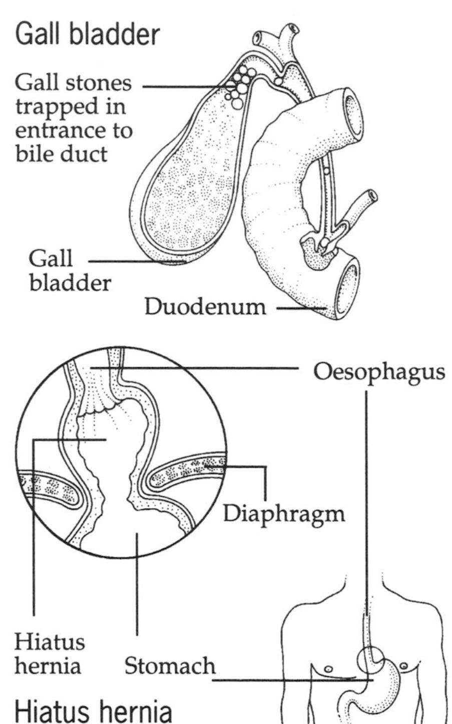

Hiatus hernia

■ PEPTIC ULCER
Excess acid leads to erosion of the lining of the stomach or of the duodenum. An ulcer can develop causing pain. If the ulcer ruptures, acid, food and blood gush into the abdomen.
* Commonest in middle-age.
* A history of upper abdominal discomfort or indigestion.
* Dyspepsia: may be waking at night.
* Severe pain in the upper abdomen, apparently radiating into the back.
* Vomit containing blood or particles looking like coffee grounds.
* Stools may be black, tarry-looking or bloody.

■ PANCREATITIS
The pancreas lies at the back of the

upper abdomen. There is usually existing gall bladder disease or a history of heavy drinking.

* Excruciating upper abdominal pain, worsening over a few hours.
* Pain in the back.
* Vomiting.
* Collapse.

Needs intensive treatment to prevent peritonitis, *page 149*.

■ GALL BLADDER DISEASE
Inflammation or obstruction of the gall bladder, usually connected with gall stones and commonest in middle-aged women.

* Pain felt in the upper right abdomen, under the ribs.
* Often a long history of discomfort on that side.
* Excruciating pain for hours at a time.
* Fever.

■ ECTOPIC PREGNANCY
If a fertilized egg lodges in a Fallopian tube, it can grow for a few weeks, eventually rupturing the tube, causing serious internal bleeding. This possibility should not be ignored in any fertile woman, even if there are no symptoms of pregnancy. Precise diagnosis is now relatively easy, thanks to ultrasound scanning.

* A missed period, tender breasts, nausea.
* Rapidly increasing lower abdominal pain, usually one-sided.
* Vaginal bleeding.

POSSIBLE

■ GASTRO-ENTERITIS
An infection of the bowels which, if severe, causes rapid dehydration as well as toxic effects from the actual infection.

* Cramping abdominal pains.
* Vomiting.
* Diarrhoea immediately, or after a few hours.

■ INFLAMMATORY BOWEL DISEASE
Typically ulcerative colitis or Crohn's disease. Associated with:

* A long history of recurrent abdominal pains, diarrhoea.
* Bleeding or mucus in stools.

RARE

■ INTESTINAL OBSTRUCTION
Most often due to a trapped hernia or a growth in the intestine.

* A trapped hernia gives a tender swelling in the groin.
* At first, cramping abdominal pains.
* Vomiting, swelling of the abdomen.
* Within hours, fever, generalized abdominal pains.

■ INTESTINAL ISCHAEMIA
A clot blocks blood supply to the intestines. Most likely in the elderly, with pre-existing heart disease.

* Sudden abdominal pain.
* Diarrhoea, vomiting, blood in motions.
* Rapid progression to collapse.

Surgical removal of the clot can be successful, but it ought to be done early.

'GENERAL' SYMPTOMS

COLLAPSE WITH SHOCK OR COMA

An emergency. Making a precise diagnosis is less important than resuscitating the individual. As a medical term, 'shock' strictly means drastic reduction in blood flow around the tissues. Here the term is used in a less technical sense, so as to include a wider range of symptoms:
* Skin clammy, cold, pale.
* Thready, weak pulse.
* Cyanosis.
* Individual reaction can vary from confusion to coma.

Coma may here be taken as unconsciousness. In trying to work out the cause of collapse with shock or coma, also consider the possibilities in the two preceding sections.

PROBABLE
STROKE
HEART ATTACK
HEART RHYTHM IRREGULARITY
BLOOD LOSS
OVERWHELMING INFECTION
SEVERE PAIN

POSSIBLE
DIABETIC COMA
ALCOHOL/DRUG OVERDOSE
LEAKING AORTIC ANEURYSM
BURNS

RARE
ANAPHYLAXIS

PROBABLE

■ STROKE
Mainly affects the elderly. Caused by a blood clot or bleeding in the brain.
* Loss of consciousness for a few minutes.
* Vomiting at first.
* Paralysis of one side of the body.
* 'Sighing', rough breathing.

The outlook depends on the reason for the stroke and the individual's overall health.

■ HEART ATTACK
A risk in the middle-aged and elderly. The treatment of heart attacks is in revolution, making quick medical help essential to maximize chances of survival.
* Sudden, crushing, central chest pain.
* Pain radiates up into jaws or down left arm.
* Breathlessness, sweating.

Not all heart attacks are so dramatic. In the elderly especially, they can occur without pain as a prominent feature.

■ HEART RHYTHM IRREGULARITY
Very rapid, very slow or very irregular heart rhythms reduce the blood output from the heart. You may notice:
* Abrupt onset of thumping or fluttering in chest.
* Breathlessness.
* Shock.

■ BLOOD LOSS

See also DEHYDRATION, page 483.

Not always obvious, but easy to recognize if the blood loss is visible, for example in vomit, motions, from the vagina. A risk after injury, especially:

* Trauma to the abdomen, which can rupture the spleen.
* Fractured thigh bone with severe bleeding into muscle.

■ OVERWHELMING INFECTION

For complex reasons, a major infection, that gets into the blood stream, causes collapse via a drop in blood pressure. There will be the general symptoms of infection, such as:

* Fever, rigors, headache.
* Spontaneous bleeding and bruising.

■ SEVERE PAIN

Severe pain from any source can cause collapse and coma as reflex actions.

POSSIBLE

■ DIABETIC COMA

Diabetics can have two types of coma. Collapse due to low blood sugar gives:

* Sweating, light-headedness, irritability.
* Rapid progression to confusion, then collapse.

If blood sugar remains high for long, another, less sudden, form of collapse — ketoacidosis — can occur:

* Usually during another mild illness.
* Onset over a few hours or days.
* Dehydration (*page 483*), intense thirst.
* Sweet smell on breath.

Both these conditions respond rapidly to the appropriate treatment.

■ ALCOHOL/DRUG EXCESS

See DRUG OVERDOSE, page 469.

■ LEAKING AORTIC ANEURYSM

The aorta is the major artery leading from the heart, and carries its whole blood output. After years of service, its walls can swell out, weaken and then split, just like a car tyre may bulge and blow out. A not uncommon cause of sudden death, but there are sometimes warning symptoms:

* Unusual pulsation in the abdomen, in time with the heart beat.
* A lump you can feel in the abdomen.
* Onset of backache as the aorta starts to leak.

Surgery is highly successful in early cases.

■ BURNS

Loss of body fluids invariably accompanies serious burns, with shock resulting both from this loss and from pain.

RARE

■ ANAPHYLAXIS

This term describes the worst form of allergic reaction.

It is an unpredictable risk, to be borne in mind whenever someone is given an injection, but anaphylaxis can happen in

response to foods and insect stings. Minor warning signs of allergic reaction are:
* Swelling of the lips.
* Itchy, raised skin wheals that come and go.

In anaphylaxis there is:
* Abrupt wheezing, progressing to cyanosis.
* Difficulty in swallowing, from swelling of the throat.
* Collapse.

Those fortunate enough to know that they are at risk should carry the appropriate medication, or a warning bracelet.

NO APPETITE, OR VERY POOR APPETITE

Brief episodes of loss of appetite accompany our changing moods and minor infections. Indeed the regaining of appetite is among the earliest signs of recovery from these minor upsets, as is the disappearance of fever. If loss of appetite is accompanied by abdominal pain or weight loss (*see these symptoms*) then more unusual disease is a possibility.

PROBABLE
MINOR FEVERISH ILLNESS
STRESS

POSSIBLE
DEPRESSION
ALCOHOLISM
INFECTIOUS HEPATITIS

RARE
CANCER OF THE STOMACH
HEART DISEASE

PROBABLE

■ MINOR FEVERISH ILLNESS
* Fever, muscle aches, sore throat or cough.
* Appetite disappears suddenly.
* The return of appetite lags a day or two behind the disappearance of fever.

■ STRESS
Or worry. This all-too-standard ingredients of modern life can either stimulate or reduce appetite.
* Tense feelings in head, neck, shoulders.
* Irritability, mild depression.

Mood and appetite recover rapidly when the source of stress is absent.

POSSIBLE

■ DEPRESSION
See page 389. Suggested by prolonged loss of appetite as well as:
* Loss of interest in general.
* Expressions of despair, crying, poor self-image.
* Apathetic mood, neglect of self and others.

* Early morning wakening (or disturbed sleep pattern).

■ ALCOHOLISM
The high carbohydrate content of alcohol satisfies hunger and causes loss of appetite for normal solid food. Of course, drink is not at all nutritious, and eventually symptoms of vitamin deficiency appear, as well as those of alcoholism. Hence such symptoms as:
* Self-neglect, smell of drink.
* Memory disturbance, swings of mood.
* Sore mouth, cracks at corners of lips, recurrent infections.
* Dilated veins over the face.

■ INFECTIOUS HEPATITIS
The combination of loss of appetite, fever for five to seven days, plus muscular aches and abdominal pains should arouse suspicion.
* Jaundice appears with yellowed eyes, dark urine.
* As the jaundice clears up, you begin to feel better.

RARE

■ CANCER OF THE STOMACH
For reasons not understood, early cancer, especially of the stomach, can cause loss of appetite before other features appear. However, it is rare for loss of appetite alone to continue for long without the other symptoms described under *NO APPETITE, LOSING WEIGHT, this page and NO APPETITE, LOSING WEIGHT AND CHEST PAIN, page 476.*

Most common in the 45-plus age group.
* Persistent, otherwise unexplained, loss of appetite.
* Feeling of fullness very soon after eating a small amount.
* Otherwise unexplained symptoms, such as generally feeling unwell, tiredness, unusual bleeding, unusual pains.

■ HEART FAILURE
In certain forms of heart failure, loss of appetite is a noticeable symptom, probably related to congestion of blood in the liver. Among the many other symptoms which appear over days or weeks are:
* Breathlessness on exertion; tiredness.
* Breathlessness when attempting to lie flat.
* Pre-existing chest disease, such as chronic bronchitis, bronchiectasis or heart disease, typically angina.
* An early feature is swollen ankles, and eventually a swollen abdomen.
* Tenderness over the liver, reduction in the volume of urine.

NO APPETITE, LOSING WEIGHT

This is a worrying combination. In the under-40s, the cause is usually a prolonged feverish illness. In the middle-aged and elderly, more serious disease must be carefully considered. If you have noticed loss of appetite and weight loss, check whether you have any of the symptoms in the lists below. Then look them up elsewhere in the book, where they are featured under a heading of their own.

PROBABLE
PROLONGED FEVERISH ILLNESS
DUODENAL ULCER
ANOREXIA NERVOSA

POSSIBLE
EMOTIONAL UPSET
CANCER

PROBABLE

■ PROLONGED FEVERISH ILLNESS
In children and young adults, loss of appetite and weight loss will accompany any moderately extended illness such as a bad chest infection or prolonged gastroenteritis. Both appetite and weight are rapidly regained after a couple of weeks. In adults, a wider net has to be cast, in order to look for:
* Chills or night sweats.
* Recent abdominal surgery.
* Prolonged cough, diarrhoea, abdominal pains.
* Unusual bleeding.
* Changes in amount of urine.

Follow up these symptoms individually, looking at other pages in this book where they are discussed in detail.

■ DUODENAL ULCER
Painless ulcers, though a little unusual, can cause:
* Hunger.
* Bleeding (from the ulcer), seen in vomit or revealed by your stools turning black.

■ ANOREXIA NERVOSA
See page 424. Weight loss due to obsessional dieting.

POSSIBLE

■ EMOTIONAL UPSET
If severe enough, self-neglect may follow. Usually there is an obvious cause of stress.
* Other symptoms of emotional upset, such as swings of mood, irritability, crying, depression.

■ CANCER
In the 40-plus age range these symptoms also require a careful check for other features suggestive of cancer such as:
* Unusual pains.
* Unusual bleeding from mouth, vagina, bowel, in phlegm, in urine.
* Swellings, lumps, enlarged lymph nodes.
* Malaise, tiredness.

NO APPETITE, LOSING WEIGHT AND CHEST PAIN

Though worrying, this combination is a little less so than simple *NO APPETITE, LOSING WEIGHT*, *page 475*. Of course, any adult with these symptoms still needs careful assessment by a doctor, but there are relatively innocent causes:

PROBABLE
PEPTIC ULCER
HIATUS HERNIA
OESOPHAGITIS

POSSIBLE
GALL BLADDER DISEASE
CANCER OF THE STOMACH

RARE
MALABSORBTION
LUNG CANCER
TUBERCULOSIS

PROBABLE

■ PEPTIC ULCER
The lining of the stomach and duodenum is washed by highly corrosive acid and salts. The digestive system has mechanisms to cope with this, but if the mechanisms break down, inflammation and eventually ulceration occurs. Smoking, drinking, worry and most anti-rheumatic drugs predispose to peptic ulcers.
* Burning pains behind the breastbone and in the upper abdomen.
* Food may help or worsen the pain.
* If it worsens pain, food is avoided, causing weight loss.
* You may be woken at night by the pain.
* Simple antacids give temporary relief.

The treatment of peptic ulcers is one of the outstanding successes of modern medicine, making surgery, which used to be the only long-term cure, unnecessary.

Peptic ulcer

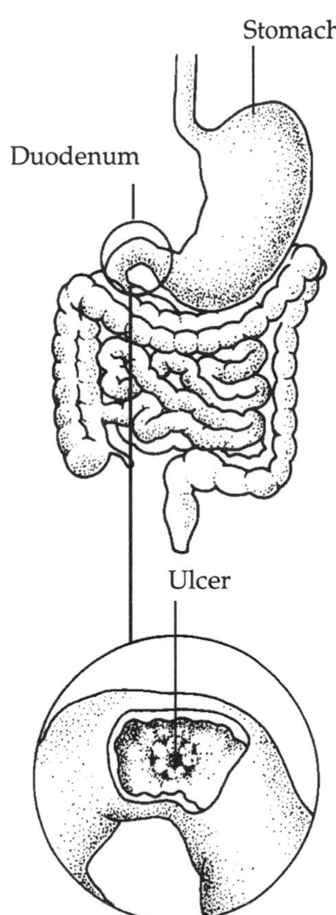

Peptic ulcers: the two types
Two types of peptic ulcer exist. *Duodenal ulcers* are four times more common than *gastric ulcers.*

Duodenal ulcers do not turn into cancers; gastric ulcers may become cancerous. Twice as many men as women have ulcers. One in ten of all people will have some ulcer-related disease during their lifetime.

'General' Symptoms

■ HIATUS HERNIA
A failure of the one-way valve mechanism that keeps stomach contents from regurgitating up into the gullet. Often just a nuisance, but if long-standing, it can cause scarring of the gullet, interfering with normal swallowing of food. Weight loss then results.

A condition of middle to later life, especially in the overweight.
* Burning pains.
* Belching, especially on bending over or lying flat.

Very commonly, the symptoms are worse during pregnancy.

■ OESOPHAGITIS
Inflammation of the gullet due to excess acid.
* Burning pain behind the breast-bone (heartburn).
* Worse after hot or acid food.
* Pain may appear to spread across the chest, and up to the jaw.

Treatment is aimed at preventing scarring and narrowing of the gullet.

POSSIBLE

■ GALL BLADDER DISEASE
This usually means gallstones, causing pain in the upper abdomen after eating, and resulting in disinclination to eat. *See GALL BLADDER, page 164.*

■ CANCER OF THE STOMACH
See page 475. This has to be checked for in anyone over the age of 40 who develops these symptoms, especially for the first time. The earlier such symptoms are reported, the earlier the diagnosis and the better the chance of successful treatment.

RARE

■ MALABSORPTION
A term covering a variety of conditions where there is interference with the way the digestive system absorbs food. Particularly a problem of childhood, with quite suggestive symptoms including:
* Failure to grow.
* Loose, greasy, bulky, offensive stools.
* Frequent chest infections.
* Swollen belly with discomfort or outright pain.

■ LUNG CANCER
In addition to the three main symptoms there may also be:
* Breathlessness.
* Coughing of blood.

See details on page 224.

■ TUBERCULOSIS
Weight loss and loss of appetite, and sweating, are general features of this disease. Chest pain results from swelling of glands inside the chest. *See details on page 447.*

ABNORMAL HUNGER

PROBABLE
INDIGESTION
LOW BLOOD SUGAR

POSSIBLE
HYPERTHYROIDISM

RARE
INTESTINAL WORMS
BULIMIA
HYPOTHALAMIC DISEASE

PROBABLE

■ INDIGESTION
Food reduces the feelings of pain or emptiness caused by excess acid present in indigestion. You feel like taking frequent snacks to relieve the discomfort.
* Burning sensation behind the breastbone.
* Burping, belching or other signs of wind.
Persistent symptoms may signify a peptic ulcer.

■ LOW BLOOD SUGAR
Very common in a mild form if you miss a meal. Diabetics, especially those on insulin, must be alert to the early symptoms.
* At first, you feel light-headed and have difficulty concentrating; also, irritability, headache.
* As it worsens, sweating, confusion, drowsiness.
* Symptoms rapidly eased by taking sugar.

POSSIBLE

■ HYPERTHYROIDISM
An overactive thyroid gland, developing over weeks or months.
* Weight loss, sweating, tremor of the hands.
* Often, bulging eyes.
* Hyperactivity, restlessness, nervousness.

RARE

■ INTESTINAL WORMS
The worm infects humans via beef, pork or fish.
* Usually no other symptoms until segments of worm appear in stools.

■ BULIMIA
Bulimia is binge eating, associated with *ANOREXIA NERVOSA*, *page 424.*
* Typically in young women worried about their weight.
* Excess dieting, interrupted by bouts of voracious feeding to the point of vomiting.

■ HYPOTHALAMIC DISEASE
Disease of the hypothalamus gland in the brain can gradually cause excess appetite and:
* Passage of enormous amounts of urine.
* Drowsiness, narrowing of visual field.

'GENERAL' SYMPTOMS

PUTTING ON WEIGHT

The 'glands' so often blamed are rarely the culprits.

PROBABLE
EATING TOO MUCH

POSSIBLE
HYPOTHYROIDISM
DRUG-RELATED

RARE
HORMONAL
CUSHING'S SYNDROME

PROBABLE

■ EATING TOO MUCH
This is not the same as overeating. Some individuals really do eat very little, yet gain weight. The reason is unknown. Overweight is a major cause of ill health, if not outright disease, including osteoarthritis, heart disease, and diabetes.
* Worsens with age.
* Fat is generally spread around the body.
* Honest, purposeful dieting achieves weight loss.

POSSIBLE

■ HYPOTHYROIDISM
* Slow, progressive weight gain.
See page 461.

■ DRUG-RELATED
Commonest culprits are the contraceptive pill; and steroids, widely used in chest and rheumatic diseases, eventually causing:
* A 'moon' face.
* Weight gain mainly in body, limbs remaining relatively thin.
* High blood pressure, diabetes.

RARE

■ HORMONAL
Several unusual hormonal disorders, mainly in boys, cause obesity.
* Obese child is unusually small or unusually tall.
* Delayed puberty.
* Under-development of penis and testicles.

■ CUSHING'S SYNDROME
Results from overproduction of natural steroids by the body.
* Gross obesity of body, with prominent purple stretch marks.
* Thin, stick-like limbs.
* 'Moon' face.
* Pronounced hump of fat on the back.
* Symptoms of diabetes (thirst, excess urine and so on, *see page 485).*
* Thin skin, easy bruising.

There are sophisticated treatments, depending on the cause.

TEMPERATURE, SUB-NORMAL

See *ABNORMALLY LOW TEMPERATURE, page 451.*

RAGING THIRST

This is the counterpart to *CRAVING FOR WATER, FEELING DEHYDRATED, page 483,* and should be read in conjunction with that topic.

PROBABLE
POOR FLUID INTAKE
SWEATING
DIARRHOEA

POSSIBLE
EXCESS OF DIURETIC DRUG
INTERNAL BLEEDING

RARE
DRUG SIDE EFFECT

PROBABLE

■ POOR FLUID INTAKE
Circumstances which could make this a possibility are:
– Prolonged vomiting.
– Disabled individual: for example, stroke victim, must rely on others for drinks.
– Obstruction of the gullet.
– Patients on intravenous drips.
The symptoms are:
* Dry mouth, low output of concentrated, dark urine.
* Skin becomes lax and loses its elasticity, eyes appear to sink.
* In babies, the soft spot on the skull becomes sunken.
* In extremes, apathy, confusion.

■ SWEATING
The fluid lost in sweat has to be replaced, otherwise thirst will follow. Fever, heavy exercise and hot weather might all cause profuse sweating. The symptoms are the same as for poor fluid intake.

■ DIARRHOEA
The body can cope with brief episodes of diarrhoea, but if it is prolonged, dehydration and thirst will follow. Babies are particularly susceptible to the effects of diarrhoea, which is also often accompanied by vomiting at that age. A careful watch must be kept for signs of dehydration.

POSSIBLE

■ EXCESS OF DIURETIC DRUGS
These medications are widely used to treat heart disease. They rid the body of fluid: even so, thirst is not often a problem, unless doses are excessive, when you may see:
* Passage of large quantities of urine for hours after taking the diuretic.
* Increasing weakness over several days or weeks.
* Constipation.

'General' Symptoms

■ BLEEDING
This has to be heavy and sustained to cause thirst. External bleeding is usually obvious, but internal bleeding may be another matter:
* Pallor, rapid pulse, collapse and thirst.

Suspicious circumstances include:
* Recent abdominal injury (for example, a ruptured spleen).
* Recent severe abdominal pain (from, say, a perforated ulcer).
* Fractured thigh.
* Abdominal distension.

RARE

■ DRUG SIDE EFFECT
Many drugs cause a dry mouth; not, strictly speaking, true thirst — but the remedy is sips of fluid. Common drugs with this side effect are anti-depressants and drugs for urinary incontinence.

RAGING THIRST, HIGH URINE OUTPUT

PROBABLE
DIABETES MELLITUS
PSYCHOLOGICAL

POSSIBLE
POTASSIUM DEFICIENCY
CHRONIC KIDNEY FAILURE

RARE
HYPER-PARATHYROIDISM
DIABETES INSIPIDUS

PROBABLE

■ DIABETES MELLITUS
See page 485. This combination of symptoms is the classical presentation of diabetes.

■ PSYCHOLOGICAL
A vicious circle of drinking to excess followed by urinating to excess. Surprisingly common, especially in children, where consuming sweet drinks becomes their main source of comfort. To diagnose, a doctor must exclude other causes.

POSSIBLE

■ POTASSIUM DEFICIENCY
Nearly always secondary to the long-term use of diuretics. Suggested by:
* Elderly person on diuretics.
* Muscle weakness, tiredness, constipation.

(In very rare cases, caused by disease.)

■ CHRONIC KIDNEY FAILURE
The passage of large quantities of dilute urine is an early sign of this problem, whose other symptoms are rather vague.
* Excessive urine day and night.
* Malaise.
* As it worsens, thirst, mild

anaemia, fatigue.

The outcome depends on the underlying cause.

RARE

■ HYPER-PARATHYROIDISM

The parathyroid glands lie next to the thyroid gland in the throat; they control calcium balance. Too much calcium in the blood gives:

* Excessive thirst and urine output.
* Pains in bones, constipation.
* Kidney stones that may be painful.
* Depression, malaise.

Summed up by generations of medical students as 'Moans, bones and abdominal groans'.

■ DIABETES INSIPIDUS

See page 485.

CRAVING FOR WATER, FEELING DEHYDRATED

Dehydration is the result of water loss exceeding water intake, remembering that water is lost not just in urine but in faeces (especially in diarrhoea), sweat (especially in heat exhaustion), blood (especially in haemorrhage) and via breathing (especially in prolonged asthma). Thirst is frequently a symptom of dehydration; other signs, in order of severity, are:

* Dry tongue (but beware mouth breathers, whose tongues are dry anyway).
* Reduced output of urine, the urine being dark and strong-smelling.
* Dry, lax skin.
* Sunken eyes.
* In babies, a sunken soft spot in the skull.
* Eventually apathy, confusion, collapse.

Depending on the cause, dehydration can develop over any length of time, from days to weeks, unless there has been a large and sudden loss of fluid. It is important to realize that babies and elderly people can dehydrate in a matter of hours, typically from diarrhoea and vomiting, and may not show any symptoms apart from restlessness until fluid loss is extreme.

PROBABLE

VOMITING
DIARRHOEA
SWEATING
DECREASED FLUID INTAKE

POSSIBLE

OVER-USE OF DIURETICS
DIABETES MELLITUS (SUGAR DIABETES)

RARE

HIGH BLOOD CALCIUM
CHRONIC KIDNEY FAILURE
KIDNEY FAILURE
DIABETES INSIPIDUS

'GENERAL' SYMPTOMS

PROBABLE

■ VOMITING
Whatever the reason for the vomiting, eventually dehydration results simply because no water is being kept down. In both children and adults, the usual cause is gastroenteritis, otherwise known as gastric 'flu or tummy upset, with:
* Abrupt onset of vomiting.
* Chills, muscular aches.
* Diarrhoea may accompany these, or begin a few hours later.

After two or three days, gastroenteritis can cause significant dehydration, but it is unusual for both the diarrhoea and the vomiting together to last so long. So, dehydration is actually a remote risk except in babies, who should be carefully watched.

■ DIARRHOEA
A few episodes of diarrhoea cause no harm. Profuse, watery diarrhoea is a different matter because if that continues for more than a day or two dehydration becomes a real risk, especially in the very old and the very young.

■ SWEATING
In a hot, dry atmosphere it is possible to lose large amounts of fluid by sweating without noticing. Those who run for pleasure should also remember this and take fluids regularly, even when on the move. Early features would be:
* Muscle cramps.
* Thirst, but not as a prominent symptom.
* Weakness, vomiting.

■ DECREASED FLUID INTAKE
If disease interferes with swallowing, dehydration, and indeed starvation, are a risk unless arrangements are made to enable feed to be taken some other way.

Similarly, with anyone unable to take sufficient fluid because of confusion, stroke or unconsciousness. The symptoms of dehydration can become confused with the symptoms of their disease leading to a vicious circle. Look for:
* Low urine output.
* Increasingly lax skin.
* A tongue so dry it begins to crack.
* Increasing confusion.

POSSIBLE

■ OVER-USE OF DIURETICS
These invaluable and widely-used drugs cause an increased output of urine. They are used to treat heart failure or high blood pressure; also to relieve fluid retention such as swollen ankles or swollen breasts before a period. When they are used over long periods, they can cause a slow dehydration. You may come to accept as normal a dry mouth or increased thirst.

It is rare for diuretics to cause rapid dehydration except through deliberate overdose, for instance, if used as a slimming aid, or when used in high dosage to relieve serious heart failure, when it is normal to monitor their effect with blood tests. The symptoms would

be those of dehydration, as listed above, with:
* General weakness, also muscle weakness.
* If very severe, apathy and vomiting.

■ DIABETES MELLITUS (SUGAR DIABETES)
In this condition, excess sugar in the blood stream starts to 'leak' through the kidneys, dragging large quantities of water with it. This leaves the body as large quantities of urine, day and night, giving the combination of thirst and dehydration. Other features might include:
* Vague feeling of ill-health.
* Weight loss.
* Frequent skin infections, especially thrush.
* A sweet smell on the breath.
* Eventually, confusion.

In teenagers and young adults, diabetes does tend to show itself in the above dramatic way, appearing over just a few days. In elderly people, the onset is usually less dramatic: the main symptoms are passing larger-than-usual amounts of urine, and very severe thirst.

RARE

■ HIGH BLOOD CALCIUM
Occurs mainly in association with diseases that affect the bones and tends to be part of a rather vague, gradually developing picture which might include:
* Weakness, drowsiness, nausea, vomiting.
* Pains in the abdomen, constipation.

Diagnosis of this condition constitutes a medical detective story.

■ CHRONIC KIDNEY FAILURE
Among the many functions of the kidneys is the job of concentrating the urine so that only enough is made as is needed to carry off waste products. One of the earliest features of kidney failure is loss of efficiency in this task, resulting in increased output of dilute urine, plus:
* Mild dehydration.
* Vague weakness, tiredness.

The disease is more likely in diabetics or those with high blood pressure.

A more severe condition, when kidneys suddenly stop working altogether, is dealt with below.

■ KIDNEY FAILURE
In serious kidney failure, usually after months or years of illness, there comes a stage of many distressing symptoms including:
* Severe dehydration.
* Dry, brown tongue with the smell of urine on the breath.
* Weakness, anaemia, hiccoughs, nausea.

■ DIABETES INSIPIDUS
This results from damage — typically as a result of head injury, tumours or meningitis — to the part of the brain that controls water balance (the pituitary gland).
* Passage of gallons of urine a day.
* A huge compensating thirst.

If you have this condition, now readily treatable, every medical school for miles around will be asking you to appear as a case in their students' examinations.

'General' Symptoms

HICCUPS

Hiccups result from a sudden contraction of the diaphragm, the sheet of muscle which separates the chest from the abdomen. It is an uncontrollable reflex action, like blinking. The chance of hiccups being the only symptom of illness is remote, even if hiccups are unusually persistent

The diaphragm

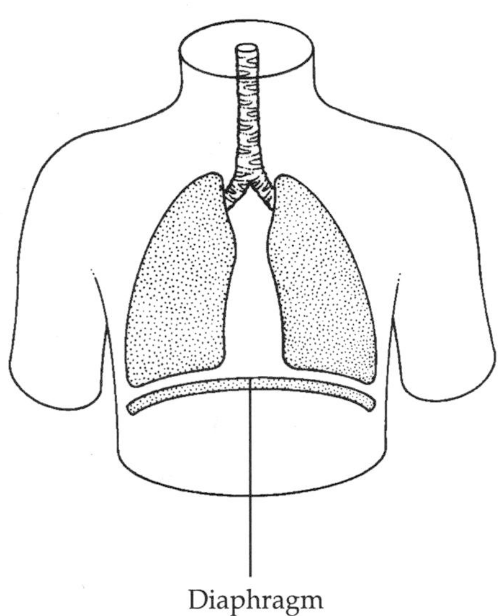

PAINS IN VARIOUS PARTS OF THE BODY

A precise definition is essential. Considered here is *recurrent, generalized pain* as opposed to pain in a specific part of the body. Such generalized pains can include the vague aches and pains which plague most people from time to time, and which may well have a psychological origin. Generally speaking, pain as a symptom of serious underlying disease is obvious when it strikes.

PROBABLE
DEPRESSION
HYPOCHONDRIA

POSSIBLE
DIABETES MELLITUS
POLYMYALGIA RHEUMATICA
PERNICIOUS ANAEMIA

RARE
SICKLE CELL DISEASE
SYPHILIS

PROBABLE

■ DEPRESSION
The pains tend to be the same minor ones everyone experiences, but they take on an exaggerated significance for the depressed person who has a lower tolerance of irritation.
* Flat, apathetic mood.
* Poor sleep, appetite and concentration.
* Crying, negative feelings.

■ HYPOCHONDRIA
If you have bought a copy of this book, you probably need no one to define for you the agonies of occasional hypochondria. It is a universal human condition, and if

you do automatically think the worst of every symptom, this book ought to give you some relief. Persistent hypochondriacs — the ones who see their doctors as often as once a week — are another matter, characterized by:
* Lack of insight.
* Resistance to reasoned explanation or proof, after investigation, that they are healthy.
* Often, a long history of neurotic behaviour.

Hypochondria is sometimes not as benign, or as funny, as it seems. Those who constantly complain of sundry symptoms can be so preoccupied that they neglect the early symptoms of true disease.

POSSIBLE

■ DIABETES MELLITUS
Sugar diabetes affects the working of nerves all over the body and can cause widespread nerve disturbance. This is usually a late complication: the disease should have been diagnosed long since on grounds of thirst, weight loss and excess urine production.
* Pain, tingling of lower limbs.
* Pain worse at night.
* Muscle tenderness.

Unfortunately this complication is possible even in well controlled diabetes.

■ POLYMYALGIA RHEUMATICA
A not uncommon illness mainly affecting women in their 60s. It comes on over a period of a few weeks giving pains in any muscles, but particularly:
* Across the shoulders.
* Tenderness at the temples.
* Vague malaise, occasional fever.

Easily and effectively treated, though treatment has to continue for a year or two.

■ PERNICIOUS ANAEMIA
General features of anaemia, *page 419*, plus:
* Tingling, numbness of limbs, hands or feet.
* Unsteady walking.
* Sore tongue.
* A hint of jaundice or yellowed skin.

Vitamin B12 injections treat both the anaemia and the pains.

RARE

■ SICKLE CELL DISEASE
In which haemoglobin, the blood's oxygen carrier, is abnormal. Found in people of African origin.
* Normal, pain-free existence interrupted by bouts of pain in limbs, abdomen.
* Pains set off by infection, surgery under anaesthetic, pregnancy.
* Screening is simple.

■ SYPHILIS
This sexually transmitted disease is now relatively rare in developed countries, but it is still worth considering if there is any odd or otherwise unexplained neurological disturbance. Years after the actual infection, syphilis can affect nerves in the spine, giving widespread nerve disorders such as:
* Severe, knife-like stabbing pains in the limbs.
* Pins and needles in hands or feet.

'General' Symptoms

* Unsteady gait.
* Painless ulcers on limbs.
* Distorted but painless joints.

Though treatment will prevent any further disease, it will not reverse these symptoms.

PUFFINESS

See SWOLLEN BODY, page 429.

FEELING THE COLD

PROBABLE
NATURAL TENDENCY

POSSIBLE
RAYNAUD'S PHENOMENON AND DISEASE
HYPOTHYROIDISM

RARE
ADDISON'S DISEASE

PROBABLE

■ NATURAL TENDENCY
In the great majority of cases, sensitivity to cold is a natural feature of your constitution: you may well have always suffered from numb and/or bluish fingers and toes *(see also BLUISH SKIN, page 424)*. The elderly often find that they 'feel the cold'. Similarly, babies have a reduced ability to compensate for low temperature, making adequate room temperature and warm clothing essential.

POSSIBLE

■ RAYNAUD'S PHENOMENON and RAYNAUD'S DISEASE
Common conditions in which the circulation of the fingers and toes over-reacts to changes in temperature.
* Fingers and toes always feel cold; go white or blue easily.
* Pain and redness are evident as they warm up.

Severe forms of Raynaud's can cause ulceration of fingers and toes. The problem may occasionally arise as a side-effect of taking beta-blockers for high blood pressure, or of working with vibrating equipment; it might also be a complication of a connective tissue disorder.

■ HYPOTHYROIDISM
Slowly increasing sensitivity to the cold is one of the classic features of this easily treated disorder. *See page 461.*

RARE

■ ADDISON'S DISEASE
A gradually developing hormone deficiency causing generalized weakness and lack of resistance to physical stress, including low temperature. People with Addison's look strikingly pale.

SWOLLEN LYMPH NODES

The lymphatic system, comprising the lymph nodes, liver and spleen, is in the front line of defence against infection and, indeed, other threats to the system. Temporary swelling for a week or two is, therefore, of little significance, being a feature of many minor viral illnesses and injuries.

However, there is no escaping the fact that prolonged swelling of lymph nodes can be a sign of several serious conditions. Frequently, these conditions are treatable, especially at an early stage, making it essential to report persistently swollen lymph nodes. Blood tests and lymph node biopsy are usually needed to confirm the diagnosis.

PROBABLE
GLANDULAR FEVER
TONSILITIS

POSSIBLE
HODGKIN'S DISEASE
LYMPHOMA
CANCER
TOXOPLASMOSIS
TUBERCULOSIS
LEUKAEMIA

RARE
SARCOIDOSIS
SECONDARY SYPHILIS
YAWS
CAT SCRATCH FEVER

Lymph nodes sites

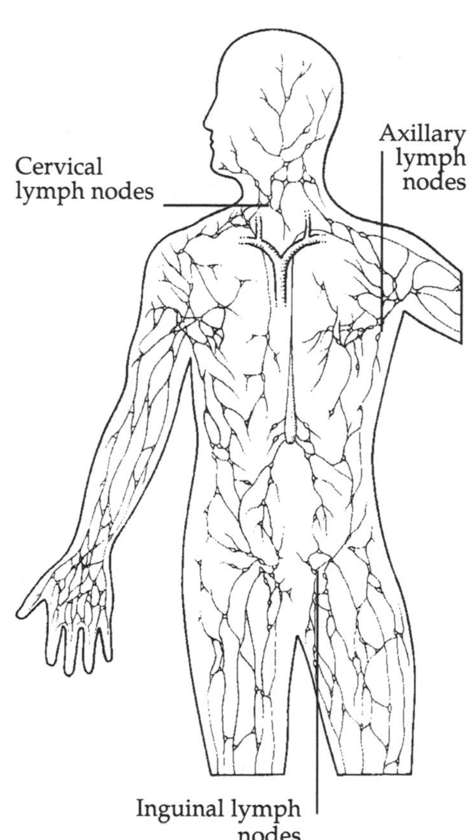

PROBABLE

■ GLANDULAR FEVER
An extremely common infection, with a combination of severe sore throat, swollen glands and tiredness. No specific treatment, but be reassured that you will eventually make a full recovery. *See also page 462.*

■ TONSILLITIS
Just a sore throat can cause massive swelling of lymph glands

'GENERAL' SYMPTOMS

below the chin. This can be particularly dramatic in children; *see page 442.*

POSSIBLE

In most of the following, the lymph nodes gradually enlarge and remain enlarged:

.

■ HODGKIN'S DISEASE
* Painless.
* Rubbery feel to lymph nodes.
* Lymph nodes grow steadily over a few weeks.
* Tiredness, sweats at night.

Swelling of the neck glands is the most likely to be noticed. The feel of the glands in this disease is characteristic, but diagnosis requires biopsy of a gland.

■ LYMPHOMA
Another form of cancer of the lymphatic system, but in an older age group — 35-plus. Symptoms are similar to those in Hodgkin's disease, with:
* Widespread, painless swollen lymph nodes.
* Weight loss, sweats at night.

Treatment depends on the type of lymphoma — determined by blood test, plus bone marrow and lymph node biopsy.

■ CANCER
By the time it causes generalized swelling of nodes, the cancer will be so advanced that it is bound to be obvious from other features. More important from the point of view of early diagnosis is enlargement of a single group of lymph nodes, which may signal the presence of an early cancer in such sites as the breast or the thyroid gland before there other obvious features.

The sites most noticeable are:
* Neck (cancers of lung, thyroid, nose and stomach).
* Groin (cancer of bowel, womb, prostate).
* Armpit (breast cancer).

■ TOXOPLASMOSIS
An infection acquired through eating infected meat, or sometimes via cat droppings. There is much current interest in screening for the disease since, if caught during pregnancy, it causes brain and eye damage in the baby.
* In mild cases, generalized, painless, swollen lymph nodes.
* Possibly fever, weakness as well.

■ TUBERCULOSIS
The usual glands involved are those around the neck. The swelling is painless and accompanied by general features of TB such as:
* Prolonged malaise.
* Weight loss.
* Cough, possibly with blood in sputum.

See also page 447.

■ LEUKAEMIA
Both childhood and adult forms of leukaemia can present with widespread swollen nodes. The childhood form tends to be dramatic, with:
* Abnormal bleeding, sore throat, malaise.
* Fever, anaemia.

* Enlarged liver, spleen.
In adults the disease tends to have a much slower onset, with:
* Enlarged lymph nodes as a main feature.
* Possibly effects of anaemia, and recurrent infections.

Treatment of childhood leukaemias is good and improving. Outlook in adults depends on the form of leukaemia.

RARE

■ SARCOIDOSIS

A condition of unknown origin, often picked up by chance from seeing enlarged glands deep inside the chest on an X-ray. Usually benign, but may cause:
* Rashes, joint pains.
* Malaise.
* Large, painful red lumps on shin.
* Painful, red eye.

■ SECONDARY SYPHILIS

Though now rare in developed countries, this remains globally a widespread disease.
* The initial sign is a painless sore on the genitalia.
* General lymph node swelling after several months.
* Wart-like growths around genitalia.
* Vague malaise.

Diagnosis is by blood test; antibiotic treatment is effective and essential in order to prevent progression to serious nerve disorders, possibly years later.

■ YAWS

A syphilis look-alike found in the tropics. Unlike syphilis, it is spread by poor hygiene, rather than sexually transmitted.
* Ulcerating skin rash, mainly on palms and soles of feet.
* Widespread enlargement of the lymph nodes.

Treatment prevents disfiguring destruction of bone.

■ CAT SCRATCH FEVER

An interesting, and probably under-recognized, reason for enlarged glands. Said to be one of the commonest causes of persistently swollen glands in the U.S.A.
* At first, just broken skin from the scratch.
* After a week or two, a small red lump appears.
* Swollen local glands, for example, in armpit.
* Glands enlarge, and may discharge pus.
* Illness settles over a few weeks.

Sometimes there are also joint pains. The organism responsible has only recently been identified. Can be cleared up with antibiotics.

INDEX

INDEX

INDEX

Index